MW00667461

*Acupuncture Cases
from China*

Thanks to Dr J. H. Chen for the Chinese calligraphy on the front cover.

For Churchill Livingstone

Publisher: Mary C. Law
Project Development Editor: Dinah Thom
Project Editor: Valerie Bain
Senior Project Controller: Neil A. Dickson
Project Controller: Nicky S. Carrodus
Sales Promotion Executive: Hilary Brown

Acupuncture Cases from China

A DIGEST OF DIFFICULT AND COMPLICATED CASE HISTORIES

Zhang Dengbu

Associate Professor, Shandong College of Traditional Medicine;
Member of All-China Association of Acupuncture and Moxibustion;
Director, Teaching and Researching Unit of Meridian, Department of Acupuncture;
Director, Department of Acupuncture, Affiliated Hospital, Shandong College of Traditional Medicine, China

English language editor:
Oran Kivity BAc (MIROM)

Technical editor:
Richard James BSc MBBS LicAc DHP

CHURCHILL LIVINGSTONE
EDINBURGH LONDON MADRID MELBOURNE NEW YORK AND TOKYO 1994

CHURCHILL LIVINGSTONE
Medical Division of Longman Group UK Limited

Distributed in the United States of America by Redwing Book Company,
44 Linden Street, Brookline, Massachusetts 01246.

First edition published in Chinese
© Shandong Science and Technology Publishing House, 16 Yuhan Road,
Jinan, Shandong, People's Republic of China 1989
First edition in English based on the first Chinese edition, revised
© Longman Group UK Limited 1994
This edition of A Study of Abnormal Medical Cases in Acupuncture is
published by arrangement with Shandong Science and Technology Publishing House.

First Chinese edition published 1989
First English edition published 1994

ISBN 0 443 04788 X

British Library of Cataloguing in Publication Data
A catalogue record for this book is available from the British Library.

Library of Congress Cataloging in Publication Data

Produced by Longman Singapore Publishers (Pte) Ltd.
Printed in Singapore

Contents

Preface xi

Part one
GENERAL MEDICINE

Part two
GYNAECOLOGY

Part three
PAEDIATRICS

Part four
DISEASES OF THE EAR, EYE, NOSE AND THROAT

Part five
DISEASES AFFECTING THE CHANNELS

Preface

In modern TCM hospitals in China doctors are usually expected to make three diagnoses: the Western medical diagnosis, the TCM diagnosis and the differential diagnosis according to syndrome. It is worth noting that some TCM disease classifications sound exactly the same as the Western ones, and others are very different. Thus a case of haemoptysis may be classified in the following way:

Western diagnosis: Left-sided lobar pneumonia
TCM diagnosis: Cough with dyspnoea
Differentiation: Phlegm Heat in the Lung
Treatment principle: Clear Phlegm Heat, stop cough.

In the following case histories the Western medical diagnosis of each disease is given as the heading, except in Part five, which covers diseases affecting the channels. To avoid repetition, the diagnosis which follows the examination section of each case is therefore the TCM diagnosis, usually followed by a differentiation according to syndrome.

This book is a collection of abstracts from many different journals, and not all the contributors followed this protocol. In some cases doctors treat without reference to pulse and tongue, and prescribe points according to the Western diagnosis of the disease. Some of the case histories do not include a TCM diagnosis or treatment principle, but nevertheless contain useful point prescriptions and details. A wide variety of needle techniques are mentioned by name in the book, for example, 'Reinforcing by obtaining sensations of heat'. For detailed descriptions of many of these needle manipulations the reader is referred to *Acupuncture and Moxibustion: A Guide to Clinical Practice* by B. Auteroche et al (Churchill Livingstone 1992). All the names of the needle techniques mentioned here are consistent with those described by Auteroche.

1993   Oran Kivity

Part One
GENERAL MEDICINE

RESPIRATORY DISORDERS

1. Pulmonary tuberculosis

Zhang, male, age 34, worker

Case registered: 5 March 1953

History: The patient had been in hospital for 11 months with pulmonary tuberculosis, but had not responded to treatment. He had a cough, white sputum tinged with blood, and occasional haemoptysis with a lot of blood. He also suffered from pain and discomfort in the chest, low grade fever which was worse in the afternoon, night sweats, fatigue, poor appetite, gradual weight loss, diarrhoea, anxiety and five palm heat.

Examination: The patient was listless and underweight. *Temperature:* 37.8°C, with pallor, malar flush and weak voice. *Tongue body:* pale and thin. *Tongue coating:* yellow in the middle and white at the edges. *Pulse:* deep, thin and weak.

Diagnosis: Cough with dyspnoea.

Treatment: Nourish and reinforce Deficient Lung Yin to protect the Lung and reduce Deficiency Heat. Strengthen Spleen to promote digestion.

Principal Points: Bailao (Extra), Gaohuangshu BL 43, Taodao Du 13, Feishu BL 13, Zhongfu LU 1. The points were all reinforced with light manipulation followed by strong moxibustion.

Secondary points: Shanzhong Ren 17, Zhongwan Ren 12, Zusanli ST 36, Taixi KID 3, all with reinforcing technique.

Treatment was given daily for 20 days, then every 2nd day for 30 days, then every 3rd day for another 30 days.

After the first five treatments, the afternoon fever had diminished. After 10 more treatments it was markedly reduced, and the patient expectorated less, though the sputum was still slightly bloody. His appetite and spirits improved.

After 20 treatments, there was substantially less sputum, which was also free of blood, and his appetite improved.

After 35 treatments he was in good spirits, gaining weight and passing normal stools.

After 45 treatments, the cough, expectoration, pain and distress in the chest had gone, and his temperature was normal. Chest X-rays revealed that the foci had been mostly absorbed.

The patient was advised to try and avoid getting worried and angry, to be cautious with sex and wine, and to take a complete rest.

Du Dewu, ACUPUNCTURE AND MOXIBUSTION SECTION, SHANDONG TCM COLLEGE HOSPITAL

Editor's Note: Pulmonary tuberculosis is caused partially by the bacterium Mycobacterium tuberculosis, and partially by weak and Deficient Qi. The disease starts in the Lung, then affects the Spleen and Kidneys, eventually progressing to all the Zang. In this case the disorder was caused by Deficient Lung and Kidney Yin, with Deficiency Fire burning the collaterals, and weakness in the Spleen and Stomach.

Bailao (Extra) is a specific for tuberculosis. Gaohuangshu BL 43 is an important point in all consumptive diseases, particularly with moxibustion. When Feishu BL 13 and Zhongfu LU 1, the Back-Shu and Front-Mu points of the Lung are used together, they invigorate the Lung and treat consumption. Moxibustion at Taodao Du 13 and Shanzhong Ren 17 strengthens Upright (Zheng) Qi, eliminates pathogenic factors, and regulates the flow of Qi by stopping cough and reducing Phlegm. Zhongwan Ren 12 and Zusanli ST 36 reinforce the Spleen and Stomach (Earth), which strengthen the Lung (Metal). Reinforcing Taixi KID 3, the Source point, nourishes Kidney Yin and eliminates Deficiency Heat.

2. Asthma

CASE 1

K, female, age 43, foreigner

History: The patient had suffered from paroxysmal asthma for 3 years, which was brought on by fatigue, cold or menstruation. On this occasion it was triggered by fatigue. Her condition was diagnosed in a Beijing hospital as bronchial asthma. At first her symptoms fluctuated, then became steadily worse, responding neither to Western nor Traditional Chinese Medicine.

Symptoms included continuous gasping for breath and rattling of sputum in the throat. She was unable to lie on her back, and expectorated large amounts: approximately 100 ml of phlegm each hour. She had been unable to eat or sleep for 5–6 days, and had drunk only a little fruit juice or hot water. Her waist was painful, and she passed dry stools and scanty reddish urine.

Examination: The patient had a pale and shrivelled complexion, cyanosed lips, and a sweaty forehead. Her voice was weak and she felt tired. She had to sit still to be able to breathe. *Tongue coating:* white and moist. *Pulse:* deep, thin and weak.

Diagnosis: Asthma: Lung and Kidney Deficiency, and Deficient Qi in the Middle Burner.

Treatment: Strengthen Kidneys and Spleen, and regulate the flow of Qi to relieve asthma.

Principal Points: Tianxi (Extra)[1], Shenshu BL 23, Qihai Ren 6, Guanyuan Ren 4, Feishu BL 13, Shufu KID 27, Sanyinjiao SP 6, Pishu BL 20, Zusanli ST 36.

Moxibustion was given after acupuncture. After the first treatment the asthma improved, and the sputum was slightly reduced.

Treatment continued once a day for 5 days, by which time the cough had cleared and the sputum was markedly reduced. The patient was able to sleep for 7 hours at a time, and walk about in the corridors of the hospital, although she was still weak and short of breath.

After the sixth treatment the cough and asthma were gone, the patient could sleep for 8–9 hours at a time. She was taking normal meals and was able to walk for longer periods.

After a further week's treatment she was completely well, and regaining her appetite and strength.

Zheng Yugui, SHANDONG TCM COLLEGE HOSPITAL
(see proceedings of the Annual Conference of Shandong Traditional Medicine Society)

Editor's Note: Asthma is a stubborn chronic disease. It is important to differentiate the Excess and Deficiency components of the condition. Treatment aims during acute episodes should be to relieve urgent symptoms, and during remission to strengthen Upright (Zheng) Qi to restore normal body function.

In this case the disease arose from deficiency in both the Lung and Kidneys, and deficiency of Qi in the Middle Burner. 'Asthma and shortness of breath develop from Cold invading Feishu BL 13, which causes

---

[1]Locate by dividing the distance between Shenzhu Du 12 and Tianzong SI 11 into 8 units. The point is 6 units lateral to Shenzhu. Insertion depth 0.8

curdling of Phlegm in the Stomach collateral channel. If this condition persists, the Lung deficiency will affect the Kidneys, which will in turn affect the Spleen. The Spleen is the source of Phlegm, the Lung stores Phlegm. Retention of Phlegm obstructs Qi, and asthma will arise any time there is Wind or Cold. Treatment should be directed up to the Lung and Stomach, and down to the Spleen and Kidneys: to the upper during acute phases and to the lower during remission' (Wang Xugao).

In this case, by strengthening the Kidney and Stomach and regulating the flow of Qi to relieve asthma, Doctor Zheng correctly recognized treatment of the Spleen and Kidney as the primary aim. Shenshu BL 23, Qihai Ren 6 and Guanyuan Ren 4 reinforce Kidney Yang and invigorate Qi in the lower Dan Tien. Sanyinjiao SP 6, Pishu BL 20 and Zusanli ST 36 strengthen the Spleen and Zheng Qi. Feishu BL 13 and Shufu KID 27 strengthen the Kidneys and regulate the flow of Qi to relieve asthma. Tianxing (Extra) enhances the effects of the other points.

CASE 2

Li, female, age 52

Case registered: 24 September 1980

History: The patient had had bronchial asthma for 8 years, with attacks brought on by fatigue or cold. She had difficulty in breathing, was unable to lie flat, and was coughing white sputum. Her waist and knees were painful and weak, and her limbs were cold. Other symptoms were dislike of cold, dizziness, tinnitus and frequent urination. She had come for acupuncture and moxibustion after failing to respond either to Western drugs or to Chinese herbs.

Examination: The patient was panting and had to lift her shoulders to breathe; she was unable to lie flat and there was a gurgling sound in her throat. Her legs were slightly swollen. *Tongue body:* swollen, pale, scalloped. *Tongue coating:* greasy white. *Pulse:* deep and thin.

Diagnosis: Asthma: Spleen and Kidney Yang Deficiency.

Treatment: Warm the Spleen and reinforce the Kidneys; send down Rebellious Qi and relieve the asthma.

Principal Points: Zhaohai KID 6 (bilateral), Gongsun SP 4 (bilateral), Qihai Ren 6.

The points were needled with reinforcing technique, followed by moxibustion. The needles were retained for 15 minutes, then the points were massaged for 1 minute after removal.

Treatments were given once every other day. After seven sessions her asthma was relieved, and she was able to work. She experienced no relapse the following winter.

Explanation: The patient's Kidney and Spleen Qi were both deficient, and therefore could not warm Chong Mai and bring Qi to the Kidneys. The Qi of Chong Mai flowed the wrong way with Phlegm, affecting the chest and throat and causing the attacks.

Zhaohai KID 6 warms the Kidneys, astringes Chong Mai and clears the air passages in the throat to benefit inhalation.

Gongsun SP 4 is one of the Eight Confluent points, and meets Chong Mai in the Stomach, the Heart and the chest. It is therefore used to treat problems in these areas. With acupuncture and moxibustion applied together it warms the Spleen, strengthens Qi and astringes Qi in Chong Mai.

Qihai Ren 6 invigorates Kidney Yang, reinforces the Kidney and relieves asthma.

Li Licheng, JINAN CENTRAL MUNICIPAL HOSPITAL, SHANDONG PROVINCE
(see Heilongjiang Traditional Chinese Medicine, Issue 3, 1983)

3. Haemoptysis

Wang, female, age 54, worker

Case registered: June 1984

History: For the previous 22 years this patient had had episodes of coughing up blood. This had become worse over the last 4 months. After admission to hospital, she coughed up 30–50 ml of blood with clots every morning. The colour of the blood varied from fresh to dark. She had scanty white sputum, joint pain, palpitations and dyspnoea which was worse on exertion. Her appetite was poor and her stools were sometimes loose and sometimes very dry.

Examination: The patient was emaciated and her complexion was yellow. *Temperature:* normal. *Tongue coating:* thin and white. *Pulse:* deep, thin and rapid.

Diagnosis: Haemoptysis: Spleen and Kidney Deficiency; Heat in the Lung damaging the collaterals.

Treatment: Reinforce Kidney Qi, clear Heat from the Lung.

Principal Points: Kongzui LU 6, Yuji LU 10, Fenglong ST 40, Zusanli ST 36.

Kongzui LU 6 and Yuji LU 10 were reduced, Fenglong ST 40 and Zusanli ST 36 were reinforced. All the points were needled bilaterally. The needles were retained for 30 minutes and manipulated at 10-minute intervals. Treatment was given daily. After 6 days the haemoptysis had stopped, but some dark blood clots could still be seen in the patient's sputum. The dyspnoea from the Kidneys failing to grasp Qi remained.

Secondary Points: Shenshu BL 23 (bilateral) and Qihai Ren 6 were added.

After 14 treatments all the patient's symptoms had gone, and she was discharged in good health. The case was monitored for 5 months, during which time she had no relapse.

Explanation: Haemoptysis is caused by damage to the channels and collaterals. Kongzui LU 6 was needled to treat the urgent symptoms. Yuji LU 10, the Yong-Spring point purges Lung Heat. Zusanli ST 36, the He-Sea point and Fenglong ST 40, the Luo-Connecting point, together strengthen the Spleen and tonify Qi to hold Blood in the channels, with the added benefits of resolving Phlegm and sending down Turbid Qi. Shenshu BL 23 and Qihai Ren 6 tonify the Kidneys, enabling them to grasp Qi. This approach thus treated both the symptoms and the cause.

Yang Yongnian, QIANJIANG SANATORIUM OF SHANGHAI RAILWAY BUREAU
(*see Shanghai Journal of Acupuncture and Moxibustion, Issue 3, 1986*)

4. Pneumonia

CASE 1

Huang, female, age 22, student

Case registered: July 1965

History: The patient had high fever, shortness of breath and chest pain. She was coughing up rust-red sputum. Her lips were cyanosed and she suffered delirium and convulsions.

Examination: The patient looked seriously ill. *Temperature:* 40°C. Her neck was soft and her thorax symmetrical. Diminished breath sounds and a thin wet rale could be heard in the right lung. Heart rate regular at 120/min. A first degree blowing murmur could be heard in the apex area of the heart. Her liver and spleen were not palpable. Knee reflex was hyperfunctional. *Total WBC:* $17.8 \times 10^9/1$ ($17.8 \times 10^3/mm^3$), neutrophils 89%, lymphocytes 10%, eosinophils 1%. Chest X-rays showed a thickened shadow at the upper lobe of the right lung. *Tongue body:* red. *Tongue coating:* yellow and greasy. *Pulse:* full and rapid.

Diagnosis: Right-sided lobar pneumonia: cough with dyspnoea, Phlegm Heat in the Lung.

Treatment: Purge Lung Heat and Phlegm.

Principal Points: Dazhui Du 14, Jugu L.I. 16, Quchi L.I. 11, Neiguan P 6, Zhongwan Ren 12, Zusanli ST 36, Sanyinjiao SP 6, Yunmen LU 2, Shufu KI 27.

All the points were reduced, and the needles were retained for 30 minutes. After this treatment the patient's chest pain improved markedly, her breathing became easier and the cyanosis cleared. Her temperature dropped to 38°C.

The prescription was repeated the next day, after which her coughing and spitting got markedly better, her temperature dropped to 37°C, and her spirits improved.

The prescription was repeated 2 days later, and all her symptoms improved further.

The patient was discharged in good health after a period of rest and nursing.

Zhang Taoqing, GANSU PROVINCIAL TCM HOSPITAL
(*see Chinese Journal of Acupuncture andMoxibustion, Issue 1, 1982*)

CASE 2

Chen, male, age 25, peasant

Case registered: January 1975

History: The patient had had a fever for 4 days, and was coughing up rust-red sputum, with pain in the chest, asthma and dyspnoea.

Examination: Temperature: 40.9°C. BP 16.3/8.0 kPa (122/60 mmHg). His breathing was rapid, percussion sounds dull at the middle and upper parts of the right lung. Respiration sounds were thinner, with moderate amount of wet rales and bronchial breathing Left lung was normal, with no heart murmur, and the liver and spleen were not palpable. WBCs totalled $9.5 \times 10^9/1$ ($9.5 \times 10^3/mm$), neutrophils 83%. X-rays on the 4th day after admission revealed extensive mottled patchy shadows of uneven density on the middle and lower portion of the right lung.

Diagnosis: Lobar pneumonia: cough with dyspnoea, Phlegm Heat in the Lung.

Treatment: Relieve asthma by clearing Lung Heat and facilitating the flow of Lung Qi.

Principal Points: Feishu BL 13 (bilateral).

Water was injected into the points with the patient sitting upright. After sterilization and accurate location a needle was inserted deep into the muscle. Lifting and thrusting method was used to obtain local sensations of soreness, numbness and distension, after which the needle was withdrawn. 2 ml. of water was then injected into the point, starting from the maximum insertion depth and continuing as the needle was slowly withdrawn. The patient was asked to lie down immediately after the treatment in case he fainted. Treatment was given twice a day for 3 days, then once a day thereafter. After 16 days chest X-rays proved normal and the patient was discharged as cured.

Explanation: These two cases arose from Phlegm and Heat in the Lung. The treatment aims were to clear Heat and facilitate the flow of Qi to relieve asthma. In the first case, conventional needling was used; multiple points were selected on the basis of correct analysis of the signs and symptoms. The second case was treated with hydro-acupuncture. This therapy has several advantages: it is easy to administer, requires few points and has a long-lasting effect.

Zhang Shengli, ZHONGXIAN PEOPLE'S HOSPITAL, SICHUAN PROVINCE
(see Chinese Acupuncture and Moxibustion, Issue 6, 1983)

5. 'Flu-like' illness

Liu, male, age 58, doctor.

Case registered: Autumn 1958.

History: The patient had a headache, had a high fever of 40°C and was aching all over. After 4 days in intensive care the fever was unabated. By this stage his symptoms were fever, aching and soreness in the head and whole body, sore throat, constipation of several days' duration, and scanty reddish urination.

Examination: Temperature: 40°C. *Tongue body:* crimson red. *Tongue coating:* central; thick and yellow. *Pulse:* full and tight.

Diagnosis: Common cold: autumn warmth syndrome.

Treatment: Cool Heat and induce sweating to release the Exterior.

Principal Points: Fengchi GB 20, Fengfu Du 16, Baihui Du 20, Touwei

ST 8, Tai Yang (Extra), Dazhui Du 14, Hegu L.I. 4, Zhongwan Ren 12, Yanglingquan GB 34 and Sanyinjiao SP 6.

After Qi was obtained at each point, birdpecking reducing method[1] was used for 1 minute, then the needle was withdrawn. The next morning the patient's family reported that the fever and aching had gone after the acupuncture and that he had managed to sleep well. His appetite was still poor, however, and he was generally quite weak.

The treatment aims were now adjusted to clear the head and eyes, strengthen the bone, tendon and muscle and regulate the Qi of the Middle Burner.

Secondary Points: Fengfu Du 16, Sishencong (Extra), Touwei ST 8, Tai Yang (Extra), Yintang (Extra), Dashu BL 11, Geshu BL 17, Shenshu BL 23, Shanzhong Ren 17, Zhongwan Ren 12, Qihai Ren 6, Yanglingquan GB 34, Zusanli ST 36 and Xuanzhong GB 39. Reinforcing method was used by twirling the needles.

After this treatment the patient's appetite and strength recovered so well he was able to teach that afternoon.

Du Dewu, ACUPUNCTURE AND MOXIBUSTION SECTION, SHANDONG TCM COLLEGE HOSPITAL

Editor's Note: This was a case of invasion by External Heat pathogens, causing an unbroken fever for 4 days. The fever and all the other symptoms subsided after one acupuncture treatment, which demonstrates its rapid effectiveness in acute febrile diseases.

DIGESTIVE SYSTEM DISORDERS

6. Oesophagitis

Jiang, male, age 53

Case registered: 9 February 1985

History: On 29 January the patient felt difficulty and pain on swallowing, with sensations of obstruction in the oesophagus and distress in the chest.

Examination: Examination revealed hyperaemia of the throat with bleeding. Two barium X-ray examinations confirmed a diagnosis of oesophagitis. *Tongue body:* red. *Tongue coating:* thick. *Pulse:* wiry and slippery.

---

[1]Birdpecking: rhythmically lifting and thrusting the needle repeatedly with a small amplitude.

Diagnosis: Dysphagia.

Treatment: Clear Heat from the Middle Burner, remove Blood stasis, regulate the diaphragm and clear collaterals.

Principal Points: The Jiaji (Extra) points at C4–C6.

The needles were inserted to a depth of 1 cun and retained for 20 minutes, and manipulated three times at intervals. Afterwards the points were cupped, then the patient was given some water to drink. He felt no obstruction, but some discomfort, which improved the next day after a repeat treatment.

The points were needled a final time on the 3rd day and the disorder was completely cured.

> Case treated by Chen Keqin, case study by Wu Yan, SHENXI TCM INSTITUTE
> *(see Jianxi Traditional Chinese Medicine, Issue 5, 1985)*

Editor's Note: The sensation of obstruction when swallowing is called *Ye*; the sensation of fullness and obstruction in the chest and diaphragm is called *Ge*. These are two different symptoms, but they usually occur together. Thus dysphagia is known in TCM as *Yege*.

Yege can be differentiated into Excess or Deficiency types. The Excess type is usually caused by emotional depression causing Stagnation of Qi in the chest. In addition there may be coagulation of Body Fluids into Phlegm, which eventually stagnates the flow of Qi and Blood. Dysphagia results from obstruction of the Upper Burner by Phlegm and Blood.

The Deficiency type arises from weakness of the Stomach and Spleen leading to Deficiency of Qi and Blood, and damage to the fluids. This leads to a lack of Blood and Body Fluids with Deficiency Fire burning and drying the oesophagus.

This case was an Excess condition and was completely relieved after three treatments by needling the Jiaji (Extra) points.

7. Oesophageal carcinoma

Yan, male, age 43

Case registered: 11 March 1978

History: From the end of 1977 the patient had had difficulty in swallowing, and phlegm, which had cleared without treatment. Barium X-ray revealed carcinoma of the lower oesophagus and cardia, and his symptoms thereafter got steadily worse. By the time he came for treatment he was suffering from pain and a feeling of fullness in the chest, had been unable to eat or drink for 3 days and had had no bowel movement for 6 or 7 days.

Examination: A barium X-ray showed oesophagectasis, obstruction near the diaphragm and retroperistalsis.

Diagnosis: Dysphagia.

Treatment: Open the chest and diaphragm, regulate Rebellious Qi.

Principal Points: Tiantu Ren 22, Zhongwan Ren 12, Zusanli ST 36, Gongsun SP 4, Fenglong ST 40, Dachangshu BL 25, Tianshu ST 25.
   The points were needled for 20–30 minutes using the twirling method of reinforcing and reducing equally. At the same time the patient was encouraged to swallow, and given 30–50 ml of water. After this treatment he was able to eat about 300 ml of millet porridge, and that night he passed about 50 g of dry pellet-like stool.

Secondary Points: Geshu BL 17, Geguan BL 46, Weishu BL 21, Daling P 7 and Neiguan P 6, added to Fenglong ST 40, Dachangshu BL 25, and Tianshu ST 25.
   Following treatment the patient was able to eat about 500 ml of millet porridge.
   After two courses of treatment the obstruction was mostly cleared, the patient's spirits improved and his stools became normal. He died on 17 December 1978 without recurrence of the obstruction.

Explanation: This treatment is generally quite effective as an adjunct to a systemic approach if obstruction has occurred. It works better in cases of adeno-carcinoma than for squamous carcinoma. It has little or no effect in cases of obstruction occurring during or after radiotherapy. The acupuncture could not cure the root disease, but complemented the systemic treatment by relieving the patient's distress, clearing the obstruction and enabling him to eat.

Feng Ruzhen, ANYANG PREFECTURE CANCER HOSPITAL, HENAN PROVINCE
(see Journal of Traditional Chinese Medicine, Issue 8, 1982)

8. Achalasia of the cardia

Li, female, age 24

Case registered: 23 February 1981

History: The problem had started a year ago when the patient had started to feel sick and uncomfortable when eating, and had progressed quickly till she had difficulty in swallowing. For the past 4 months her nights had been troubled by vomiting; at first this was only in reaction to food, but more recently even a drink of water would make her sick.

Her hospital had diagnosed achalasia of the oesophagus after barium X-ray examination, and she was given Chinese herbs to regulate Qi and dissolve Phlegm, as well as injections of atropine, all with no effect.

Examination: She was emaciated and weak, intolerant of cold, with cold limbs and loose stools. *Tongue body:* pale and swollen. *Tongue coating:* thin and white. *Pulse:* thin and weak.

Diagnosis: Vomiting.

Treatment: Warm and regulate the Middle Burner, invigorate the Spleen, send down Rebellious Qi.

Principal Points: Neiguan P 6, Zhongwan Ren 12, Qimen LIV 14, Zusanli ST 36, Dushu BL 16, Pishu BL 20, Weishu BL 21.

Four of these points were used at a time, with reinforcing method followed by moxibustion. Treatment was given daily.

After three treatments the patient felt an improvement in the sensation of obstruction, but she continued to vomit food and water at night.

Secondary Points: Auricular points: Diaphragm, Stomach, Oesophagus, Cardiac orifice.

The principal points were reinforced with ear acupuncture, retaining 0.5 cun needles for 30 minutes. Treatment was given daily, alternating left and right ears.

After the first of these combined treatments the patient's symptoms improved, and the vomiting stopped after the second. After 15 treatments she had no symptoms at all.

Liu Mingyi, ACUPUNCTURE AND MOXIBUSTION SECTION, GUIYANG TCM COLLEGE HOSPITAL

Editor's Note: The main symptoms in this case were difficulty in swallowing and vomiting, so this case was classified in TCM as 'vomiting'. The signs and symptoms indicate Deficiency Cold in the Spleen and Stomach, with obstruction of both Phlegm and Qi. Neiguan P 6, Zhongwan Ren 12, Qimen LIV 14 and Zusanli ST 36 regulate the Qi of the Middle Burner and the functions of the Stomach. Pishu BL 20 and Weishu BL 21 strengthen and invigorate the Qi of the Middle Burner. Dushu BL 16 relieves fullness in the chest and diaphragm.

Acupuncture followed by moxibustion at these points warms and invigorates the Middle Burner, and enhances their effects of regulating Qi and sending down Rebellious Qi. This persistent condition was thus cured in 14 days.

9. Food poisoning

Zhang, male, age 13

Case registered: 12 December 1958.

History: The patient ate some donkey meat for lunch and 2 hours later started to feel some pain in the abdomen, which got steadily worse. He began to vomit continuously, with diarrhoea and cold limbs, and felt faint and weak.

Examination: The patient's abdomen was tender and painful, and his limbs were cold. Obvious dehydration. *BP:* 6.67/3.33 kPa (50/25 mmHg). *Tongue coating:* none. *Pulse:* deep, thin and weak and a little rapid.

Diagnosis: Food poisoning: vomiting and diarrhoea.

Treatment: Invigorate the Qi of the Middle Burner and regulate the function of the Stomach to suppress vomiting and stop diarrhoea.

Principal Points: Zhongwan Ren 12, Neiguan P 6 (bilateral), Tianshu ST 25 (bilateral), Guanyuan Ren 4, Zusanli ST 36 (bilateral), Weizhong BL 40 (bilateral), Chengshan BL 57 (bilateral).
   Weizhong BL 40 was needled with a three-edged needle and bled. 15 minutes after this prescription was given the abdominal pain, vomiting and diarrhoea were all alleviated. Blood pressure remained low however.

Secondary Points: Shenque Ren 8. Moxibustion was given for 1 hour. The patient's blood pressure gradually returned to 13.3/9.33 kPa (100/70 mmHg). His hands and feet grew warmer, his pulse became strong and he was discharged from hospital after a period of rest.

Explanation: This case of food poisoning is classified in TCM as vomiting and diarrhoea. The *Ling Shu* says, 'Disordered Qi in the Stomach and intestines creates vomiting and diarrhoea ... treat the Spleen and Stomach channels'. Disordered Qi in the Stomach and Intestines affects the functions of descending and ascending energy, so treatment should reinforce the Qi of the Middle Burner and regulate the functions of the Stomach.
   Zhongwan Ren 12 is the Front-Mu point of the Stomach; it regulates and nourishes the Stomach and Middle Burner.

Neiguan P 6, the Luo-Connecting point, is one of the eight Confluent points and connects with Yin Wei Mai (Linking Vessel). It regulates the Qi of the Middle Burner, normalizes the functions of the Stomach and sends down Rebellious Qi.

Tianshu ST 25 is the Front-Mu point of the Large Intestine channel, and Guanyuan Ren 4 is the Front-Mu point of the Small Intestine channel. Together they restore the functions of the Intestines, remove stagnation and obstruction by sending down the Turbid and clearing space for the Clear.

Zusanli ST 36, the He-Sea point, is an important point for stomach and intestinal diseases. It regulates and nourishes the Stomach and Spleen, clears the Intestines by removing obstruction and strengthens the whole body.

Moxibustion at Shenque Ren 8 reinforces Source Qi, warms the Qi of the Middle Burner and readjusts the Intestines.

Bleeding Weizhong BL 40 clears poison from the Blood, and Chengshan BL 57 alleviates urgency and spasm.

Zang Yuwen, ACUPUNCTURE AND MOXIBUSTION SECTION, SHANDONG TCM COLLEGE HOSPITAL
(see Journal of Acupuncture and Moxibustion, Issue 2, 1966)

10. Vomiting

CASE 1

Wei, male, age 28, cadre

Case registered: 15 February 1958

History: The patient had been belching and vomiting water for 5 years. The problem started in 1953, when he had been working in the countryside and eating badly and irregularly. He had oppression in the upper abdomen, dull pain, belching, vomiting after eating or drinking water. He would also vomit if exposed to wind or cold, and retch if his stomach was empty. This had persisted day and night for 5 years, and had not responded to Chinese or Western medication.

Examination: The patient was emaciated, with thin and shallow respiration. His voice was thin, and he spoke little. *Tongue body:* pale. *Tongue coating:* thin and white. *Pulse:* thin and slow.

Diagnosis: Vomiting: Deficiency of Spleen and Stomach, Rebellious Stomach Qi.

Treatment: Strengthen Yang, send down Rebellious Qi, regulate the functions of the Stomach.

Principal Points: Three groups of points were selected, and one group was needled each day, with reinforcing manipulation followed by moxibustion.

1. Zusanli ST 36, Zhongwan Ren 12, Pishu BL 20, Qimen LIV 14, Guanyuan Ren 4.
2. Shangwan Ren 13, Qihai Ren 6, Neiguan P 6, Gongsun SP 4, Riyue GB 24.
3. Juque Ren 14, Weishu BL 21, Jianshi P 5, Zhangmen LIV 13, Tianshu ST 25.

The original intention was to treat the patient in this way for a month before reviewing the procedure, but after three sessions his symptoms improved dramatically. After 20 days he stopped vomiting, and his appetite, strength and spirits were much better.

At this point the acupuncture was stopped and he was advised to rest and follow a more regular lifestyle. This he did, and he was well within a month. The case was followed up and there was no relapse.

Explanation: Vomiting can arise from Excess or Deficiency patterns. In both kinds Rebellious Qi affects the Stomach, which fails to send Qi down.

Irregular eating impaired this patient's Stomach Qi, and he had 5 years of stomach trouble as a result. This weakened him, so it was necessary to strengthen his Yang, as well as regulate the Stomach to send down the Rebellious Qi.

Yang Jiebin, CHENGDU TCM HOSPITAL
(see Correspondence Journal of Acupuncture and Moxibustion, Issue 1, 1987)

CASE 2

Zhang, male, age 35

Case registered: 26 May 1979

History: This patient had been healthy and strong until 5 April 1979, when after a 10-minute bus journey he became faint and nauseated and began to vomit continuously. He was so weak he had to be carried home, and from that time on vomited whenever he ate. Various investigations including EEG, spinal puncture, barium meal X-ray and oesophagoscopy were normal, so he was given a diagnosis of 'neurogenic dysphagia'. The vomiting continued, and he was fed nasally and with glucose drips. After 50 days he was very distraught, and came to Shanghai for treatment.

Examination: The patient was restless, thin, yellow and exhausted. *Tongue body:* red. *Tongue coating:* thin. *Pulse:* thin and slightly wiry.

Diagnosis: Vomiting: Hyperactive Liver Qi invading the Stomach, failure of Stomach to send Qi down.

Treatment: Reinforce Yin and nourish the Blood, relieve the chest and Qi of the Middle Burner, strengthen the Spleen and regulate the function of the Stomach.

Principal Points: Weishu BL 21 (bilateral), Tiantu Ren 22, Danzhong Ren 17, Liangmen ST 21 (bilateral), Neiguan P 6 (bilateral), Zhongwan Ren 12, Zusanli ST 36 (bilateral), Sanyinjiao SP 6 (bilateral).

Weishu BL 21 was reinforced to contract the Stomach, then Tiantu Ren 22 was gently reduced until needle sensation spread to the chest. These needles were not retained. Reinforcing and reducing equally method was used at Danzhong Ren 17, Liangmen ST 21 and Zhongwan Ren 12, and the remaining points were reinforced. These needles were retained for 30 minutes and manipulated at intervals, while the patient was encouraged to swallow.

After this the patient was able to swallow, but still felt nauseated. He was advised to drink a lot of water.

After two more treatments he stopped vomiting and began to eat and drink. The case was followed up for a year and there was no relapse.

Situ Hansun and Zhu Wenying, ACUPUNCTURE AND MOXIBUSTION SECTION, SHANGHAI PEOPLE'S HOSPITAL 1
(see Shanghai Journal of Acupuncture and Moxibustion, Issue 2, 1983)

Editor's Note: This patient had been healthy and strong until the sudden onset of faintness and nausea, which arose from Stagnant Liver Qi invading the Stomach (Wood invading Earth). The Spleen is Yin Earth, and raises Qi; the Stomach is Yang Earth, and sends Qi down. When the Liver does not smooth the flow of Qi, the Spleen cannot send Qi up and the Stomach cannot send Qi down so it rebels upwards causing vomiting. Vomiting depletes the Stomach and Spleen, so the disease becomes Deficient in character, which is why reducing techniques were barely used.

Reinforcing Weishu BL 21, Neiguan P 6, Zusanli ST 36 and Sanyinjiao SP 6 nourishes and strengthens the Stomach and Spleen. Reducing Tiantu Ren 22 sends down Rebellious Qi. Reinforcing and reducing equally at Danzhong Ren 17, Liangmen ST 21 and Zhongwan Ren 12 relieves the chest and the Qi of the Middle Burner, and invigorates the Middle Burner.

11. Epigastric fullness

Shao, male, age 68

Case registered: 18 September 1980

History: The patient had upper abdominal fullness with reduced appetite for 3 years. His symptoms were intermittent, but although he took medication continuously, he always relapsed. Examinations revealed no sign of organic disease. Over the last month he had fullness and distress in the chest and upper abdomen, with poor appetite and disturbed sleep. Occasionally he had a sensation of hot gas rushing upwards to the chest, and burning pains in the upper abdomen. These symptoms occurred about three times a day and caused the patient severe discomfort.

Examination: The patient was restless, and had a bitter taste in his mouth. Electrical current was measured at the Yuan-Source points. *Pulse:* thin, wiry and rapid.

Diagnosis: Rushing Piglet syndrome: Liver Qi Stagnation transforming into Heat, Rebellious Qi rushing up.

Treatment: Soothe and redirect Rebellious Qi downwards, clear Pathogenic Liver Heat.

Principal Points: Taichong LIV 3, Chongyang ST 42, Zhaohai KID 6, Shangjuxu ST 37, Xiajuxu ST 39.

All the points were needled bilaterally. Taichong LIV 3 and Chongyang ST 42 were reduced, and the other points were needled with reinforcing and reducing evenly method. Treatment was given once every other day. After 10 treatments the disease was cured. Electrical current at the 12 Yuan-Source points was remeasured.

Table of electrical resistance

Before treatment			
Taichong LIV 3		Chongyang ST 42	
Left	*Right*	*Left*	*Right*
64 µA	66 µA	74 µA	80 µA
Comparison to average of resistance at 12 Source points			
+26 µA	+30 µA	+36 µA	+44 µA
After treatment			
30 µA	32 µA	38 µA	40 µA
Comparison to average of resistance at 12 Source points			
+2 µA	+3 µA	+10 µA	+11 µA
Individual changes			
–34 µA	–34 µA	–36 µA	–40 µA

Explanation: The *Jin Gui Yao Lue* (Prescriptions from the Golden Chamber) describes Rushing Piglet syndrome: 'Gas rises like a rushing piglet from the lower abdomen up to the throat. It can cause severe discomfort and is due to fright'. The *Wai Tai Mi Yao* (Medical Secrets of an Official Vol. 12) quotes the *Xiao Pin Fang* (Simple Prescriptions) to give the following description: 'Rushing Piglet Gas is caused by fright. The patient is restless and nervous. The organs are disturbed causing sickness in the stomach and distress in the chest. Mental disturbance is also possible. The disorder can come and go dramatically. The patient may present with distress, shortness of breath and cold limbs'.

Rushing Piglet syndrome can be differentiated into three types, a Heat pattern and two Cold patterns. *Heat:* Emotional disturbance can cause Liver disharmony, which stops promoting the free movement of Qi and becomes Stagnant. Stagnant Liver Qi transforms into Fire, and Fire and Heat rise with the Liver Qi to cause the disease. *Cold:* i) Excessive perspiration causes Deficiency of Yang and invites attack by exterior pathogens. These induce cold Qi in the organs to rise upwards; ii) If there is Stagnation of Water in the Lower Burner, invasion of external pathogens causes Water to move inside after perspiration.

The *Su Wen* says, 'The Chong and Kidney channels travel alongside each other, and ascend along both sides of the navel. If the Kidney Qi is deficient, Chong Mai is damaged, and the Qi rises rebelliously causing sensations of contracture' (Gu Kong Lun, Bones chapter). Chong Mai is the supplementary vessel of the Kidney. If the Kidney is Deficient, the Qi in Chong Mai is liable to break loose and rush upwards, impairing the digestion. The manifestations of disease in Chong Mai are Rebellious Qi, contracture, fullness and pain in the abdomen, pain in the sides, faintness, and a wiry, long pulse. It is most severe in people who are very emotional.

The syndrome can be differentiated into Heat, Cold and Cold Water patterns. It can also be differentiated into Kidney, Liver and Stomach types. For all of these, however, it is the Rebellious Qi in Chong Mai which causes the sensations of gas rushing upwards like a piglet.

To treat the Heat type, purge the Heat and redirect the Rebellious Qi downwards. To treat the Cold type, disperse the Cold by warming the Yang and soothe the Rebellious Qi. To treat the Cold Water type, warm the Yang, move the Water and soothe the Rebellious Qi. In all of these types, soothing and redirecting the Rebellious Qi in Chong Mai downwards is paramount. To conclude, the key to successful treatment is correct differentiation and treating Chong Mai.

Li Licheng, JINAN CENTRAL MUNICIPAL HOSPITAL, SHANDONG PROVINCE

12. Gastric dilatation with cardiospasm

Zhang, female, age 67

History: The patient had suffered for 9 years from a feeling of fullness in the abdomen after eating. This had got gradually worse, and was especially bad if she ate rice. A year ago she had turned to semiliquid foods like porridge, oatmeal and milk, which she found easier to digest. Treatment at the local district hospital had not helped, and for the past month she had not even been able to keep her semiliquid food down. She also had palpitations, a heavy feeling in her stomach and felt faint. By this point she was refusing to eat at all because she would vomit immediately afterwards. She had not responded to any treatment and she and her family had lost hope of a cure. She was near death.

Examination: The patient was pale and emaciated. She looked exhausted and very ill. Her voice was weak and her eyes dull. Her limbs were slightly cold and she could not stand still. *Hypotension:* BP 10.7/6.67 kPa (80/50 mmHg), RBC $2.3 \times 10^{12}/1$ $(2.3 \times 10^6/mm^3)$ Haemoglobin 60 g/1 (6 g%). Weight 30 kg. Barium meal X-ray of stomach and intestines on 18 August 1979 revealed ptosis of the stomach, with the lowest point being 12 cm below the iliac crest, slow evacuation, and oesophagectasis cardia like a bird's beak (sic). *Tongue body:* pale. *Tongue coating:* thin and greasy. *Pulse:* thin and weak.

Diagnosis: Abdominal distension and vomiting.

Treatment: Readjust Qi of Stomach and Spleen.

Principal Points: Zhongwan Ren 12, Tianshu ST 25, Zusanli ST 36, Sanyinjiao SP 6 and Neiguan P 6.

Secondary Points: Xiawan Ren 10, Liangqiu ST 34, Xuehai SP 10, Shuiquan KID 5, Diji SP 8, Shangjuxu ST 37, Pishu BL 20, Weishu BL 21 and Shenshu BL 23.

To prevent vomiting, no medication was given by mouth, but points were needled with reinforcing method and injected with Angelica to nourish the Blood and facilitate the flow of Qi. Treatment was given once daily, and a course of treatment lasted 15 days. Two principal and two secondary points were used each time, acupuncture alternating with injections of Angelica. After the first course the patient felt an improvement in the sensation of fullness and heaviness in the stomach, so she could tolerate a little liquid food, but the vomiting persisted. She felt less faint and was able to come to hospital unassisted.

After another two courses of the same treatment she no longer vomited after eating and regained her appetite: she was able to tolerate porridge, oatmeal and milk. Her spirits gradually improved, her pallor disappeared, her tongue became normal, her pulse slowed down and became strong, and she no longer fainted. She could look after herself and even do some housework.

Barium meal X-ray of the stomach and intestines on 12 January 1980 revealed that the stomach was 8 cm higher, there was only slight cardiac spasm, an improvement in oesophagectasis and better evacuation. RBCs were up to $2.8 \times 10^{12}/1$ $(2.8 \times 10^6/mm^3$, haemoglobin 90 g/l (9 g%). Her weight had increased to 37 kg, and all her symptoms had eased. Treatment was stopped to observe the effect, but there was no relapse.

Explanation: According to TCM theory gastric dilatation arises from Deficiency of Spleen and Stomach Yang. Cardiospasm arises from disorders in Stomach and Spleen Qi. In this case points on the Stomach and Spleen channels and the related Back-Shu points were reinforced. Point injection with Angelica was added to invigorate and adjust the functions of the Stomach and Spleen.

Digestion is supported by Yang Qi and essential substances from the Kidneys. The proper functioning of the Spleen is rooted in the Kidneys. Shenshu BL 23, the Back-Shu point of the Kidneys, was therefore used to promote the function of the Spleen and Stomach.

When harmony between Yin and Yang was re-established and the Stomach Qi was raised, the disease was cured.

Wang Xiuyun, ACUPUNCTURE AND MOXIBUSTION SECTION, GUANGDONG PROVINCIAL TCM HOSPITAL
(*see New Chinese Medicine, Issue 7, 1984*)

13. Gastroptosis

Tan, female, age 55, cadre

Case registered: 12 May 1974

History: For the past 2 years the patient had had frequent abdominal pain which was aggravated by eating. Her appetite was poor and she got progressively thinner. She also had insomnia and amnesia, and felt weak and faint. She had taken 30 doses of Chinese herbs, but without effect.

Examination: The patient was thin and old. Her stomach area was slightly tender. Barium X-ray revealed that the lesser curvature of the angular notch of the stomach was 6 cm below the iliac crest. *Tongue body:* pale red with teethmarks. *Pulse:* deep and thin.

Diagnosis: Abdominal distension.

Treatment: Reinforce Qi of the Middle Burner and raise Spleen Yang.

Principal Points: Zhongwan Ren 12, Tiwei (Extra), Weishang (Extra), Qihai Ren 6, Zusanli ST 36 and Neiguan P 6.[1]

Zhongwan Ren 12 and Qihai Ren 6 were needled perpendicularly to a depth of 1–1.2 cun and reinforced by rotation method. Other points were needled bilaterally. Tiwei (Extra) and Weishang (Extra) were needled at an angle of 45° towards the navel.

Electro-acupuncture was also given, with the negative pole at Zhongwan Ren 12 and the positive poles at Tiwei (Extra), Weishang (Extra) and Qihai Ren 6. Intensity of stimulation was adjusted to be tolerable for the patient, and sparse–dense waves were used for 20–30 minutes.

Treatment was given daily, and a course was 12 days long. 3–5 days were left between courses.

After three courses of treatment the abdominal fullness and pain were alleviated, and the patient's faintness, weakness and poor appetite had improved. After two more treatments these symptoms had virtually disappeared. Reexamination by barium meal X-ray revealed no abnormalities in the digestive tract, and she was discharged as cured.

Explanation: TCM theory classifies gastroptosis as abdominal distension. This is caused by Sinking of Central Qi arising from weakness after protracted illness, especially chronic diseases of the stomach and intestines. When the Spleen and Stomach Qi are Deficient the stomach and related tissues become loose and flaccid and begin to prolapse. Neither Western medicines nor traditional Chinese herbs are effective in this condition, so in this case the methods of the late Dr Chen Xingtian from this hospital were used.

Zhongwan Ren 12, Tiwei (Extra), Weishang (Extra), and Qihai Ren 6 invigorate Central Qi to raise the depressed Yang. Zusanli ST 36 and Neiguan P 6 reinforce the Stomach and regulate the Qi of the Middle Burner. Electro-acupuncture was used to enhance the overall therapeutic effect.

Zhang Dengbu, SHANDONG TCM COLLEGE HOSPITAL

---

[1]Tiwei (Extra): 4 cun lateral to Zhongwan Ren 12. Weishang (Extra): 4 cun lateral to Xiawan Ren 10

14. Volvulus of the stomach

CASE 1

Jin, male, age 24, worker

Case registered: 19 May 1984

History: 5 years previously the patient had had an appendicectomy after acute appendicitis. About a month later he developed intestinal obstruction which was treated with Chinese herbs, but he suffered from fullness and pain in the upper abdomen ever since. In January 1982 he suddenly became nauseated and developed abdominal pain; intestinal obstruction was once again diagnosed and he was treated with Western drugs. The condition recurred in 1983. He came to this hospital in April 1984 still suffering from fullness and pain in the abdomen and dry stools. His condition was diagnosed after barium X-ray examination as volvulus of the stomach and he was referred for acupuncture and moxibustion.

Examination: The patient was young, thin and yellow in appearance. His abdomen was flat and soft. The liver and spleen were not palpable, and his upper abdomen was not tender on palpation. *Tongue body:* red. *Tongue coating:* thin, yellow.

Diagnosis: Stomach pain.

Treatment: Clear Qi and regulate the function of the Stomach and Intestines.

Principal Points: Neiguan P 6, Zhongwan Ren 12, Zusanli ST 36 and Gongsun SP 4.
   The points were needled bilaterally with reinforcing and reducing equally method, and the needles were retained for 30 minutes. Treatment was given daily, with a 1-day interval between courses. A course lasted 6 days.
   After 18 treatments the abdominal fullness and pain improved. After 12 more treatments the patient's symptoms had mostly cleared, and a barium X-ray showed no organic disease in the upper digestive tract. He was discharged as cured one month after admission.

Explanation: This case of volvulus of the stomach is classified in TCM as stomach pain. The patient had had abdominal surgery and repeated abdominal fullness and pain arising from Stagnation of Qi in the Stomach and Intestines. As the disease persisted, his digestive function became weaker and he became thin.
   The treatment aim was to regulate and clear the Qi of the Stomach

and Intestines. Neiguan P 6 is the Confluent point of Yin Wei Mai, which governs the internal organs and is used to treat diseases of the heart, chest and stomach. Zhongwan Ren 12 is the Front-Mu point of the Stomach, and clears and regulates Stagnant Qi in the Stomach and Intestines. This effect is enhanced when it is used in combination with Zusanli ST 36, the He-Sea point. Gongsun SP 4, the Luo-Connecting point of the Spleen channel, regulates the Qi of the Spleen and Stomach, and is especially good for fullness and pain of the upper abdomen.

Zhang Dengbu, SHANDONG TCM COLLEGE HOSPITAL

CASE 2

Jia, male, age 20.

History: The patient had had pain in the upper abdomen for about 2 months. The pain was worse after eating. He had a past history of haemoptysis, and his condition had been diagnosed some years previously as gastric ulcer.

Examination: Barium X-ray showed the stomach was raised and rotated, and the fundus and duodenal bulb were twisted caudally.

Diagnosis: Stomach pain: Spleen Qi Deficiency, Liver Stagnation transformed into Fire, Rebellious Stomach Qi.

Treatment: Regulate and send down Stomach Qi, strengthen Spleen Qi, regulate the Intestines, clear Stagnation and send down the Turbid.

Principal Points: Zusanli ST 36 (bilateral), Zhongwan Ren 12, Weixia (Extra)[1], Xiawan Ren 10, Hegu L.I. 4.

Weixia (Extra) was punctured with a 5 cun needle towards Shenque Ren 8 at an angle of 15° After obtaining Qi the needle was rotated, lifted and thrust with a large amplitude. All the needles were retained for 30 minutes and manipulated at 5 minute intervals. 3–5 large moxa cones on medicated plaster were also burned on Zhongwan Ren 12.

Treatment was given daily. After 20 days the fullness and pain were completely gone and the patient's appetite improved. Barium X-rays revealed that the stomach had returned to normal shape. The case was followed up for 6 years and there was no relapse.

Luo Wei, QINGHAI PROVINCIAL PEOPLE'S HOSPITAL
(see Shanghai Journal of Traditional Chinese Medicine, Issue 1, 1980)

---

[1]Weixia (Extra): located 0.5 cun lateral to Shuifen Ren 9.

15. Acute gastric perforation

Li, male, age 23, worker

Case registered: 30 July 1984

History: Earlier in the day the patient suddenly felt severe piercing pain in his upper abdomen. The pain was continuous, but got worse paroxysmally. Initially the pain was worse in the upper right abdomen, but it spread and became so severe he was unable to breathe normally. He was given symptomatic treatment at his work unit clinic, but this did not help and he was admitted to the surgery department of this hospital at 11.30 p.m.

Examination: Temperature: 38°C. *BP:* 14.7/9.33 kPa (110/70 mmHg). The patient was pale and sweating. His abdomen was rock hard and very tender, especially in the upper and lower right area. There was no visible peristalsis or peristaltic wave. No hepatic dullness. Diminished bowel sounds. Haemoglobin 125 g/l (12.5 g%). WBC 20.4×10^9/l (20.4×10^3/mm³). Lymphocytes 8%. Neutrophils 92%. Abdominal X-ray: there was free gas below the diaphragm, and large quantities of gas in the intestinal cavity. *Tongue coating:* yellow. *Pulse:* wiry and rapid.

Diagnosis: Abdominal pain: Accumulation of Heat, Stasis of Qi and Blood.
    The patient was not allowed food or water. He was given gastro-intestinal decompression, antibiotics and fluid infusion for 12 hours, but his symptoms did not change. After 12 hours he was prescribed acupuncture.

Treatment: Clear Heat, relieve inflammation.

Principal Points: Zhongwan Ren 12, Tianshu ST 25, Liangmen ST 21, Neiguan P 6, Zusanli ST 36.
    All the points were reduced. Electro-acupuncture was given at Zusanli ST 36 with a G6805 unit, at an intensity tolerable to the patient. The needles were retained for an hour. The pain was markedly reduced, with softening of the abdomen. The tenderness became more localized on the upper and lower right hand side. The treatment was repeated after 3 hours. Afterwards the tenderness was only moderate. Bowel sounds could be heard and the patient was able to pass wind. Treatment was then given every 6 hours. By 1 August most of the patient's symptoms had gone. There was slight tenderness below the xiphoid process and in the upper right abdomen. Treatment was continued twice a day. By 2 August there were no more abdominal symptoms. At this point the acupuncture and gastrointestinal decompression were stopped

for observation, but the fluid infusion and anti-inflammatory treatments were continued. After 4 August the patient was on a liquid diet, passing stools regularly and in better spirits. He was discharged as cured from hospital. The case was followed up 6 months later: he was still healthy and had had no adverse reactions.

Explanation: Acupuncture can be very effective in some cases of acute gastric perforation. This case was caused by accumulation of Heat in the Interior and Stagnation of Qi and Blood resulting in obstruction of the Organic Qi. Stagnation of Heat and Blood leads to impaired gastrointestinal peristalsis. The treatment principle is to clear away Heat.

Using Zhongwan Ren 12, the Front-Mu point of the Stomach, and Tianshu ST 25, the Front-Mu point of the Large Intestine, readjusts the function of the stomach and intestines. All these points in combination restore these functions and relieve the inflammation in the abdominal cavity.

Liu Xuilian, ACUPUNCTURE AND MOXIBUSTION SECTION, KUITUN 127TH REGIMENT HOSPITAL, XINGJIAN
(see Xingjian Traditional Chinese Medicine, Issue 1, 1986).

16. Appendiceal abscess

Yan, male, age 52, peasant

Case registered: 18 July 1982

History: 7 days previously the patient was exposed to cold. He developed fever, aversion to cold and periumbilical pain. The pain was dull and paroxysmal, and became worse the next day. After 6 days the pain shifted to his right lower abdomen and an extremely tender mass about the size of a fist emerged there. He was treated in the outpatients' ward for one day without success, and then hospitalized.

Examination: Temperature: 38.1°C. The patient's abdomen was flat with marked muscular tension, tenderness and rebound tenderness in the lower right region. The lump was fist-sized and extremely tender on palpation. *Blood test:* WBC 9° 10^9 (9000 mm³), neutrophils 84%.

Diagnosis: Acute appendicitis.

Treatment: Auricular point injection therapy.

Auricular Points: New Appendix point (Xinlanweidian)[1].

---

[1]New Appendix point is located on the lower margin of the inferior antihelix crus, superior to Kidney and Pancreas/Gall Bladder.

The points on both ears were used. Each point was injected with 0.2 ml of water, or until a 1 cm lump had formed. Treatment was given twice a day.

After 3 days the patient's temperature was normal. After 4 days blood tests were normal. After 5 days treatment was given once a day, on the affected side only. After 7 days the abdominal mass was reduced in size to 3 cm × 4 cm, and the tenderness and abdominal tension disappeared. After 14 days the mass had also disappeared, and the patient was discharged as cured. The case was followed up for 2 months and there was no relapse.

Zhang Shengli, ZHONGXIAN COUNTY PEOPLE'S HOSPITAL, SICHUAN PROVINCE
(see Sichuan Traditional Chinese Medicine, Issue 1, 1987)

Editor's Note: In TCM appendicular abscess is classified as acute appendicitis. This case was cured quickly by auricular point injection. The therapy is simple and easy to administer. If body acupuncture had also been used, the results would have been even quicker.

17. Postoperative intestinal paralysis

Mao, male, age 47

Case registered: 28 September 1978

History: The patient had a chronic stomach ulcer, which had not responded to treatment. He was finally given a successful partial gastrectomy. Following this operation, however, he had abdominal fullness, diminished bowel sound and was unable to pass wind or stool. He was given gastrointestinal decompression, and large quantities of fluid were aspirated. His condition was diagnosed as postoperative gastrointestinal paralysis and he was given Da Cheng Qi Tang (Major Order the Qi Decoction) enemas, acupuncture at Zusanli ST 36 and point injection with neostigmine, but after a week he had not improved so specialists from the Acupuncture and Moxibustion Section were invited for a joint consultation.

Examination: The patient was pale, weak and spoke little. His voice was weak. *Tongue body:* pale. *Pulse:* empty.

Diagnosis: Postoperative exhaustion of Vital Qi, Yang Qi failing to circulate, Large Intestine failing to transport.

Treatment: Nourish and reinforce Vital Qi, warm the Yang and stimulate intestinal movement.

Principal Points: Qihai Ren 6, Guanyuan Ren 4.

Secondary Points: Fujie SP 14 (bilateral).

Five moxa cones were burnt at each point. The cones were placed on medicated biscuits containing Fu Zi (prepared aconite root), Rou Gui (cinnamon bark) and other herbs to warm the Yang. Immediately after treatment the patient felt refreshed and felt an urge to defaecate, but he was not yet strong enough to do this. The treatment was repeated four times. His bowel movements became regular and he was able to eat porridge and noodles. Later he recovered well and was discharged.

Explanation: In Traditional Chinese Medicine the Large Intestine is said to be 'in charge of transportation'. Stagnation of Heat, Deficiency of Body Fluids or Qi can all affect this function. In some cases of intestinal paralysis, non-surgical treatments such as acupuncture, point injection or herbal enemas are the optimum treatments. They are indicated for Excess conditions presenting with abdominal fullness, dry mouth, restlessness, dry yellow tongue coat, and a deep and strong pulse. Acupuncture at Zusanli ST 36 or point injection therapy can also be used for Stagnation of Qi in the Yang Ming channels, presenting with disturbance of the gastrointestinal functions, abdominal fullness, pain and difficulty passing stool, white greasy tongue coating and tight and wiry pulse.

This case did not respond to these treatments because they were applied inappropriately. From the symptoms and pulse it is clear that this was a Deficiency disease. The Yang was exhausted, leading to disturbance of the intestinal function of transporting. Moxibustion at Qihai Ren 6 and Guanyuan Ren 4 with medicated biscuits warms the Yang and restores intestinal peristalsis.

Zhang Yuanlong, Acupuncture and Moxibustion Section,
SHANGHAI TCM COLLEGE HOSPITAL, LONGHUA
(*see Shanghai Journal of Traditional Chinese Medicine. Issue 1, 1980*)

18. Volvulus of the intestine

CASE 1

Song, male, age 24

Case registered: 14 July 1978

History: The patient suddenly developed abdominal pain at 4.00 p.m. when carrying bricks at work. The pain came in bursts, with sensations of abdominal fullness and nausea. As it passed he would be unable to have a bowel movement or pass wind. He had previously been healthy, and had no history of abdominal pain. He was transferred from the county hospital to this one at 8.30 p.m. that day.

Examination: The patient appeared to be in great pain. *Temperature:* 36°C. *Pulse rate:* 76/min. *BP:* 17.3/12.0 kPa (130/90 mmHg). His abdomen was very swollen, and the upper part was distended higher than his xiphoid process. There was high-pitched resonance on percussion. During the bouts of pain strong peristalsis was visible below the navel. There were excessive bowel sounds and sounds of gas. WBC $6.7° × 10^9/1$ ($6.7 × 10^3/mm^3$), neutrophils 61%, monocytes 2%, eosinophils 9%, lymphocytes 28%. X-ray: in the right upper abdomen there was a large liquid filled cavity about 20 cm wide, and many gas-filled intestinal loops around the navel.

Diagnosis: Abdominal pain: Stagnation of Liver Qi, failure of Stomach and Intestines to send Qi down.

Treatment: Relieve Stagnation of Liver Qi, activate and regulate Qi and Blood, regulate Stomach and Intestines.

Principal Points: Zhangmen LIV 13 (bilateral).

The points were needled at 9.45 p.m.. The needles were inserted perpendicularly to a depth of 0.5 cun, then connected to a G6805 electro-acupuncture unit. Sparse-dense wave stimulation was given, at frequency 16, at an intensity tolerable to the patient. Seven minutes after the current was turned on the patient broke wind with an explosive sound. The sensations of fullness improved, the visible peristalsis disappeared and the abdominal pain was relieved. He was peacefully asleep 40 minutes after the current was applied. During the night he was able to pass first dry and then loose stools. The next morning all his symptoms had gone and his abdomen was flat. X-rays showed that the liquid filled cavity had disappeared. He was discharged as cured after one day's observation.

Shan Cuirong, RUSHAN COUNTY HOSPITAL, SHANDONG
(see Shandong Journal of Traditional Chinese Medicine, Issue 3, 1979)

Editor's Note: Volvulus can be classified in TCM as abdominal pain, abdominal fullness or nausea. It is an acute abdominal disease and quite hard to treat. It is usually due to Stagnation of Liver Qi, and failure of the Stomach and Intestines to send down Qi. The Clear and the Turbid interfere with each other, causing obstruction of the intestinal Qi.

Zhangmen LIV 13 is the Front-Mu point of the Spleen, the Hui of the Five Zang, and a meeting point of the Liver and Gall Bladder channels. When reduced it relieves Stagnation of Liver Qi, activates and regulates

Qi and Blood, regulates the Stomach and Intestines. Electro-acupuncture enhances this effect.

CASE 2

Liu, male, age 17

History: 2 hours previously the patient was playing basketball when he developed sudden severe paroxysmal pain in the abdomen, especially in the lower abdomen and around the navel. He was nauseated and vomited frequently. This was diagnosed as intestinal obstruction, and surgery was suggested.

Examination: The patient was well built. He appeared to be in considerable pain and was sweating all over his head. He lay in fetal position. Heart and lungs negative. Visible peristalsis and peristaltic waves. Tension and tenderness around the navel. No rebound tenderness. Excessive bowel sounds.

Auricular Points: Small Intestine, Sympathetic.
   The points were needled bilaterally. The patient felt severe pain when needled, which seemed to travel like a thread from his ear to his navel. The pain improved immediately, then disappeared altogether. Re-examination found all his symptoms had gone.

Explanation: The patient was a young man. His symptoms were abdominal pain, sickness, visible peristalsis and peristaltic wavs, with a palpable abdominal mass. These point conclusively to a diagnosis of intestinal obstruction. The presentation suggests strangulated intestinal obstruction and volvulus.
   This is caused by reversal of the ansa intestinalis on the long axis of the mesentery, leading to obstruction of the intestinal cavity and the blood circulation of the intestinal canal. There are many causative factors: increased gravity in the intestinal canal, i.e. a heavy meal, roundworm entangling in the intestinal cavity, tumours, constipation, megacolon, abnormal intestinal dynamics or external pressure. In this case the pain began whilst the patient was playing basketball. The movement of his body during the game caused abnormal dynamics in the intestinal tract and unbalanced pressure in the intestines. This was a mild volvulus, and could be treated with acupuncture.
   In TCM intestinal obstruction is classified as 'Intestinal Knot' (Chang Jie) or 'Intestinal Blockage' (Chang Ge). In this case the disease was in the initial stages of development, with slight abdominal distension and no signs of peritonitis poisoning. Auricular therapy is easy to administer,

and should therefore be the first choice for intestinal obstruction, especially for volvulus. In serious cases, however, this therapy would not be effective.

Zhang Zhizhu, LIAOCHENG PREFECTURAL HOSPITAL, SHANDONG PROVINCE

19. Abdominal pain, chronic

Li, female, age 27, teacher

Case registered: 25 July 1978

History: The patient had had recurrent dull periumbilical pain for 10 years. For the previous month or so the pain had got worse, and was occasionally accompanied by sensations of fullness and oppression. The pain would move around and extended to her back and waist. The most common times for it to start would be 2.00 p.m.–3.00 p.m. and 7.00 p.m.–9.00 p.m. The condition had been diagnosed as 'gastric neurosis', but protracted treatment with Western drugs and Chinese herbs had had no result.

Examination: Barium X-ray and ultrasound examinations found no organic disease. The patient was pale, thin and emaciated and spoke in a weak voice. Her appetite was poor, and her stools were loose. Her abdomen was not tender on palpation. *Tongue body:* swollen, pale, scalloped. *Tongue coating:* thin, white and moist. *Pulse:* weak and wiry.

Diagnosis: Abdominal pain: Stomach and Spleen Deficiency.

Treatment: Strengthen Spleen and Stomach, promote the circulation of Qi to relieve pain.

Principal Points: Dazhui Du 14, Zusanli ST 36.

Dazhui Du 14 was needled to a depth of 0.8 cun, until the doctor could feel a sensation of tightness and heaviness around the needle, and the patient could feel soreness and distension extending to Fengfu Du 16. The needle was initially manipulated with slowly advance/slowly withdraw method, propagating sensation to the fingers and toes. Zusanli ST 36 was alternated from left to right with each treatment and needled with the same technique, propagating Qi down to the toes and up to the index finger. The points were needled once a day at 2.00 p.m.–3.00 p.m., and the needles were retained for 20 minutes. During this time they were manipulated with slow/fast method.

The pain improved during treatment, then disappeared altogether. It recurred between 7.00 p.m. and 9.00 p.m. that evening, but was not as severe.

The treatment was repeated the next day, with a similar response from the patient. She also felt mild sensations of warmth around the needles.

The next day she felt considerably better and the sensations of warmth during treatment were more evident, extending to the extremities.

After two more treatments the abdominal pain had gone, her appearance was robust, her appetite was better and her pulse was strong. An obstinate disease of 10 years' duration was cured just with acupuncture.

Explanation: This disease arose from Deficiency of the Spleen and Stomach. The Spleen Qi goes into the abdomen and around the navel, which is why the pain was most severe around that area. Dazhui Du 14 is the meeting point of Du Mai with the three hand Yang channels, and tonifies the Qi of the whole body. Zusanli ST 36, the lower He-Sea point, is where the Stomach channel goes deep. 'The He-Sea points control the Interior.' In combination, these two points stimulate and regulate Spleen and Stomach Qi. The first manipulation was used to obtain Qi, to activate and regulate it. The second reinforcing manipulation strengthened the body's resistance. If the Qi flows, and the body's resistance is strong, the disease will be cured.

Li Pulang, TAISHANG TCM COUNTY HOSPITAL, GUANGDONG PROVINCE
(see the New Chinese Medicine, Issue 8, 1983)

20. Borborygmus

Li, female, age 27, teacher

Case registered: 25 July 1978

History: Over the last 2 years the patient had suffered from several abdominal lumps which would appear at night, particularly after midnight. The lumps would appear one after the other accompanied by loud continuous borborygmus. She had been to several hospitals for treatment, but neither Chinese herbs nor Western drugs had helped.

Examination: The patient had undergone many examinations including blood, urine and stool analyses, barium meal and barium enema examinations and rectoscopy, but all the findings were normal.

Diagnosis: Borborygmus: Deficiency of Spleen and Stomach.

Treatment: Reinforce the Spleen and regulate the Stomach and intestines.

Principal Points: Acupoint injection of Zusanli ST 36 (bilateral).

Treatment was given every other day. After two treatments the symptoms improved. After 10 treatments the case was cured.

Liu Jingping, JI'AN TEACHER'S SCHOOL HOSPITAL, JIANGXI PROVINCE
(see Forum for Traditional Chinese Medicine, Issue 1, 1987)

21. Constipation, chronic

Liu, male, age 79

Case registered: 4 June 1987

History: The patient had been constipated for over 25 years. Initially he had a bowel movement every 3–5 days, but the interval had increased to 8-10 days over recent years, with feelings of abdominal fullness and some mild pain. He was also weak, short of breath and had pruritis all over his body. Chinese herbs and Western medication had provided only temporary relief; the symptoms would return if he stopped taking the medication.

Examination: The patient was old, and in good spirits. *BP:* 21.3/13.3 kPa (160/100 mmHg). Heart and lungs were normal, abdomen flat and soft, and the liver and spleen were not palpable. There was slight tenderness on his lower left abdomen, but no rebound tenderness. *Tongue body:* pale. *Tongue coating:* thin and white. *Pulse:* thin and weak.

Diagnosis: Constipation: Deficiency of Qi and Blood.

Treatment: Reinforce Qi and Blood and relax the bowels.

Principal Points: Tianshu ST 25, Zusanli ST 36, Shangjuxu ST 37, Qihai Ren 6, Guanyuan Ren 4.
  Qihai Ren 6 and Guanyuan Ren 4 were needled alternately with reinforcing method followed by moxibustion for 15 minutes. The other points were needled bilaterally with reinforcing method.
  Treatment was given daily. After the first session the patient was able to feel some movement in his abdomen, and was able to pass stool during the night. After 15 sessions he passed stool every 5–6 days.

Auricular Points: Large Intestine, Lower Part of Rectum, Sympathetic and Constipation joined to Subcortex.
  The needles were retained with plasters and renewed every 5 days, alternating between the two ears.
  After another 15 days of treatment the patient was passing stools every 2–3 days with ease. His pruritis also disappeared.

Explanation: The patient was weak and old, and his Qi, Blood and Body

Fluids were Deficient. There was insufficient Qi in the Large Intestine to move the stools, and the Body Fluids were Deficient because the Blood was Deficient.

Tianshu ST 25 is the Front-Mu point of the Large Intestine on the Stomach channel. Shangjuxu ST 27 is the lower He-Sea point of the Large Intestine. In combination, these points activate and regulate the Qi of the Large Intestine.

Acupuncture and moxibustion at Qihai Ren 6 and Guanyuan Ren 4 builds Original Qi of the Lower Burner, and nourishes the Middle Burner, the source of Qi and Blood. When the Middle Burner was strengthened, the function of the Intestines was restored. The auricular points were added to reinforce the effects of the channel acupuncture and moxibustion.

Hou Fengqin, ACUPUNCTURE AND MOXIBUSTION SECTION, SHANDONG TCM COLLEGE HOSPITAL
(see Sichuan Traditional Chinese Medicine Issue 3, 1988)

22. Hepatoptosis

Zheng, male, age 53, cadre

History: The patient had had pain in the liver area for 10 years. Over the past 2 years it was worse if he stood for a long time or travelled by bus or train, but better when he lay down. His appetite was poor and he was losing weight, and he had occasional abdominal fullness and belching. His condition had been diagnosed as chronic hepatitis, but had not responded to treatment.

Examination: Ultrasound scans in July 1981 revealed that when standing his liver extended 6 cm below the costal margin. Lying down it reached 2.8 cm. below the costal margin. X-rays revealed that the anterior 9th rib crossed the diaphragm at the outside edge. The rear 11th rib could not be seen.

Diagnosis: Abdominal distension: Deficiency of Central Qi.

Treatment: Invigorate Qi of the Middle Burner and raise depressed Yang.

Principal Points: Zhongwan Ren 12, Guanyuan Ren 4 and Zusanli ST 36.
The points were needled with strong stimulation and the needles were not retained. A course consisted of seven daily treatments, and 3 days' rest was allowed between courses.

After 2 months of treatment the symptoms were alleviated. After 3 months of treatment the pain and other symptoms had largely disappeared.

Ultrasound scans after 4 months revealed that the liver was positioned normally both when the patient was lying down and when he was standing up. X-rays showed that the diaphragm had raised.

Li Jun, 852 STATE HOSPITAL, HEILONGJIANG PROVINCE
(see Chinese Acupuncture and Moxibustion, Issue 5, 1982)

23. Hepatitis, infectious, with jaundice

Ji, male, age 32, worker

Case registered: 4 September 1961

History: The patient had had contact with a hepatitis carrier and had felt weak and nauseous for two weeks. His appetite was poor, he had pain and fullness in the liver area and was passing reddish urine.

Examination: Slight yellowing of the sclera and skin. Heart and lung negative, abdomen flat and soft, liver 3 cm below costal margin, texture slightly dull, with tenderness on pressure and percussion. It was not possible to palpate the spleen below the ribs. *Liver function:* SGPT 320 u, TTT 8 u. Sulphuric acid turbidity test 12 u. Bilirubin 4.2 mg/dl. *Tongue coating:* thin and yellow. *Pulse:* wiry, thin and rapid.

Diagnosis: Yang jaundice: Damp Heat in Liver and Gall Bladder.

Treatment: Clear Damp Heat, soothe the Liver and normalize the Gall Bladder.

Principal Points: Dazhui Du 14, Zhiyang Du 9, Ganshu BL 18, Danshu BL 19, Pishu BL 20.
    The points of Du Mai were needled in the direction of the flow of Qi in the channel, and the Bladder points were needled against the flow. Fast-slow reducing technique was used, and the needles were retained for 15 minutes.
    Treatment was given daily. After a week the symptoms had markedly improved: SGPT 116 u, bilirubin 2.2 mg/dl.

Secondary Points: Treatment was continued once every other day with the addition of Yongquan KID 1, Zusanli ST 36 and Yanglingquan GB 34, with the same needle manipulation as before.
    After 12 treatments the patient's symptoms had mostly disappeared: SGPT was normal, bilirubin 0.8 mg/dl. He was discharged after a period of consolidating treatment.

Explanation: Acute infective hepatitis with jaundice (icteric hepatitis) is classified in TCM as Yang jaundice or 'side pain'. Many texts, ancient and modern, stress the importance of Zhiyang Du 9 as a specific for this condition. Reducing Dazhui Du 14 activates Yang and clears Damp Heat. The Back-Shu points enhance these effects.

Yongquan KID 1 is a Jing-Well Wood point and therefore related to the Liver and Gall Bladder. These two organs are implicated in feelings of fullness below the heart. The *Tong Xuan Zhi Yao Fu* (Songs to the Essential and Mysterious) says, 'Use Yongquan KID 1 for oppression of the chest and jaundice'. Reducing Yongquan KID 1 clears Heat and removes Stagnation.

Yanglingquan GB 34 is the He-Sea point of the Gall Bladder channel, which is paired to the Liver. Zusanli ST 36 is the He-Sea point of the Stomach channel, which is paired to the Spleen. The *Nei Jing* says, 'He-Sea points affect the Yang organs'. Reducing these points therefore clears Damp Heat in the Stomach and Spleen, and Heat and Stagnation in the Gall Bladder and Liver.

> Case treated by Xi Yongjiang, case study by Pu Yunxing and Xi Depei, YUEYANG HOSPITAL, SHANGHAI TCM COLLEGE
> *(see Correspondence Journal of Acupuncture and Moxibustion, Issue 1, 1987)*

24. Ascites from cirrhosis

Meng, male, age 34, cadre

Case registered: 11 January 1960

History: The patient was admitted to hospital in June 1959 after he suddenly became jaundiced. His condition was diagnosed as cirrhosis. He developed ascites, with varicose veins on the abdomen, and became bedbound. His appetite disappeared and he began to lose weight. He was only able to pass 500 ml of urine per day, and the ascitic fluid was drained off 10 times.

Examination: The patient was thin, but still conscious. Abdominal circumference 103 cm.

Diagnosis: Tympany: Kidney and Spleen Deficiency with retention of water.

Treatment: Reinforce Kidney and Spleen, clear Triple Burner channel to reduce swelling and promote urination.

Principal Points: Renzhong Du 26, Hegu L.I. 4, Shuidao ST 28, Zusanli ST 36.

The next day the patient was able to pass 1000 ml of urine.

Secondary Points: Yongquan KID 1, Shuifen Ren 9, Yinjiao Ren 7.

These points were added to the principal points on the second day. Urination increased to 1080 ml after treatment. After the third treatment urination was 1020 ml. On the sixth treatment Shuifen Ren 9 and Yinjiao Ren 7 were given moxibustion after needling. A course of treatment consisted of 10 daily sessions, and after the first course it was clear that there had been some improvement, with urination up to 1800 ml. After a break of 10 days for observation the patient was given another course, after which urination increased to 2000 ml. Abdominal circumference dropped to 93 cm. 6 days after the course it had dropped to 88 cm and urination was holding steady at about 1400 ml. During the fourth course moxibustion was applied to Shenshu BL 23 in addition to the other points, and abdominal circumference dropped to 75 cm. Urination held steady at 1400 ml.

After the fourth session in the fifth course, however, the patient complained of feeling thirsty, and had difficulty passing water. The moxibustion was discontinued, and only Yangchi TB 4 on the left and Weiyang BL 39 on the right were needled. The next day these two points were needled again on the opposite sides. The symptoms continued to improve, with abdominal circumference down to 68 cm and urination ranging from 1500–2800 ml. By this time the patient was in much better spirits with improved appetite, and was more or less cured.

Xie Linyuan, WENDENG COUNTY BONE SETTING HOSPITAL, SHANDONG PROVINCE
(see Proceedings of the Symposium for Jing-Luo and Acupuncture and Moxibustion in Traditional Chinese Medicine, Shandong Province, 1960)

Editor's Note: Ascites due to cirrhosis is classified in TCM as tympany, and usually arises from Stagnation of Liver Qi, Spleen Deficiency, Blood stasis and retention of water. Doctor Xie took the approach of strengthening the body's resistance to eliminate pathogenic factors: reinforcing the Kidney and Spleen, clearing the Triple Burner channel and inducing diuresis to drain oedema. He got good results by using acupuncture and moxibustion in combination.

Renzhong Du 26 (Water Drain) is a meeting point of the Stomach and Large Intestine channels and drains fluids. Hegu L.I. 4, the Yuan-Source point, clears Heat, relieves thirst and restlessness. Shuidao ST 28 (Water Pathway) is where the Qi of the Stomach channel originates, and removes obstruction in the water passages. Zusanli ST 36, the He-Sea point, relieves fullness in the abdomen, strengthens Spleen and Kidney, regulates the Qi of the Middle Burner and sends down Rebellious Qi.

Moxibustion at Shuifen Ren 9 and Yinjiao Ren 7 enhances the effect of inducing diuresis to drain oedema. Moxibustion at Shenshu BL 23 nourishes Kidney Qi. When Kidney Qi is full and active, the Bladder function of removing water by Qi transformation is reinforced.

NEUROLOGICAL DISORDERS

25. Post-viral pain syndrome

Sun, female, age 15

History: The patient had caught a cold 6 weeks previously, which had improved after treatment, but she still had a sore throat. Two weeks after the cold she began to suffer from severe prickling pains, first at the hips, then the knees, legs, shoulders, elbows and feet, with the worst pain in her right leg. The pain came about three times a day, for 3–4 hours at a time, and was triggered or made worse by fatigue. Before an attack her hands and feet would become cold. During an attack she would become intolerant of warmth and heavy bedclothes, and would feel more comfortable if the painful limb was elevated. There was no fever.

The patient had a previous history of headache and systemic pain going back 2 or 3 years; each episode was triggered by fatigue and relieved by rest.

Examination: The patient's hands and feet were sweating, and the skin on her palms and soles was flaky, especially on her palms. Electromyography was normal.

Diagnosis: Wind Bi syndrome.

Treatment: Expel pathogenic Wind, invigorate the Blood, relieve pain by removing obstruction from the channels.

To start with, the patient was given acupuncture and far-infrared treatment, but her symptoms got worse. Next, acupuncture and moxibustion were given together, but these provided only temporary relief, and soon the pain was back with increased severity. A final prescription was used.

Principal Points: Hegu L.I. 4, Xuehai SP 10 (bilateral).

Hegu L.I. 4 was palpated and needled where it was most tender. Xuehai SP 10 was stimulated by laser. The pain was relieved instantly, and the patient was able to walk after the treatment. The pain recurred in the evening, however, although it was not as severe. This treatment was repeated daily for 10 days, and the patient was taught some exercises. At this point she had one very mild 15-minute attack.

This case was observed for a month. There were no further attacks during this time, but the outside of the patient's thigh was painful when palpated strongly (in the area where electromyography had been performed). Another 7-day course was given and the pain disappeared, as well as the tenderness at Hegu L.I. 4. The patient's sweating was markedly reduced, and the flaking on her hands and feet much improved.

Explanation: The pain was caused by Stagnation of Blood. The migration of the pain arose from a very strong pathogenic Wind.

Hegu L.I. 4 is the Source point of the Large Intestine channel, which is rich in Blood and Qi. It therefore regulates the vessels of the whole body. Xuehai SP 10 has the same effect.

When treating Wind, treat the Blood first; Wind is subdued when the Blood flows. These two points expelled the pathogenic Wind and relieved the pain.

Liang Yiqiang, ACUPUNCTURE AND MOXIBUSTION SECTION, SINO-JAPANESE FRIENDSHIP HOSPITAL
(see Shanghai Journal of Acupuncture and Moxibustion, Issue 2, 1987)

26. Numbness

Pang, female, age 30, peasant

Case registered: 22 July 1982

History: Several days previously the patient had been distressed and preoccupied. Later her body and limbs had suddenly become numb. Various therapies were tried unsuccessfully at her local hospital, and here she was given diazepam orally and intramuscular injections of meperidine, also with no effect.

Examination: The patient complained of an unbearable feeling of numbness all over her body. She looked as if she was in considerable pain, and moaned constantly. *Tongue body:* red edges. *Tongue coating:* white and dry. *Pulse:* wiry, rapid and slightly irregular.

Diagnosis: Liver Qi Stagnation, Stagnation of Qi and Blood.

Treatment: Regulate Qi by relieving mental depression, activate the circulation of Blood, invigorate the channels and readjust Yin and Yang.

Principal Points: Geshu BL 17, Ganshu BL 18, Yamen Du 15, Danzhong Ren 17, Qimen LIV 14.

The needles were manipulated with reducing technique for 5 minutes and then withdrawn.

Secondary Points: Neiguan P 6, Zhongdu LIV 6, Shuigou Du 26 and Qimai TB 18.

These points were needled with reinforcing and reducing evenly method, and retained for several hours.

During the first hour the patient's symptoms gradually improved, and after 3 hours she was sleeping quietly. After treatment with medication for another 2 days she was discharged, completely cured. There has been no relapse.

Explanation: The traditional name for this disease is *mamu:* it manifests with tingling (*ma*) and numbness (*mu*). It is rare for tingling to appear on its own. The pain is severe and the disease is hard to treat.

In this case, examination by the four diagnostic methods showed the cause to be mental depression impairing the Liver and Jue Yin. The True Qi was disordered, Yin and Yang were unbalanced and the circulation of Blood and Qi was obstructed. Points on Jue Yin were therefore indicated. Geshu BL 17 is the Gathering point of Blood. Danzhong Ren 17 is the Gathering point of Qi and the Front-Mu point of the Pericardium. Ganshu BL 18 and Qimen LIV 14 are respectively the Back-Shu and Front-Mu points of the Liver. Neiguan P 6, the Luo Connecting point of hand Jue Yin, leads through to the Shao Yang channels and to the Yin Wei Mai. Zhongdu LIV 6 is the Xi-Accumulation point of the Liver. Yamen Du 15 and Shuigou Du 26, together with Danzhong Ren 17, regulate Yin and Yang. Qimai TB 17 is on the hand Shao Yang channel and is an empirical point for calming pathogenic Wind and relieving convulsion.

Liu Leigeng, ACUPUNCTURE AND MOXIBUSTION SECTION, DAXIAN PREFECTURE TCM HOSPITAL, SICHUAN PROVINCE
(see Shenxi Traditional Chinese Medicine, Issue 7, 1984)

27. Itching, tingling and spasm in the upper body

Zhou, female, age 23

Case registered: 5 April 1984

The patient complained of itchiness, numbness and heaviness above the chest. The problem had started 6 months previously in December 1982, when she gave birth to her first baby. At first she felt hot and cold; later the itchiness and numbness became worse, and the muscles in her upper body, arms and hands became very tight. When the symptoms were severe the heaviness would go down as far as her pelvis, and there would be slight pain in her chest and back, especially on the left, and when she turned her body.

Examination: The patient seemed emotionally well balanced. When touched, she had itching and tingling sensations above the chest, in the elbows, upper arms and the fingers. *Pulse:* deep, slow and weak.

Treatment: Regulate the Nutritive and Defensive Qi, eliminate pathogenic factors and activate the channels.

Principal Points: Dazhui Du 14, Fengfu Du 16, Waiguan TB 5.

Fengfu Du 16 was first reduced then reinforced. The other points were needled with reinforcing and reducing evenly method. The needles were retained for 30 minutes and twirled at 5 minute intervals. Treatment was given once every 2 days.

After two treatments the patient's symptoms had improved. After another four they had almost completely disappeared. The case was followed up for 2 years and there was no relapse.

Dazhui Du 14 is the point where the hand and foot Shao Yang channels meet with Du Mai. It relieves Exterior syndromes, activates the Yang and expels pathogenic Wind and Cold. Fengfu Du 16 expels pathogenic Wind from the brain. Used together, these two points activate the Yang Qi of the channels, expel Wind, Cold and Damp. Waiguan TB 5 regulates the Nutritive and Defensive Qi, and also activates the Yang Qi and the channels.

Shi Mingxue, BEIJI DISTRICT HOSPITAL, BINXIAN COUNTY, SHENXI PROVINCE

28. Trigeminal neuralgia

CASE 1

Li, female, age 71

Case registered: 21 October 1981

History: The patient had had hypertension for 10 years. After a period of worry and anger in March 1981, she suddenly started to have severe paroxysmal burning pains in the right side of her face. The pain was worse when she was feeling emotional. The attacks would start with a sudden feeling of soreness, heaviness and burning in her right eye. The pain would then spread to the right temple and gums. The right side of her mouth would become stiff, with severe burning pain. The duration of each attack varied from a few seconds to a few minutes, and would be most severe at mealtimes or just before bed. She also had a bitter taste in her mouth and very bad breath. She felt thirsty, with a preference for cold drinks, but after drinking she would need to urinate frequently or would develop diarrhoea. Her vision was occasionally blurred.

Examination: The patient was thin and old, with red cheeks and a tendency to sigh a lot. Point palpation revealed tenderness at Qihai Ren 6, which when pressed would refer to Zhongwan Ren 12 and Qugu Ren 2. Qimen LIV 14 and Danzhong Ren 17 were slightly tender, Yutang Ren 18 was more tender, and Riyue GB 24 was more tender still. *Tongue body:* dark. *Tongue coating:* thin and yellow. *Pulse:* slippery and rapid at both Guan positions, but the right Guan was also wiry. The cun and chi pulses on both sides were deep, small and weak.

Diagnosis: Facial pain: Qi stagnation turning into Fire, stirring of Liver Wind.

Treatment: Soothe Liver Qi, cool Fire to calm pathogenic Wind.

Principal Points: Three prescriptions were used:
1. Qiuxu GB 40, Ligou LIV 5, Lieque LU 7 on the right, Hegu L.I. 4 on the left.
2. Zhiyin BL 67, Jingming BL 1, Guangming GB 37 on the right, Zhongdu LIV 6.
3. Three Root points and three Branch points on the right foot. Taichong LIV 3 on the left, Guangming GB 37, Gongsun SP 4.
   13 treatments were given from October to November 1981, at intervals of 2 or 3 days. At the end of the course the pain was gone and the patient was cured. The case was followed up for a year and a half and there was no relapse.

Explanation: Qiuxu GB 40 is the Source point of the Gall Bladder channel, which is rooted in Qi and governs Fire; it is effective for both Excess and Deficiency diseases. Ligou LIV 5 is the Luo-Connecting point of the Liver channel, which has its root in Qi and governs Wind; it is effective for diseases of both the Interior and Exterior channels. In this case the Stagnation of Qi in the Liver and Gall Bladder had turned to Fire and induced Wind. Using the Source and Luo-Connecting points together soothes suppressed Liver Qi, removes Heat and calms Wind.

Hegu L.I. 4, the Source point, clears Dryness and Heat and activates Qi and Blood to affect the tightness in the mouth and toothache. Lieque

LU 7, the Luo-Connecting point of the Lung channel, goes through the Large Intestine channel and through to Ren Mai. It opens the Lung to the Exterior to disperse ascending Dryness and Heat, and nourishes Lung Yin.

Zhiyin BL 67 is the Jing-Well point and root of the Bladder channel. It pulls the Qi of the Tai Yang channels down, and therefore controls the rising pathogenic Wind, Dryness and Heat. Jingming BL 1 is a junction (jie) point of the Large Intestine, Stomach, Small Intestine, Bladder and the Yin and Yang Qiao Mai and was used to disperse the rising Dryness and Heat.

Zhongdu LIV 6, the Xi-Accumulation point, relieves Stagnation of Liver Qi. Guangming GB 37, the Luo-Connecting point, clears Heat from the Gall Bladder and Wind from the Liver.

The Root and Branch Points of the three leg Yang are:

	Root	Branch
Bladder	Zhiyin BL 67	Jingming BL 1
Gall Bladder	Qiaoyin GB 44	Tinggong SI 19
Stomach	Lidui ST 45	Touwei ST 8

The Root points are also Jing-Well points. They can be used to pull down the Qi of the channels to prevent Wind, Heat and Dryness from rising upwards. The Branch points remove Dryness and Heat to stop Wind. The combination of Root and Branch points reinforces the body's resistance and removes pathogens by regulating the upward and downward movement of Qi.

The combination of Taichong LIV 3, the Source point of the Liver channel, with Guangming GB 37, the Luo-Connecting point of the Gall Bladder, removes Stagnation of Liver Qi, and clears Heat and Wind.

Gongsun SP 4, the Luo-Connecting point of the Spleen channel, leads to Chong Mai. It lifts the Clear Qi and sends down the Turbid, strengthens the Earth to help control Wood, sends down Rebellious Qi and relieves pain and other acute symptoms.

Xia Shouren and Kong Xianfen, BEIJING MUNICIPAL TCM HOSPITAL
(see *Journal of Traditional Chinese Medicine*, Issue 8, 1984)

CASE 2

Guo, male, age 56, cadre

Case registered: July 1982

History: In 1976 the patient had developed severe shocking pain in his right cheek after overworking for 3 days. It was diagnosed as trigeminal neuralgia, and he was treated with local blocking injections of procaine, vitamin B_1 and vitamin B_{12}, and oral phenytoin sodium. The pain improved, but from that time on he would have relapses. In 1980 he had severe pain once again and the above treatment was repeated, with the addition of a local blocking injection of absolute ethyl alcohol, and some Chinese herbs. These treatments were not effective and in 1981 a posterior rhizotomy was performed, which gave some relief. 5 months later, however, the pain returned worse than ever. He would have about 10 attacks a day, which would be triggered by meals, brushing his teeth, washing his face or any sudden movement.

Diagnosis: Migraine.

Principal Points: Xiaguan ST 7, Yangbai GB 14 through to Yuyao (Extra), Zanzhu BL 2, Taiyang (Extra), Touwei ST 8, Chengjiang Ren 24, Hegu L.I. 4.

Electro-acupuncture was applied to all the points, at a frequency of 250/minute. The needles were retained for 1 hour.

The pain improved after three treatments. After 15 treatments the attacks only occurred 2–3 times a day. 45 treatments were given in total, and the length of time the needles were retained was increased to 80 minutes. The pain was cured.

Explanation: The causes of trigeminal neuralgia are unclear. It is classified in TCM as migraine. For example, in the *Zhong Yi Lin Zheng Bei Yao* (Essentials for Practitioners of Traditional Chinese Medicine) by Qim Bomo, it is called Three Yang Channel Migraine. The *Zheng Zhi Zhun Sheng* (Standards of Diagnosis and Treatment) by Wang Kentang says that the disease arises from obstruction by Phlegm Damp of the Shao Yang and Yang Ming channels, which circulate over the face and head. The point prescription was therefore mostly on these two channels, and the points also intersect with the pathway of the trigeminal nerve. Needling and electrical stimulation improve the blood circulation by dilating the local vessels, thus reducing the pain.

> Yang Yu-en, QINGDAO RAILROAD SANATORIUM
> *(see Shanghai Journal of Acupuncture and Moxibustion , Issue 2, 1984)*

29. Headache, parietal

Dong, male, age 26, peasant.

Case registered: October 1987

History: In May 1987 the patient had been caught in the rain and developed a cold. He was treated with Chinese herbs, which cleared all his symptoms except headache. For the last 5 months he had had paroxysmal parietal headaches, in an area the size of a small coin centred around Baihui Du 20. The headaches would come every 1–3 days, usually at night, accompanied by restlessness, faintness and sensations of heaviness. After 2–3 hours these symptoms would recede to be replaced by a feeling of exhaustion. For the last 2 months the patient had been treated with both Chinese and Western medication, but with no results.

Examination: The patient mentioned that he liked to cover his head when sleeping during or after an attack. *Tongue body:* pale. *Pulse:* tight and irregular.

Diagnosis: Headache: Cold Damp invading the channels.

Treatment: Warm Du Mai and disperse Cold, ease pain by activating the collaterals.

Principal Points: Dazhui Du 14, and two extra points, one 5 mm above Dazhui, the other 5 mm below.

A triangular needle was inserted to a depth of 5 mm into each point, and five drops of blood were squeezed out. The points were then cupped with a medium sized glass jar for 15 minutes.

There was no pain for 3 days after the first treatment. The prescription was repeated three times and the disorder was cured. The case was followed up and there was no relapse.

Explanation: The illness was caused by invasion of external pathogens from exposure to the cold rain. Illness from Cold Damp is Yin in nature, coagulating and contracting, causing obstruction of the channels and pain by stagnating Qi and Blood.

Du Mai passes through the affected area, so Dazhui Du 14 was selected to dredge the Qi of the channel. The points above and below were added to reinforce the effect.

Bleeding the points activates the channels and removes Stagnation of Cold Damp. Cupping warms and activates the channels, and disperses Cold and Damp.

Zhang Weihua, ACUPUNCTURE AND MOXIBUSTION SECTION, SHENXI TCM COLLEGE

30. Headache, recurrent following fever

Zhu, male, age 14, student

History: 7 days previously this boy suddenly became pale and faint with a low grade fever. He was nauseated and vomited. The illness lasted 3 days but after treatment at his local clinic, which included fluid infusion, the fever receded and the vomiting stopped. He then started to get severe headaches at 8.00 a.m. each morning. During an attack, which would last for about 30 minutes, he would turn pale, cry out loud and sweat all over. Afterwards he would feel slightly faint. The boy had previously been fit and active, with no relevant family history.

Examination: The boy was well developed both mentally and physically. General tests were normal, heart and lungs negative, neck movement normal, blood test: WBC $9.5 \times 10^9/1$ ($9.5 \times 10^3/mm^3$), neutrophils 32%, lymphocytes 56%, eosinophils 12%. *Tongue body:* pale, scalloped. *Tongue coating:* thin and white. *Pulse:* thin and slightly rapid.

Diagnosis: Deficiency of Stomach Qi, malnourishment of brain by Qi and Blood.

Treatment: Dredge and regulate Du Mai, lift and nourish Yang, reinforce the brain and calm the mind.

Principal Points: Baihui Du 20 through to Sishencong (Extra), Yintang (Extra), Dazhui Du 14, Shanxing Du 23, Hegu L.I. 4, Fengfu Du 16, Neiguan P 6, Taichong LIV 3.

Treatment was given once a day, using 2–4 points from the above in rotation.

The first treatment, on 7 April, used electro-acupuncture at Baihui Du 20 through to Sishencong (Extra), Dazhui Du 14, and Yintang (Extra). After obtaining sensation the needles were connected to a G6805 therapeutic unit using continuous wave stimulation for about 15 minutes. The intensity was adjusted so that the needles vibrated slightly and produced a bumping sensation.

The next day the patient had a headache an hour earlier, at 7.00 a.m., but the duration and severity were less. The second treatment consisted of Baihui Du 20, Yintang (Extra), Shanxing Du 23 and Fengfu Du 16. He had another very mild headache that afternoon.

There was no headache the next day. The third treatment consisted of Baihui Du 20 through to Sishencong (Extra), Dazhui Du 14, Yintang (Extra) and Neiguan P 6.

The seventh treatment was given on 16 April. The patient had had no headache for 4 days, but that morning he had a mild one for about 10 minutes. Electro-acupuncture was given at Baihui Du 20 through to Sishencong (Extra), Yintang (Extra), Shenting Du 24 and Hegu L.I. 4. After this treatment he had no headaches for 8 days.

On the afternoon of 25 April the patient was scolded, and developed a mild headache afterwards. He cried out, but did not sweat and the pain stopped after a few minutes.

To consolidate the treatment another course of daily acupuncture was given, using the same points. A total of 20 treatments was given and the case was cured. The case was followed up for 2 months and there were no relapses, even at times when the patient was upset.

Zheng Huaiyue, ACUPUNCTURE AND MOXIBUSTION SECTION, YUQIAN
COUNTY PEOPLE'S HOSPITAL, JIANXI PROVINCE
(see Jianxi Traditional Chinese Medicine, Issue 6, 1983)

Editor's Note: In children the Yang is not full and strong. In this case, 3 days of sickness and low grade fever had weakened the Qi of the Stomach channel. According to the theory of Zi Wu Liu Zhu, 8.00 a.m. is Chen (Branch 5) time, when the Stomach Qi is predominant. If the Stomach Qi is weak and Qi and Blood are Deficient, the vessels of the brain will not be nourished. This is why the severe headache persisted after the fever and vomiting were cured. The treatment was effective because it lifted and nourished the Yang Qi, invigorated the brain and calmed the mind.

31. Paralysis, facial

Ma, female, age 18, peasant

Case Registered: August 1979

History: The patient had been paralysed on the right side of her face since she was 1 year old. She was unable to close her right eye, which teared constantly, and her mouth and eyes were pulled over to the left. This made eating and drinking difficult. The disease had never been treated consistently.

Examination: Frontal crease and nasolabial groove shallow on the right. Unable to close right eye. Mouth inclined to the left. Unable to purse lips to whistle. *Tongue body*: dark red. *Pulse*: wiry.

Diagnosis: Pathogenic Wind and Cold.

Treatment: Expel Wind, invigorate the Blood.

Principal Points: Yingxiang L.I. 20, Sizhukong TB 23, Dicang ST 4, Jiache ST 6, Yifeng TB 17, Fengchi GB 20, Hegu L.I. 4.

The points were all needled on the right with reinforcing and reducing evenly method. 2–3 minutes after insertion she began to sweat on the right hand side, and then all over her face. She felt a warm comfortable feeling on the right. The needles were withdrawn after 30 minutes, and the sweating stopped. The next day there was a marked improvement in her symptoms. She was given 12 treatments in total. Each time she would sweat on her face, and this phenomenon was most noticeable between the second and sixth treatments. At the end of the course her symptoms were mostly cured.

Explanation: Fengchi GB 20 and Yifeng TB 17 expel Wind and dredge the collaterals. Dicang ST 4 and Jiache ST 6 regulate the channel Qi in the face, activate the circulation of Blood and relax the muscles and tendons. Sizhukong TB 23 and Yingxiang L.I. 20 activate and regulate the vessels around the eyes and nose. Hegu L.I. 4, the Yuan-Source point, is selected as a distal point. It activates and regulates Qi and Blood, and dredges the channels and collaterals.

The sweating was an indication of fullness of Qi and Blood in the face. The Wind Cold was expelled by the sweating, and the tendons and muscles were nourished when the Qi and Blood were activated.

Zhang Zihan, ACUPUNCTURE AND MOXIBUSTION SECTION, JINAN MUNICIPAL TCM HOSPITAL, SHANDONG PROVINCE

32. Collapse

Ma, male, age 68, peasant

Case registered: 22 April 1960

History: The patient had been feeling weak. On 22 April his limbs became cold, he sweated profusely all over his body and fell to the ground unconscious.

Examination: The patient was lying on the floor, his face pale and sunken. His body was stiff and cold, and he had wet himself. His breathing was imperceptible and he was close to death.

Diagnosis: Collapse of Original Qi.

Treatment: Resuscitate the patient.

Principal Points: Shidou SP 17 on the left (Mingguan)[1], Guanyuan Ren 4. 'Suspended moxibustion' was applied at Mingguan SP 17. After 5 minutes the patient moved his lips slightly and exhaled some cold and foul-smelling air. Next moxibustion was applied to Guanyuan Ren 4 to

---

[1]Shidou SP 17 on the left is near the apex of the heart and so is also known as Mingguan, 'the key to life', and considered to be a very important point.

connect the Qi of the Dan Tien. The patient suddenly swung his left hand and groaned; his cheeks regained their shape and he started to breathe normally. The entire rescue procedure lasted 2 hours and cost no more than the price of four moxa sticks.

Explanation: Mingguan or Shidou SP 17 on the left is in the 5th intercostal space 6 cun lateral to the midline of the chest. *The Bian Que Xin Shu* (Bian Que's Accumulated Clinical Experience) says this point 'connects the real Spleen Qi and cures 36 kinds of Spleen disease. In severe disease, when life is hanging by a thread, moxibustion at this point with 200–300 moxa cones will assure the patient's survival. Use this point in any major Spleen disease'.

The Spleen and Stomach have an Interior/Exterior relationship; the major Luo-Connecting point Xuli ST 18 (Rugen) lies just medial to Mingguan. Moxibustion at Mingguan is thus effective for resuscitation. Guanyuan Ren 4, Zhongwan Ren 12 or Danzhong Ren 17 can be added to reinforce the effect.

Li Quanshi, HEZE CITY TCM HOSPITAL
(see Shandong Journal of Traditional Chinese Medicine, Issue 2, 1982)

33. Stroke

CASE 1

Li, female, age 55, peasant

Case registered: 8 July 1972

History: The patient was overweight and had suffered from faintness for years. She had a history of hypertension and occasional tingling in her fingers. One morning she suddenly lost consciousness and fell down, making gurgling sounds. She was brought to hospital immediately.

Examination: The patient was paralysed on the right with facial hemiplegia which affected her speech. *BP:* 21.3/13.3 kPa (160/100 mmHg). *Tongue body:* pale. *Tongue coating:* white. *Pulse:* slippery and rapid.

Diagnosis: Excess-type stroke.

Treatment: Resuscitate the patient, activate the channels and calm Liver Wind.

Principal Points: Renzhong Du 26, the 12 Jing-Well points, Fenglong ST 40, Taichong LIV 3 through to Yongquan KID 1, Hegu L.I. 4 through to Laogong P 8.

Secondary Points:
1. Jianyu L.I. 15, Quchi L.I. 11, Waiguan TB 5, Zusanli ST 36, Dicang ST 4 through to Jiache ST 6, Yongquan KID 1, Quanliao SI 18, Hegu L.I. 4, Fengfu Du 16.
2. Yanglingquan GB 34, Kunlun BL 60, Neiting ST 44, Huantiao GB 30, Yingxiang L.I. 20 through to Sibai ST 2, Tongziliao GB 1, Chengqi ST 1, Yamen Du 15.
3. Shousanli L.I. 10, Fenglong ST 40, Hegu L.I. 4, Tongli HT 5, Jiexi ST 41, Juegu GB 39, the associated Jiaji (Extra) points, Fengshi GB 31.

The principal points were for emergency use to revive the patient. The secondary points were for the sequelae. These points were needled bilaterally, and the needles manipulated with reinforcing and reducing equally method. Each group of points was needled in rotation, one group per day.

When the patient's blood pressure became normal, moxibustion was added to the treatment. Each course of treatment lasted 7–10 days, with a 3-day gap between courses. The acupuncture was supplemented with massage and rehabilatory exercise.

After 3 months the patient could walk without a stick and was able to look after herself.

Explanation: The patient was in her 50s and her body resistance was poor. Her Liver and Kidney Yin were Deficient, leading to Yang Wind rising upwards; this had been the cause of her faintness in previous years. She was overweight, and this had led to the formation of internal Phlegm Damp. When she had become fatigued, the Wind and Fire had combined with the Phlegm to rise upwards and obstruct the seven orifices; she fell down gurgling in her throat and lost consciousness as a result. The collaterals were malnourished and weak, and the circulation of Blood and Qi was impeded, causing the paralysis and aphasia. Her clenched mouth, red face, restlessness, gasping, red tongue and slippery pulse were all manifestations of Wind, Phlegm and Fire.

It was clear that this was an Excess-type stroke (i.e. Excess-type coma accompanied by Heat). The first treatment priority was resuscitation and calming of the Liver Wind. Later, treatment was aimed at activating the Blood circulation and strengthening Qi to deal with the sequelae.

Yang Jiebin, CHENGDU COLLEGE OF TCM
(see Correspondence, Journal of Acupuncture and Moxibustion, Issue 1, 1987)

CASE 2

Zhang, male, age 66

Case registered: 10 November 1984

History: 3 days previously the patient had felt faint after getting up in the morning. He experienced headache, numbness, heaviness and difficulty in movement. By noon the symptoms were much worse. The headache was severe and he was unable to move his right arm and leg. There was no nausea or vomiting but his speech was impaired and he choked and coughed if he drank. The condition was diagnosed in hospital that afternoon as cerebral thrombosis. After one day's observation and treatment he was transferred to this hospital.

Examination: The patient was conscious but his speech was impaired. His right arm and leg were paralysed, with grade 3 muscle power. Deep and superficial reflexes present. Extensor plantar response on right. Impaired superficial sensitivity on right side. *BP:*18.7/12 kPa (140/90 mmHg). *Cholesterol:* 7.02 mmol/l (270 mg/dl). *Tongue body:* dark red with ecchymosis. *Tongue coating:* dry and yellow. *Pulse:* wiry.

Diagnosis: Wind Stroke involving the channels and collaterals.

Treatment: Activate circulation of Blood by reinforcing Qi and invigorating the channels and collaterals.

Principal Points: Tianchuang SI 16 on the left, Baihui Du 20.
   Indirect moxibustion with a moxa stick was applied to both points for 15 minutes, twice a day. After 20 days the symptoms had improved; the patient was able to walk by himself, bend and stretch his right hand easily, with an improvement in muscle power. He felt a deep sense of relaxation after the moxibustion and also discovered black hairs growing on his head where he had previously been bald. EEG before and after moxibustion showed obvious improvements after 30 minutes treatment. *Cholesterol:* down to 6.19 mmol/l (238 mg/dl).
   After treatment lasting 62 days, the patient was discharged from hospital, almost completely cured.

Explanation: Moxibustion at Baihui Du 20 and Tianchuang SI 16 for hemiplegia and loss of speech from apoplexy was recorded in the Tang dynasty, in Sun Simiao's *Qian Min Yao Fang* (Essential Prescriptions Worth a Thousand Gold Pieces) and *Qian Jin Yi Fang* (A Supplement to the Essential Prescriptions Worth a Thousand Gold Pieces), in which he said, 'For hemiplegia, first apply moxibustion at Tianchuang ... and when the hands and feet are paralysed, at Baihui'. He also said, 'For loss of speech, first apply 50 moxa cones at Tianchuang then 50 cones at Baihui'.
   We modified this to indirect moxibustion to minimize the pain. Out of 33 cases treated with this therapy, the rate of effectiveness was 97%. We

have observed the immediate and longer term therapeutic effects of this therapy and found that indices of EEG, blood pressure and serum cholesterol all improved. We conclude that moxibustion at these points can improve cerebral circulation and is effective in reducing blood pressure and serum cholesterol.

Zhang Dengbu, Yin Jinghai et al, SHANDONG TCM COLLEGE HOSPITAL
(see Shandong Journal of Traditional Chinese Medicine, Issue 4 1987)

CASE 3

Pang, female, age 68, homemaker

Case registered: 2 March 1981

History: The patient had a history of hypertension and atherosclerosis. Recently she had been feeling faint and having headaches, but had not thought her discomfort severe enough to warrant treatment. 5 days previously, however, she began to feel weak in the waist, legs and knees. If she walked quickly she would stumble. Soon her legs were useless and she could not stand. She also developed tinnitus and felt thirsty, with a preference for cold drinks. Her bowels moved only once every 3 days, and she passed scanty reddish urine. Her condition was diagnosed as cerebral thrombosis.

Examination: The patient's face was red. Her speech was impaired. *BP:* 26.7/16.0 kPa(200/120 mmHg). Electrical resistance was tested at the 12 Source points and Zhaohai KID 6 with an electronic channel detector. Taixi KID 3: left 15 A, right 18 A, respectively 11 A and 8 A lower than the average value of the electrical resistance at the 12 Source points on the same side. Zhaohai KID 6: left 10 A, right 11 A, respectively 16 A and 5 A lower than the average value of the electrical resistance at the 12 Source points on the same side. *Tongue body:* red, swollen and dry, with no coat. *Pulse:* 82/min, wiry, big, but weak when pressed firmly.

Diagnosis: Aphasia and paralysis: Deficiency of Kidney Qi and Yin.

Treatment: Nourish Kidney, Liver and Stomach Yin.

Principal Points: Zhaohai KID 6, Taixi KID 3, Gongsun SP 4, Sanyinjiao SP 6, Taichong LIV 3, Shangjuxu ST 37, Xiajuxu ST 39.
   All the points were needled bilaterally, and the needles retained for 20 minutes. Zhaohai KID 6, Taixi KID 3, Gongsun SP 4, Sanyinjiao SP 6 were reinforced, and the remaining points were needled with reinforcing and reducing evenly method. A course consisted of 6 daily treatments, and an interval of 1 day was left between courses.

By the beginning of the second course the patient was already able to get out of bed and walk. Her pulse was no longer big and wiry, but rapid and wiry at 102 beats per minute. Her tongue was now red and moist. The point prescription seemed effective and was repeated for another course, after which her pulse and tongue became normal and her legs were mobile. She could now walk steadily without a stick.

Her electrical resistance was remeasured. Taixi KID 3: left 30 µA (up 15 µA on the previous reading), right 32 µA (up 14 µA on the previous reading), 3–5 µA higher than the average value of electrical resistance at the 12 Source points on the same side. Zhaohai KID 6: left 20 µA (up 10 µA on the previous reading), right 20 µA (up 9 µA on the previous reading), 7 µA lower than the average value of electrical resistance at the 12 Source points on the same side. These changes demonstrate that the Kidney Qi was now strong, the circulation of Qi and Blood in Chong Mai was good and that the circulation of Blood was normal. The case has been followed up and there has been no relapse.

Table of electrical resistance

Before treatment			
Zhaohai KID 6		**Taixi KID 3**	
Left	*Right*	*Left*	*Right*
10 µA	11 µA	15 µA	18 µA
Comparison to average of resistance at 12 Source points			
–16 µA	–5 µA	–11 µA	–8 µA
After treatment			
20 µA	20 µA	30 µA	32 µA
Comparison to average of resistance at 12 Source points			
–7 µA		+3–5 µA	
Individual increases			
+10 µA	+9 µA	+15 µA	+14 µA

Explanation: The *Su Wen* says, 'Aphasia and paralysis are caused by Deficiency in the Interior. When the Kidney is Deficient and the Qi of the Shao Yin meridians fails to come, the result will be fainting' (Mai Jie, *Familiar Conversations*, Pulse chapter). Wang Bing says in his commentary on this that, 'The Kidney channel comes with Chong Mai from the Qijie (Qichong ST 30), passing through the medial aspect of the leg obliquely into the popliteal fossa, down into the medial aspect of the tibia and fibula into the inside of the ankle and the sole. Thus, if the Kidney Qi is Deficient and stagnant, the result will be aphasia and paralysis of the feet. The disease arises from Deficiency of Kidney Qi'.

The term 'Deficiency' means lack of essential substances. If the body lacks essential substances, the Qi is Deficient also, resulting in fainting. The disease originates from the Kidney, which goes up to govern the tongue and down to the middle of the sole, leading to symptoms of aphasia and paralysis. If the doctor treats the Kidney channel and Chong Mai as the origin of the disease, he or she will succeed.

Li Licheng, JINAN MUNICIPAL CENTRAL HOSPITAL, SHANDONG PROVINCE

CASE 4

Wang, female age 68, homemaker

Case registered: 18 July 1987

History: The patient had been through an emotionally trying time a few months previously. Afterwards she had become faint and nauseated. Her blood pressure at that time was 25.3/13.3 kPa (190/100 mmHg). The hypertension was treated in her local clinic but the next day, although her faintness improved, her speech became slurred and difficult, her motor coordination degenerated and she had difficulty walking. She was nauseated and vomited, choked and coughed when drinking, and had faecal and urinary incontinence. She was treated in one hospital for cervical spondylopathy, but after 5 days without improvement was sent to a municipal hospital, where CAT scans revealed cerebral thrombosis and cerebellar arterial embolism. The patient was treated with low molecular weight dextran and Venoruton (troxerutin), and her symptoms gradually improved. The patient's motor coordination was poor and she was still unable to walk properly. Her speech was slurred and difficult. She occasionally choked and coughed when drinking. Faeces and urine normal.

Examination: Pupils equal. Muscle power normal. Reflexes normal. Finger to nose test positive. Heel to knee test positive. *BP:* 21.3/10.7 kPa (160/80 mm Hg). *Tongue body:* red. *Tongue coating:* thin and white, peeled in the centre. *Pulse:* wiry and thin.

Diagnosis: Wind Stroke involving the channels and collaterals.

Treatment: Activate the Blood, invigorate the collaterals and open the sense organs.

Principal Points: Lianquan Ren 23, Tongli HT 5 (bilateral), Fenglong ST 40 (bilateral), Zhaohai KID 6 (bilateral).

The needles were manipulated with reinforcing and reducing evenly method, and retained for 30 minutes. Treatment was given once a day, and a course lasted 12 days.

Scalp acupuncture: Balance area. Electro-acupuncture was given bilaterally with a G6805 unit for 40 minutes. A course consisted of 12 daily treatments. These two therapies were given concurrently for 2 weeks and the patient's condition improved considerably. She was able to walk by herself and eat normally, but her speech was still indistinct. Treatment was resumed for another 2 weeks, by which time her speech was almost normal. After another 2 weeks' consolidating treatment the patient was discharged, completely cured.

Explanation: This case of cerebellar arterial embolism, manifesting with impaired speech, swallowing and cerebellar ataxia, is classified in TCM as apoplexy involving the channels and collaterals.

Lianquan Ren 23, Tongli HT 5, Fenglong ST 40 and Zhaohai KID 6 were chosen to open the sense organs, restore speech and proper swallowing. These points also nourish the Yin, calm Excessive Yang, remove Wind and eliminate Phlegm.

Scalp acupuncture at the Balance area restores the functions of the cerebellum by activating the circulation of Blood, invigorating the collaterals and removing Stagnation.

Zhang Dengbu, SHANDONG TCM COLLEGE HOSPITAL

CASE 5

Xia, female, age 52, homemaker

Case registered: 15 July 1987

History: The patient had had high blood pressure for 10 years. In March 1987 her speech suddenly became slurred, and her mouth deviated to the left. This got steadily worse until she was unable to speak, and she became paralysed on the right. CAT scans at a provincial hospital revealed cerebral thrombosis. She was treated with low molecular weight dextran, persantine (dipyridamole) and Benol (thiamine hydrochloride), and her paralysis improved to the point where she could walk, but her arm remained useless and her aphasia was unchanged.

Examination: The patient had grade 3 muscle power, and was unable to flex and extend her right arm. Her right leg was slightly flexible, with grade 4 muscle power. Right side extensor plantar response. Complete loss of speech. No problems with swallowing. Bowels once every 2 days, with dry stool. Urine normal. *BP:*16.0/10.7 kPa (120/80 mmHg). *Tongue body:* red, with cracks. *Tongue coating:* thin and white.

Diagnosis: Aphasia from Wind Stroke.

Treatment: Strengthen Qi, activate the circulation of Blood and invigorate the collaterals.

Principal Points: Lianquan Ren 23, Tongli HT 5 (bilateral), Zhaohai KID 6 (bilateral), Yongquan KID 1 (alternating from one side to the other with each treatment), Tianchuang SI 16 and Baihui Du 20.

The needles were manipulated with reinforcing and reducing equally method, and retained for 30 minutes. At Yongquan KID 1 the needle was twirled for 1–2 minutes. A course consisted of 12 daily treatments.

Moxibustion was given at Tianchuang SI 16 and Baihui Du 20, and the patient was given rehabilatory physical exercises and speech therapy. These courses were given concurrently.

After a month she was able to lift her upper arm more easily and her speech had improved to the point where she could make some distinguishable syllables.

Secondary Points: Fenglong ST 40 (bilateral).

Fenglong ST 40 was added to the formula and treatment continued for another month. She could now say a few simple words, and her mobility improved. After another month of treatment she was discharged, as she had regained most of her mobility and speech.

Explanation: This was a difficult case. Two different approaches, ancient and modern, were used together because they have both been found to be effective. Moxibustion at Tianchuang SI 16 and Baihui Du 20 benefits the cerebral circulation. The Kidney points were needled because the channel pathway goes through the throat, and they are therefore effective for restoring speech. Fenglong ST 40 eliminates Phlegm and invigorates the collaterals.

Zhang Dengbu, SHANDONG TCM COLLEGE HOSPITAL

34. Paralysis following stroke

Sun, male, age 62, worker

Case registered: 18 December 1980

History: The patient had had high blood pressure for many years. On 3 December 1980 he collapsed and was rushed to hospital, where his condition was diagnosed as hypertension and haemorrhage. His life was saved by emergency intervention, but he was left paralysed on his left side. He was given 10 acupuncture treatments at Jianyu L.I. 15, Quchi L.I. 11, Hegu L.I. 4, Huantiao GB 30, Yanglingquan GB 34, Zusanli ST 36, Kunlun BL 60, Dicang ST 4 and Jiache ST 6, but without any improvement. He was then referred to this hospital.

Examination: The patient was conscious. He was flushed, his face was paralysed on the left and his speech was impaired. His left arm and leg were useless. His muscles were flaccid and sagging. His mouth was dry but he was not thirsty. His appetite was normal. Urine test negative. Electrical resistance at the 12 Source points; Taixi KID 3: left 14 A, right 24 A; Taichong LIV 3: left 45 A, right 30 A. *BP:* 24.0/17.3 kPa (180/ 130 mmHg). *Tongue body:* dark red and peeled. *Tongue coating:* thin and white. *Pulse:* thin, wiry and rapid.

Diagnosis: Paralysis from Kidney obstruction (Shenyong).

Treatment: Nourish the Yin and suppress Excess Yang.

Principal Points: Zhaohai KID 6 (left), Taixi KID 3 (left), Taichong LIV 3 (left), Baihui Du 20.
    Zhaohai KID 6 and Taixi KID 3 were reinforced, Taichong LIV 3 and Baihui Du 20 were reduced. Treatment was given once every 2 days. After 20 treatments the patient's blood pressure was down to 18.7/12.0 kPa (140/90 mmHg). *Electrical resistance:* the previous test had shown clear differences in the values of left and right Source points. The left Taixi KID 3 had been 10 µA lower than the right, and the left Taichong LIV 3 had been 15 µA higher than the right. These values were now the same. The paralysis was greatly improved and the patient was already walking without a stick.

Secondary Points: Jiache ST 6, Dicang ST 4, Jianyu L.I. 15.
    These points were needled to activate the channels and regulate Qi and Blood. After another 12 treatments the patient was cured.

Explanation: The *Su Wen* says, 'The signs of Shenyong (Kidney Obstruction) are fullness of the feet and abdomen, unequal legs, and problems with the thigh, tibia and fibula. The most likely outcome is paralysis of one side' (Da Qi Lun, *Familiar Conversations*, Most Peculiar Diseases Chapter). The origin of Shenyong (Kidney obstruction) is in Stagnation of the Kidney channel which affects the lower limbs, so the legs become unequal and mobility is impaired. If the limbs are left untreated and malnourished, one-sided paralysis will set in. Wang Bing observed that Chong Mai runs alongside the Kidney channel. If the Kidney channel is obstructed, then Chong Mai will also be obstructed. If both channels are affected there will be one-sided paralysis. To cure this disease, both channels must be regulated.

Li Licheng, JINAN CENTRAL MUNICIPAL HOSPITAL,SHANDONG PROVINCE

35. Sequelae of brain trauma

CASE 1

Chen, male, age 22, student

Case registered: 5 October 1987

History: The patient was in a car accident and received serious injuries to his head. He lost consciousness and was rushed to hospital where he received emergency treatment to remove an intracranial haematoma. He gradually revived, but developed severe headaches which were worse at night, especially on the right side. He felt faint and his head felt heavy. He had difficulty sleeping, even with sedatives, and his memory was noticeably impaired. He was able to move his limbs, but felt weak when holding things or walking.

Examination: The patient was conscious but looked lacklustre and flat. Temperature, pulse rate and blood pressure were all normal. Appetite poor, bowels and urination normal. Speech normal. The five sense organs were normal and located correctly. There were scars on his right forehead and temple. Heart, lungs, liver and spleen normal. Physiological reflexes normal, no pathological reflexes induced. Muscle power in the limbs normal. He was able to extend his tongue without deviation. *Tongue body:* red. *Tongue coating:* greasy. *Pulse:* wiry.

Diagnosis: Stagnation of Qi and Blood in the vessels and collaterals.

Treatment: Activate Qi and Blood and invigorate the channels and collaterals.

Principal Points: Baihui Du 20, Fengchi GB 20, Xinshu BL 15, Geshu BL 17, Zusanli ST 36, Sanyinjiao SP 6.

All these points were given indirect moxibustion for 5 minutes on both sides. A course consisted of treatment twice a day for 6 days. After two courses the patient's spirits and appetite got better, and the faintness and heaviness improved slightly. His headache, however, remained severe and his memory was not restored. He was given another four courses of treatment which led to further improvements. As his headache still persisted, acupuncture was given on the right side only to Tai Yang (Extra) and Waiguan TB 5. The needles were retained for 20 minutes and treatment was given daily, in conjunction with moxibustion. Two more courses were given: the headache nearly disappeared and his memory improved. Two more courses of consolidating treatment were given; and the patient was discharged from hospital, completely cured.

Explanation: In this case trauma to the brain was causing headache, faintness and impaired memory. The classics state that, 'The head is the house of intelligence' (*Su Wen*, Mai Yao Jing Wei Lun, The Essentials of Pulse Taking chapter), and, 'The Brain is the Sea of Marrow' (*Ling Shu*, Hai Lun, The Seas chapter). The injury caused Blood Stagnation and obstruction in the collaterals, so the brain was not nourished. The *Ling*

Shu goes on to say that, 'When the Sea of Marrow is Deficient the brain revolves and the ear rings, the leg is sore and the vision is blurred. The man is lazy and inclined to lie down'. These symptoms occur because the brain is malnourished.

In this case moxibustion was given with a moxa stick, using warming and activating method. Baihui Du 20 and Fengchi GB 20 activate the channel Qi of the head area, calm the mind, subdue Wind and nourish the brain. Xinshu BL 15 and Geshu BL 17 promote Blood circulation and resolve Blood Stagnation, calm the mind and improve hearing. Zusanli ST 36 and Sanyinjiao SP 6 strengthen the Middle Burner and reinforce Qi and Blood, at the same time tonifying the Kidney, Liver and Spleen. All the points work together to activate Qi and Blood, dredge and invigorate the channels and collaterals.

> Zhang Dengbu, ACUPUNCTURE AND MOXIBUSTION SECTION, SHANDONG TCM COLLEGE HOSPITAL

CASE 2

Cao, male, age 19, peasant

Case registered: 23 July 1969

History: 1½ years previously the patient had been kicked in the head and knocked unconscious for about 30 minutes. Ever since he had suffered from headache, faintness, poor appetite and fatigue. His sleep was poor, he walked slowly, spoke with a thin voice and had cold limbs.

Examination: The patient looked thin and tired. BP normal. *Tongue body:* pale. *Tongue coating:* none. *Pulse:* deep and thin.

Diagnosis: Blood Stagnation in the channels and collaterals of the brain.

Treatment: Nourish and reinforce Qi and Blood, resolve Blood Stagnation.

Principal Points: Baihui Du 20, Dazhui Du 14, Gaohuangshu BL 43 (bilateral).
Three moxa cones were burnt at each point. Blistering moxibustion was given at Dazhui Du 14 and Gaohuangshu BL 43. After 2 weeks of daily treatment the patient's complexion turned red and he was able to sleep. His appetite, headache and faintness improved. He was also stronger and able to do some light farm labour.

After 6 months all his symptoms had gone and he could do normal farm work. The patient has been monitored for 10 years and has remained healthy.

Explanation: The headache, faintness and disturbed sleep resulted from malnutrition of the brain caused by Blood Stagnation in the vessels and collaterals of the brain. Moxibustion at Baihui Du 20 strengthens and raises Yang. Dazhui Du 14 is the meeting of the Yang. It refreshes the brain and tranquillizes the mind. Dazhui Du 14 and Gaohuangshu BL 43 are points which reinforce the body. Blistering moxibustion here greatly tonifies the vital Yang Qi and reinforces Deficiency and loss.

Han Zulian, TONGXIANG COUNTY NO 1 HOSPITAL, ZHEJIANG PROVINCE

CASE 3

Hu, female, age 17, student

Case registered: 24 August 1981

History: The patient fell off a high terrace at midday. By the time she was brought here she was comatose, with high fever and paroxysmal spasms of the whole body.

Examination: The patient was in a medium degree coma, with spasms as often as 20 times a minute. She was short of breath. Soft tissue injuries had resulted in swelling over her right hip and waist, but there were no abnormalities in the bones and no accumulation of blood. *Pulse:* deep, wiry and choppy.

Diagnosis: Tremor due to brain trauma.

Treatment: Resuscitate the patient and relieve Heat and spasm.

Principal Points: Yongquan KID 1 (bilateral), Neiguan P 6 (bilateral), Dazhui Du 20.
   Yongquan KID 1 was reduced with twirling method. The other points were needled with reinforcing and reducing evenly method. The tremor stopped after insertion, and the needles were retained for 30 minutes. 3 hours later the patient was conscious. The symptoms did not recur. She was given supplementary treatment for the swelling and discharged as cured.

Explanation: The *Nei Jing* says, 'Alarm causes disturbance of Qi inside', and 'Heat, dim vision and spasm are due to Fire'. In this case the shock and fear of the fall disturbed the circulation of Qi and Blood, and the Qi of the five Zang rose upwards to the brain. This exuberant Qi transformed into Fire, producing symptoms of fever, coma and spasm.
   Yongquan KID 1, the Jing-Well point, relieves Wind Stroke and resuscitates and tranquillizes the mind. In accordance with the principle of choosing a point in the lower part of the body to treat a disorder in the upper part, it also induces Qi and Blood to flow downwards.

Neiguan P 6, the Luo-Connecting point, goes through the Triple Burner channel and Yin Wei Mai. It calms the mind and benefits the functional Qi. Baihui Du 20 relieves Heat and Wind, invigorates the brain and tranquillizes the mind.

Shi Mingxue, BEIJI DISTRICT HOSPITAL, BINXIAN COUNTY, SHENXI PROVINCE
(*see Shenxi Traditional Chinese Medicine, Issue 5, 1985*)

36. Hydrocephalus

Jing, male, age 58, cadre

Case registered: 10 January 1983

History: In October 1982 the patient had begun to experience occipital headaches, faintness and nausea. On 25 December 1982 the headaches became severe and he vomited. All his symptoms improved after this, but at 8.00 a.m. the next day his faintness and headache got worse again, and he was unable to keep his breakfast down. The same thing happened that evening, and by the time he was admitted to hospital in the small hours of the next day he was semiconscious and found it difficult to move or speak. Initial neurological tests were negative; *BP:* 24.0/13.3 kPa (180/100 mmHg). There was a slight drop in the muscle power of the legs. Spinal puncture showed pressure of 43.3 kPa, fluid was colourless and clear, with positive test result for protein. Preliminary diagnosis: cerebral ischaemia or cerebral thrombosis. Symptomatic treatment was given to reduce intracranial pressure, which led to a slight improvement in the symptoms. Cranial X-rays on 28 December revealed no discernible intracranial hypertension, clear image of sella turcica, no discernible lesions. Examination of the fundus showed the optic disc had fairly clear borders. The next day ultrasonic examination of the brain found no mesal inversion. CAT scans on 29 December revealed hydrocephalus and narrowed cerebral aqueduct.

Examination: The patient was well developed and had had an average diet. *Temperature:* 35.5°C. *BP:* 21.3/13.3 kPa (160/100 mmHg). Pupils were equally dilated, with reaction to light. Neck soft, with no distension in jugular vein. Heart and lungs normal. Abdomen soft, liver and spleen not enlarged. Movement of spine and limbs normal. Neurological examination: deep and superficial sensitivity, no marked abnormalities. Muscle power normal. Knee jerk response weak on both sides, no pathological response. *Tongue body:* red. *Tongue coating:* thin and yellow. *Pulse:* wiry, 71/min. *Respiration:* 17/min.

Diagnosis: Headache and faintness: Hyperactive Liver Yang, Rebellious Stomach Qi.

Treatment: Suppress hyperactive Liver Yang, send down Rebellious Qi to stop vomiting.

Principal Points: Fengchi GB 20, Taichong LIV 3, Neiguan P 6.

Secondary Points: Zhongfeng LIV 4, Tianzhu BL 10, Wangu GB 12.

The local points, Fengchi GB 20, Wangu GB 12 and Tianzhu BL 10, were reinforced, twirling the needles rapidly with small amplitude. Aching and sensations of heaviness were propagated from behind the neck, spreading to the forehead along the Triple Burner channel. Treatment was given twice a day, alternating the two groups of points.

The occipital headache and nausea responded quickly, but the patient continued to feel faint if he moved his head. By 13 January his symptoms had improved markedly and he was able to get out of bed and walk around, although with difficulty. It was still very hard for him to speak. *BP:* 20.0/12.0 kPa (150/90 mmHg). *Pulse:* wiry. By 15 January the headache had completely gone but the faintness remained, especially in the mornings on rising, or if he moved his head. By 18 January the headache and faintness had completely disappeared, and he was able to move freely. *BP:* 18.7/12.0 kPa (140/90 mmHg).

After consolidating treatment the patient was discharged at the end of January. The case was followed up a year later. He was doing a full day's work, and had had no relapse.

Explanation: In TCM, this disease is attributed mainly to disorders of the Bladder and Liver channels. The usual diagnosis is headache and faintness. The *Nei Jing* says, 'The Bladder channel rises from inside the eye, up to the forehead and to the top of the head . . . into the vessels of the brain. The Liver channel . . . rises to the forehead and joins Du Mai at the top of the head'. In the section on diseases and symptoms of the Bladder channel, the *Nei Jing* says, 'so the illness goes up to cause headache'.

Tianzhu BL 10 activates the flow of Qi and the circulation of Blood in the brain. It drains out fluids accumulated in the upper part of the body through the bladder. Taichong LIV 3, Zhongfeng LIV 4, Wangu GB 12 and Fengchi GB 20 disperse hyperactive Liver Yang and ease the symptoms.

Western medicine would classify this case as hydrocephalus caused by narrowing of the cerebral aqueduct. As the patient had no history of physical trauma, it is likely that the aqueduct narrowed after adhesions of local tissue following a viral infection. Acupuncture was able to cure the condition by regulating Qi and Blood, improving 'Stagnation in the Interior and Stasis on the Exterior', improving the blood supply to the tissues and nourishing the local areas affected.

Liu Jinduo et al, TIANJIN TCM COLLEGE NO. 1 HOSPITAL
(see Hospital Journal, Issue 3 and 4, Bound Volume)

37. Muscular dystrophy

Xiu, male, age 16, schoolboy

Case registered: 9 August 1977

History: The patient had felt weak when walking since 1974. He could not run as fast as he had previously been able to and found it difficult to squat when passing stool; he would topple over backwards. These symptoms gradually got worse and he started to lose weight. His legs began to feel heavy and hard to lift, and walking became difficult and tiring, so that he had to stop frequently to rest. When standing he was unable to bring his feet together, and his back tilted forward. In bed he would feel weak in the lumbar region. He was examined at an army university in August 1977. He passed 1040 ml of urine over a 24-hour period; creatinine 1070 mg, creatine 48 mg, ESR 1 mm in 1 hour. Appetite was normal. The condition was diagnosed as muscular dystrophy and he was told to return home and have treatment with TCM.

Examination: The patient felt his legs were weak, and walking was difficult. The symptoms were getting worse. He stood with his feet apart, with no apparent pain or distortion. There was no apparent muscular dystrophy in the waist, pelvis or legs. The gastrocnemius muscles on both sides were relatively firm, with tendon reflex on both legs. No pathogenic reflex was induced. *Tongue coating:* thin and white. *Pulse:* deep and slow.

Diagnosis: Wei syndrome: Deficiency and exhaustion of Spleen and Kidney, Qi Deficiency and Blood stagnation.

Treatment: Reinforce Spleen and Kidney, activate Blood and dredge the collaterals.

Principal Points: Pishu BL 20, Shenshu BL 23, Huantiao GB 30, Biguan ST 31, Zusanli ST 36, Liangqiu ST 34, Jiexi ST 41.
   Treatment was given once a day. After a month the patient's legs were stronger and he was able to squat, though not very steadily.

Secondary Points: Pishu BL 20 through to Shenshu BL 23, Huantiao GB 30 through to Chengfu BL 36, Yanglingquan GB 34 through to Yinlingquan SP 9.

A long needle was used to join the points and treatment was given once a day. After 5 months the patient was able to run, and could walk for 2.5 km, but was still unable to stand with his feet together. A new prescription was devised following the principle of 'treating the Spleen for all conditions of Dampness, Excess and swelling'.

Revised Points: Xuehai SP 10, Shangqiu SP 5, Yinlingquan SP 9, Zhibian BL 54, Weizhong BL 40, Kunlun BL 60.

After a month the patient had gained 2 kg in weight and was able to cycle about 50 km. A second urine test at the army university showed creatinine 174 mg, creatine 0.058 mg over a 24-hour period.

Treatment was continued to consolidate the result. The above prescriptions were alternated. Altogether the patient received 130 treatments over a 7-month period. By the end of this time he was cured, with normal movement and strength in his legs. The case was followed up for 5 years and there was no relapse.

Explanation: Progressive muscular dystrophy is classified in TCM as Wei syndrome. The *Su Wen* says, 'When there is illness in the Spleen it fails to transport Body Fluids for the Stomach. The limbs are weakened because they cannot get nourishment. Qi is unable to pass through the vessels so the tendons, bones and muscles are not nourished and cannot function, and become useless' (*Familiar Conversations*, Spleen and Stomach chapter). All flaccidity disease therefore relates to the Yang Ming channels, and points on the Stomach channel were selected. As the Spleen is the Yin coupled organ of the Stomach, Spleen points were selected. In TCM the Kidney is the root of Original Qi, and dominates bone. As the Bladder is the Yang coupled organ of the Kidney, Zhibian BL 54 and Chengfu BL 36 were selected to dredge these channels, regulate Qi and Blood and nourish the tendons and vessels.

Chang Mingqi, DONGDAJIE HOSPITAL, BEILIN DISTRICT, XI'AN
(see Shenxi Traditional Chinese Medicine, Issue 7, 1984)

38. Faecal and urinary incontinence
following spinal injury

Gao, male, age 61, cadre

Case registered: 7 April 1982

History: The patient had injured his lower back in 1968 and ever since had had pain in the waist and hips. He would frequently become paralysed in the legs and lose control of his bowels and urination. Hospitals in Beijing and Guayang diagnosed the problem as a compression fracture with damage to the cauda equina, but after various treatments his condition was unchanged. He was given the same diagnosis at this hospital on 23 February 1982. Supporting treatment improved his symptoms, but they still recurred if he coughed, sneezed or moved his body. There was also a nasal mucus-like discharge from his anus. His doctors were perplexed by this problem and referred him for acupuncture and moxibustion.

The patient currently felt weakness and pain in his waist and knees. He had faecal and urinary incontinence, especially if he coughed. His limbs were cold and he was averse to cold. His appetite was poor and he was generally weak. He felt faint, could hear roaring and ringing in his ears and his vision was blurred.

Examination: The patient looked pale and lacklustre. *Tongue body:* pale. *Tongue coating:* white and greasy. *Pulse:* deep and weak.

Diagnosis: Deficiency of Spleen and Kidney Yang.

Treatment: Warm the Kidney and nourish the Spleen.

Principal Points: Pishu BL 20, Shenshu BL 23, Guanyuan Ren 4, Zhangmen LIV 13.

Gentle moxibustion was given with moxa sticks. Treatment was given once a day for 20 minutes at each point. Wrist–ankle needling at lower points 1 and 2. The needles were retained for 20 minutes[1]. After three treatments there was no improvement, but after the fourth there was less mucus secretion before and after bowel movement. At this point the wrist–ankle needling was stopped.

Gradually the patient's stools started to become drier and the secretion lessened, particularly after bowel movements. Coughing and sneezing no longer caused incontinence, and he urinated less frequently. His appetite improved and he was able to drink without fear. After 30 treatments his bowels and urination were normal and his other symptoms had improved or gone altogether. Five more consolidating treatments were given. After 4 weeks of observation the patient was discharged as cured.

Explanation: In TCM theory this disease is caused by Deficiency of the Spleen and Kidney. The Kidney is the Prenatal source of Qi and the key to the Stomach. It opens at the two Yin orifices and is in charge of faeces and urine. When Kidney Qi is sufficient it acts both on the upper part of the body and the lower part. In the upper part, Kidney Qi warms the Spleen for digestion and the movement of food and water; in the lower

---

[1]Wrist-ankle needling is a therapy which uses six points proximal to the wrist (upper 1–6) and six points proximal to the ankle (lower 1–6) to treat disease in corresponding parts of the body.

part it warms the Bladder to help Qi resolve fluids. If the Kidney Yang is deficient, the Fire of Life withers and Yin becomes Exuberant, causing faecal and urinary incontinence.

The Spleen is the Postnatal source of Qi. When the Spleen is healthy and vigorous it digests food and water, sending the Clear upwards and the Turbid downwards, so urine and stools are normal. Normal defaecation and urination are therefore dependent on the Spleen and Kidney.

Pishu BL 20 is the Back-Shu point of the Spleen, and Zhangmen LIV 13 is the Front-Mu point. Together they reinforce Spleen Qi. Shenshu BL 23 and Guanyuan Ren 4 are sources of Yang Qi. Together they reinforce the body's resistance and regulate and reinforce Yang. Moxibustion was added to 'warm what is cold'.

Warming and reinforcing the Spleen and Kidney treats the cause of the disease. The Bladder channel 'goes into the anus and spreads into the Kidney', so selecting Bladder points also addresses the symptoms, bringing Yang directly to the anus to help it open and close properly. When both the cause and the symptoms were taken into account and treated, the Yang was able to circulate properly and the disease was cured.

Liu Zuqian, under the direction of Liu Mingyi, GUIYANG SCHOOL OF TCM, CLASS OF 1977
(see *Journal of Traditional Chinese Medicine, Issue 12 1982*)

39. Paralysis following haematomyelia

Wang, female, age 31

Case registered: 19 September 1982

History: The patient became paralysed after severe pain in the lumbar area, back and legs. At the same time she lost control of both her bladder and her bowels. She was diagnosed with haematomyelia (bleeding into the spinal cord), and after 50 days in hospital her incontinence was cured, although she was still paralysed. At this point she came for acupuncture and moxibustion.

Examination: Both legs were paralysed, with muscular atrophy and flaccidity. No physiological reflex. Spinal flexion normal, with no tenderness or distortion. Grade 0 muscle power. Plantar reflex normal. Oppenheim's sign negative. Chaddock's sign negative. *Tongue body:* red. *Tongue coating:* yellow. *Pulse:* thin and rapid.

Diagnosis: Wei syndrome.

Treatment: Reinforce Kidney Yang, nourish the bones and tendons, dredge the channels and collaterals and activate the joints.

Principal Points: Zhongji Ren 3, Shenshu BL 23, Sanjiaoshu BL 22, Huantiao GB 30, Biguan ST 31, Yinmen BL 37, Futu ST 32, Yinshi ST 33, Yanglingquan GB 34, Zusanli ST 36, Shangjuxu ST 37, Xiajuxu ST 39, Diji SP 8, Xuanzhong GB 39, Kunlun BL 60, Jiexi ST 41, Qiuxu GB 40.

5–6 of the leg points were used at a time. The points were needled bilaterally, and alternated with each treatment. After sensation was obtained, the needles were retained for 30–45 minutes and connected to a G6805 unit at an intensity bearable to the patient. Treatment was given once a day and a course lasted 10 days. After 10 weeks the patient's symptoms were much better. She was able to move but she tired easily. After another 2 weeks, the disorder was cured.

Explanation: In TCM this case is classified as Wei syndrome. For the treatment of this disease the *Nei Jing* says, 'Only use points on the Yang Ming channels', because, 'Yang Ming is the sea of the organs and is in charge of nourishing the major tendons, which tie the bones and move the joints'. The Yang Ming channels are rich in Qi and Blood, so using such points regulates Qi and Blood, dredges the channels and collaterals, strengthens the bones and tendons and activates the joints. It is important to use points of Yang Ming together with points of Tai Yang and Shao Yang, e.g. points which reinforce Kidney Yang such as Shenshu BL 23, Huantiao GB 30, Yinmen BL 51 and Yanglingquan GB 34. A doctor must be able to adapt to the clinical situation and not limit himself to one channel only.

Kong Lingjiu, JILIN FARM PRODUCE SCHOOL
(*see Tianjin Traditional Chinese Medicine, Issue 5, 1985*)

40. Transverse myelitis

CASE 1

Liu, male, age 18, worker

Case registered: 11 May 1981

History: 4 days previously the patient had become weak, with fever and a sore throat. He then felt sudden discomfort and soreness at the inferior angle of the scapula, and dullness of the legs when getting out of bed. These symptoms gradually got worse. Soon he had difficulty walking, and urinary incontinence, and he was admitted to this hospital for emergency treatment.

Examination: The patient was of average build and had an adequate diet. *Temperature:* 37°C. *Pulse:* 84/min. *Respiration:* 21/min. *BP:* 10.7/5.33 kPa

(80/40 mmHg). Thyroid normal. No distortion of the limbs and spine. Heart, lungs, liver, spleen normal. Abdomen flat and soft, with no tender areas. No tenderness or pain from percussion in the kidney area. Faint bowel sound. Ankle reflex sluggish. Extensor plantar response on the right. Muscle power grade 0 in the right leg, grade 2 in the left, normal in the arms. Superficial sensitivity of the skin dulled in both legs. Cerebrospinal fluid clear and colourless. Pressure high. Protein 140 mg/dl, chloride 79 percent (sic), sugar 55 mg/dl. Cells 14. Pandy's reaction positive. Blood test showed RBC $4.15 \times 10^{12}/l$ ($4.15 \times 10^6/mm^3$), haemoglobin 12 g %. WBC $9 \times 10^9/l$ ($9 \times 10^3/mm^3$), neutrophils 77%, lymphocytes 23%, platelets 90 000/mm³. ECG normal. Waist and chest X-ray normal.

Diagnosis: Wei syndrome.

Principal Points:
1. Shenshu BL 23, Dachangshu BL 25, Zhongliao BL 33, Weizhong BL 40, Chengshan BL 57, Kunlun BL 60.
2. Huantiao GB 30, Yanglingquan GB 34, Xuanzhong GB 39, Liangqiu ST 34, Futu ST 32, Zusanli ST 36, Jiexi ST 41.
3. Renzhong Du 26, Zhongji Ren 3, Guanyuan Ren 4, Sanyinjiao SP 6, Waiguan TB 5.

These groups of points were alternated. The needles were retained for 15 minutes and electric stimulation was applied. Treatment was given daily and a course lasted for 10 days, with a 3-day rest between courses. After 10 courses the patient was much better. This was a very serious case however, and his appetite was still poor. He was weak and caught colds easily, which exacerbated his condition. He was prescribed Hu Qian Wan (Hidden Tiger Pill) and advised to do more rehabilatory exercise.

These two supplementary therapies combined with acupuncture led to a further improvement in the patient's condition. After 6 months, laboratory tests showed all indices were normal, and the patient was discharged. The case was followed up 8 months later; he was in good shape and could walk about, sometimes for a few miles. He was able to climb up and down five floors and could do some housework.

Explanation: Transverse myelitis is categorized in TCM as Wei syndrome. In the Differentiation of Syndromes According to the Eight Principles, it is a Deficiency disease and must be treated with reinforcing techniques.

Shenshu BL 23, Dachangshu BL 25 and Zhongliao BL 33 are used together to activate the Qi of the Fu organs, to strengthen the Kidney Yang and invigorate the channels and Blood.

Huantiao GB 30, Yanglingquan GB 34, Xuanzhong GB 39, Futu ST 32, Zusanli ST 36 and Jiexi ST 41 dredge the channels and collaterals and regulate Qi and Blood.

Renzhong Du 26, Zhongji Ren 3, Guanyuan Ren 4, Sanyinjiao SP 6 and Waiguan TB 5 were used for the urinary incontinence, because Renzhong Du 26 activates Du Mai and invigorates the Yang. Zhongji Ren 3, the Front-Mu point of the Bladder, and Guanyuan Ren 4 are both located in the Lower Burner. They dredge the Qi of the Lower Burner and regulate the Bladder. Sanyinjiao SP 6 regulates the Qi of the three leg Yin channels. Waiguan TB 5, the Luo-Connecting point, activates the Blood of the Triple Burner.

> Sun Changlin, LUOYANG MUNICIPAL PEOPLE'S HOSPITAL NO. 2, HENAN PROVINCE
> (see Shanghai Journal of Acupuncture and Moxibustion, Issue 3, 1985)

CASE 2

Kang, female, age 61

History: The patient had initially felt pain in her back and lumbar region. Later her feet became slightly swollen and numb, and the numbness extended up to the lumbar region. She began to have difficulty moving her legs and finally became paralysed from the waist down, losing control of her bowel and bladder. She was treated with Chinese herbs but showed no improvement.

Examination: Cerebrospinal fluid: protein 600 mg/l (60 mg/dl), lymphocyte $5.0 \times 10^7/1$ (50/mm^3), WBC $1.2 \times 10^{10}/1$ (12 000/mm^3).

Diagnosis: Wei syndrome

Treatment: Two therapies were used: body acupuncture and point injection therapy.

Point Injection: 4 ml of vitamin B$_1$ and 4 ml of vitamin B$_{12}$ were used. 0.5–1 ml of each were injected into Mingmen Du 4, Yaoyangguan Du 3 and the lumbar Jiaji (Extra) points.

Body Acupuncture: Huantiao GB 30, Yinmen BL 37, Weizhong BL 40, Zusanli ST 36, Yanglingquan GB 34, Juegu GB 39.

The points were needled bilaterally with strong stimulation, and the needles were not retained. Treatment was given daily and a course lasted for 10 days. After four courses the patient was much better; she had regained partial control of her bowel and bladder, could walk short distances and the dull feeling in her legs was reduced. After two more courses her bowel and bladder were normal and she could walk properly. Laboratory tests found blood and cerebrospinal fluid to be normal, and she was discharged as cured. The case was followed up 2 years later, and she was still well.

Editor's Note: In TCM transverse myelitis is classified as Wei Syndrome. Although the *Nei Jing* says, 'Only use points on the Yang Ming channels', for the treatment of this disease, in clinical practice the doctor should differentiate the type of disease and select methods and points accordingly. In this case the doctor combined point injection therapy with body acupuncture. Mingmen Du 4 and Yaoyangguan Du 3 nourish and reinforce the Kidney Yang, to strengthen the waist and back. Huantiao GB 30, Yinmen BL 51, Yanglingquan GB 34, and Juegu GB 39 dredge the tendons, activate the Blood and the channels. Zusanli ST 36 tonifies the digestion to generate Qi and Blood.

41. Transverse myelitis (recuperative stage)

Liu, male, age 60, cadre

History: A year previously the patient had caught a cold. He felt discomfort in the neck, but shortly afterwards he lost control of his bladder and bowels and was paralysed in all four limbs. He was diagnosed with acute myelitis and treated with hormones. His condition stabilized, and he was discharged from hospital. He did not, however, regain movement in his limbs, and he came to this hospital to try acupuncture and moxibustion.

Examination: The patient was conscious. *Temperature:* 36.3°C. Skin dry and coarse. Superficial sensitivity diminished below T4 vertebra. Grade 3 muscle power in the four limbs. Muscle tone increased. No abdominal reflex. Tendon reflexes hyperactive. Hoffmann's sign positive bilaterally. Extensor plantar response on both sides.

Diagnosis: Wei syndrome.

Principal Points:
1. Jiaji points at C3, C5, C7, L2, L4.
2. Jiaji points at C2, C4, T1, L3, L5.

Secondary Points:
1. Jianyu L.I. 15, Shousanli L.I. 10, Sanyangluo TB 8, Yanglingquan GB 34, Juegu GB 39, Sanyinjiao SP 6.
2. Indirect moxibustion for 5 minutes at Ganshu BL 18 and Shenshu BL 23. The first two groups of points were alternated and treatment was given

daily. After 3 weeks the patient felt strength returning to his limbs and was able to get out of bed. The treatment was modified and the secondary points were changed:
Neiguan P 6, Yinlingquan SP 9, Fenglong ST 40, Sanyinjiao SP 6, Zhaohai KID 6.

These points were needled bilaterally with reinforcing method. After 2 months the patient's condition was greatly improved; he was able to walk up and down stairs, make his bed and look after himself. His complexion became rosy and he looked stronger. Superficial sensitivity diminished below T7 vertebra. Muscle power grade 4 in the arms, grade 5 in the legs. Muscle tone slightly increased. Abdominal reflex normal. Tendon reflexes brisk. Hoffmann's sign negative bilaterally. Plantar responses normal.

Explanation: In TCM this case is classified as Wei syndrome. In accordance with the principle of nourishing the Postnatal Qi of the Stomach and Spleen, the *Nei Jing* says, 'Only use points on the Yang Ming channels' to treat this disease. This theory has been regarded as important and has given good results, but in clinical practice it cannot be adhered to too closely. In this case, for example, good results were obtained mainly by using the Jiaji points.

The Jiaji points are selected according to their relation with the affected area. The needles are angled slightly towards the spine, 0.5–1.2 cun deep. Reinforcing method was used till sensation was propagated towards the limbs. Initially, the treatment was supplemented with points mostly on the Yang channels. Later, supplementary points mostly on the Yin channels were used. Moxibustion at Ganshu BL 18 and Shenshu BL 23 nourishes the Liver and Kidneys, strengthens the tendons and bones and accelerates the recovery of the affected limbs.

It was also important to wean the patient off the hormones gradually, and encourage him to do appropriate rehabilatory exercise.

Han Youdong, ACUPUNCTURE AND MOXIBUSTION SECTION, SHANDONG TCM COLLEGE HOSPITAL

42. Paraplegia, traumatic

Zhao, male, age 50, worker

Case registered: 12 April 1976

History: The patient had tried to rescue some comrades from danger when he was hit by some falling sheet metal. In hospital that day he was given two lumbar punctures. 11 days later he underwent exploratory surgery, and he was found to have a comminuted fracture and transposition of thoracic vertebrae 11 and 12, which were then reinforced with a steel plate. He also required urethral catheterization. By July of the same year he had urinary infection and fever, and was constipated.

Examination: Both legs were flaccid and completely paralysed. There was loss of sensation below the level of the injury. He had some mild bed sores.

Diagnosis: Traumatic paraplegia: Kidney Yang Deficiency, Stagnation of Qi and Blood.

Treatment: Invigorate the channels and collaterals to resolve Stasis, nourish and invigorate Kidney Yang.

Principal Points:
1. Guanyuan Ren 4, Xiawan Ren 10, Qihai Ren 6, Tianshu ST 25, Fengshi GB 31, Yanglingquan GB 34, Zusanli ST 36, Sanyinjiao SP 6, Qiuxu GB 40, Taichong LIV 3.
2. Shenshu BL 23, Mingmen Du 4, Pangguangshu BL 28, Dachangshu BL 25, Ciliao BL 32, Huantiao GB 30, Weizhong BL 40, Chengfu BL 36, Chengshan BL 57, Kunlun BL 60.

Secondary Points: Hegu L.I. 4, Yangchi TB 4, Waiguan TB 5, Quchi L.I. 11, Jianyu L.I. 15, Zhongzhu TB 3, Fengchi GB 20.

The two groups of principal points were alternated, and the secondary points were added every three treatments. The patient was given rehabilatory exercises. After six treatments the urinary infection was greatly reduced. The catheter was removed and he was able to urinate with the help of massage. His bed sores improved and his temperature was normal. After 36 treatments he was standing and able to mark time on the spot with support. He was brought to this institute for further treatment in May 1977. By then he was able to walk and do squatting exercises. His bladder function was partially restored.

Comment: Recovery from traumatic paraplegia depends on early clinical examination and diagnosis, and well conceived and prompt treatment. Compression of the spinal cord should be removed as soon as possible. Acupuncture should be given during the period of spinal shock. It can not only treat pain, but is effective for shock, infection and fever. In certain conditions we believe it is possible for the spinal cord to regenerate after injury. The functions of the nervous system can be restored. The regenerative potential of the spinal cord is partially dependent on the age of the patient: it is better in younger patients because the spinal cord is more elastic.

Gao Xipeng, YUCI MUNICIPAL INSTITUTE FOR PARALYSIS, SHANXI PROVINCE
(see Chinese Acupuncture and Moxibustion, Issue 1, 1985)

43. Paraplegia, tuberculous

Liu, female, age 58, homemaker

Case registered: October 1981

History: The patient was admitted to hospital in March 1980. She had pain in the lumbar region and sides. The pain got worse and soon she was unable to move, and had urinary and faecal incontinence. She was numb below the waist. X-ray examination led to a diagnosis of tuberculosis of the thoracic vertebrae. Standard treatments did not help and she was referred for acupuncture and moxibustion.

Examination: There was spastic paralysis in both legs, and diminished sensation below the waist. Patellar reflex was excessive.

Principal Points:
1. Jiaji (Extras) from T4-T6, Shenshu BL 23, the eight sacral foramen points (optional), Yinmen BL 37, Weizhong BL 40, Kunlun BL 60.
2. Qihai Ren 6, Tianshu ST 25, Biguan ST 31, Fengshi GB 31, Zusanli ST 36, Jiexi ST 41.
3. Yanglingquan GB 34, Juegu GB 39, Qiuxu GB 40.

   The three groups of points were rotated, but the first group was used more often. Reinforcing and reducing evenly method was used. Treatment was given daily, and a course consisted of 10 treatments. Intervals of 3–5 days were allowed between courses.

   Stress was placed on getting good needle response, but care was taken to stop the needle breaking if the spastic limbs went into spasm. The routes of the three groups of points were tapped with a plum blossom needle every 5 days, alternating each group per treatment. Antituberculosis drugs were given orally. The patient began to show improvement after 2 months. After 10 months she was walking on one crutch. Recently the case was followed up. She was walking without a stick, and able to do some housework.

Comment: Acupuncture can improve the function of the bowels and bladder in cases of tuberculous paraplegia, and restore the movement of the lower limbs. Both the doctor and the patient must have confidence in the therapy, and must remain patient. In the later stages of treatment it is important for the patient to do rehabilatory exercises.

Lu Jing, GUANGYUAN TCM COUNTY HOSPITAL, SICHUAN PROVINCE
(see Chinese Acupuncture and Moxibustion, Issue 5, 1985)

44. Paralysis, functional

CASE 1

Shen, male, age 38, school teacher

Case registered: October 1980

History: In December 1979 the patient fainted while grieving over his mother's death. He was resuscitated, but had palpitations, shortness of breath and a pallid complexion. Five days later his legs began to feel weak and his mobility was impaired. By February 1980 his legs were completely paralysed. He was able to pass stool and water, but these were not regular. X-ray examinations of the chest, neck and lumbar region were all normal, as was a lumbar puncture. He was given medication and physiotherapy for 6 months, without effect. In August 1980 he was admitted to the Neurology Department of this hospital, and after a month without improvement was referred for acupuncture and moxibustion. By this time he also had palpitations, nightsweats and pain in the lumbar region.

Examination: The patient was conscious, but a little nervous and short of breath. His muscles were rigid. Reduced sensation below the 10th thoracic vertebra. Tendon reflex in the upper limbs, knee and ankle excessive. Abdominal reflex positive. Cremasteric reflex present, with active flexion of right leg before reflex. No plantar eversion. Plantor reflex normal. Rossolimo's sign negative. Hoffman's sign negative. Grade 0 muscle power in lower limbs. X-rays revealed no apparent hyperplasia or destruction of lumbar vertebrae. *Tongue body:* red. *Tongue coating:* white and greasy. *Pulse:* wiry, thin and rapid.

Diagnosis: Wei syndrome.

Treatment: Nourish the Heart, clear Heat, strengthen the Kidney and tendons.

Principal Points: Xinshu BL 15, Guanyuanshu BL 26, Zhibian BL 54, Guantiao GB 30.
   The points were first needled bilaterally, with reinforcing and reducing evenly method. The needles were then heated with three moxa cones until the warmth was felt deep in the points, then cupped. At Zhibian BL 54 and Guantiao GB 30 the needles were manipulated until sensation was propagated to the foot. Treatment was given once every 2 days. After seven treatments the patient was able to walk. The coating on his tongue was thinner and his appetite and spirits had improved. The nightsweats, however, persisted.

Secondary Points: Dazhui Du 14 and Fuliu KID 7 were added.

These points were reinforced by lifting, thrusting and reinforcing, and retained for 15 minutes. After four of these treatments the nightsweats had diminished and the patient could walk steadily. The patient was almost fully recovered and discharged. The case was followed up for a year and there was no relapse.

Explanation: In TCM paralysis is classified as Wei syndrome, but according to the *Su Wen,* 'all five organs are capable of causing flaccidity' (Wei Lun, *Familiar Conversations,* Flaccidity chapter), and the syndrome should be differentiated and treated accordingly.

The *Su Wen* says, 'Extreme Grief causes the cessation of the functions of the collaterals which in turn causes the agitation of Yang Qi inside . . . when the Heart Qi is hot the lower vessels send energy upwards, leading to Deficiency of the lower vessels. This leads on in turn to flaccidity of the tendons, and the patient is unable to walk'. In this case the flaccidity was in the vessels. It started when the patient fainted from grief. This caused agitation of the Yang, which in turn resulted in Exuberance of Yang Heat in the Upper Burner and Deficiency of the channels and collaterals of the Lower Burner. Eventually the channels became flaccid.

Xinshu BL 15 and Guanyuanshu BL 26 were selected to nourish the Heart, clear Heat and strengthen the Kidney and tendons. Zhibian BL 54 activates the circulation of Qi and Blood in the lower limbs. Huantiao GB 30 is an important point for strengthening the tendons and resolving flaccidity. Dazhui Du 14 governs the Yang of the whole body, and connects the Yin of the body. It clears Heat, invigorates the Qi and consolidates resistance on the Exterior. Fuliu KID 7 removes Fire by nourishing the Yin, and dredges and nourishes the sweat pores. Although this was a simple prescription, it yielded good quick results. In clinical practice flaccidity must be differentiated into the five types and treated accordingly. The principle of treating flaccidity by 'selecting only points on the Yang Ming channels' does not have to be followed to the letter.

Chen Weicang, ACUPUNCTURE AND MOXIBUSTION SECTION, REIJIN HOSPITAL, SHANGHAI NO. 2 MEDICAL COLLEGE
(see Journal of Traditional Chinese Medicine, Issue 6, 1985)

CASE 2

Li, female, age 26, peasant

Case registered: 1 August 1980

History: 2 months previously the patient developed occipital headache and insomnia after a traumatic and emotional childbirth. Her legs became weak, but she was able to walk, so she did not seek medical advice. A month later she began to feel dullness in her legs after stress. This time she was unable to walk or stand, though she could still move her legs when lying in bed. She lost her appetite, and felt pain and distress in the chest with headache and insomnia.

Examination: The patient kept switching from tears to laughter to sighing. Her legs were weak and paralysed. Her fingers were rigid and she had difficulty flexing or extending them. *Tongue coating:* slightly yellow and greasy. *Pulse:* deep.

Diagnosis: Wei syndrome: Stagnation of Liver Qi.

Treatment: Dredge Liver and Gall Bladder Qi, activate Qi and Blood.

Principal Points: Dazhui Du 14, Danzhong Ren 17, Fenglong ST 40, Zusanli ST 36, Yanglingquan GB 34, Taichong LIV 3, Shenmen HT 7.
Electro-acupuncture was used at Fenglong ST 40.

Secondary Points: Baihui Du 20, Fengchi GB 20, Taiyang (Extra), Hegu L.I. 4. Waiguan TB 5.

After one treatment the patient was able to get out of bed and stand, though her legs were still weak. Her hands regained their mobility, her headache was relieved and her appetite improved. The disease was completely cured after one course of treatment, but another course was given to consolidate the effect.

Explanation: The disease was caused primarily by Stagnation of Liver Qi, so treatment was directed at dredging and regulating the functional Qi. Using Danzhong Ren 17, the Hui-Converging point of Qi, and Taichong LIV 3, the Yuan-Source point, relaxes the chest and relieves Stagnation of Qi. The Heart is in charge of the mind, so Shenmen HT 7, the Yuan-Source point, was used to calm the mind. In keeping with the principle of treating flaccidity by 'selecting only points on the Yang Ming channels', Zusanli ST 36 and Fenglong ST 40 were selected to nourish Qi and Blood. Yanglingquan GB 34, the Hui-Converging point of the tendons, strengthens tendon and bone. Dazhui Du 14, the meeting of all the Yang channels, invigorates the Yang of the whole body, and dredges the channels and collaterals.

Of the secondary points, Baihui Du 20 and Fengchi GB 20 were used to send down the rising Liver and Gall Bladder Yang, and Taiyang (Extra) was added to relieve headache. Hegu L.I. 4 and Waiguan TB 5 were used to dredge the channel Qi in the local area.

Li Fujun, ACUPUNCTURE AND MOXIBUSTION SECTION, ZHANGJIAKOU MUNICIPAL TCM HOSPITAL, HEBEI PROVINCE
(see Journal of Traditional Chinese Medicine, Issue 12, 1981)

45. Paraplegia, idiopathic

Chu, male, soldier

Case registered: April 1953

History: A year ago the patient began to feel numb and weak in both legs. This became worse until he was completely paralysed. He had no previous history of trauma. He was given treatment in a hospital in the North East, but did not improve. His doctors were unable to give him a definite diagnosis, and thought perhaps this might be syringomyelia or tuberculosis of the lumbar spine. He was brought to a convalescent home in Lanzhou but did not improve, and finally came here for acupuncture and moxibustion.

Examination: The patient looked thin and pale, and felt cold. He was paralysed in both legs, with muscular atrophy and no sensation. *Tongue body*: pale. *Tongue coating:* white and greasy. *Pulse:* deep and weak.

Diagnosis: Wei syndrome.

Treatment: Nourish the Liver and Kidney.

Principal Points: Jinsuo Du 8, Jizhong Du 6, Mingmen Du 4, Yaoyangguan Du 3, Shenshu BL 23, Ganshu BL 18, Huantiao GB 30, Weizhong BL 40, Yanglingquan GB 34, Zusanli ST 36, Sanyinjiao SP 6, Kunlun BL 60, below Shiqizhui (Extra).

   10 to 12 points were selected at a time. The points not on the midline were needled bilaterally. All the points were reduced strongly and the needles were retained for 20 minutes. The needles were manipulated 2–3 times during retention with medium strong stimulation, and reduced once again before withdrawal. Moxibustion was given on the back points. Treatment was given once every other day. After three treatments the patient could sit on the edge of his bed and move his legs a little. After 7 months treatment he was able to walk without a stick.

Explanation: In TCM paraplegia is classified as Wei syndrome. It is usually due to extreme Heat in the Lung and Stomach, Invasion of Damp Heat or Kidney and Liver Yin Deficiency. In the Excess type, Pathogenic Heat impairs the Yin, so the tendons and muscles are malnourished. In the Deficiency type, long-term consumptive disease causes Deficiency of the Liver and Kidney Yin and the Sea of Marrow, so the tendons and muscles are malnourished.

   Zhou Zhijiu said, 'The core of Wei syndrome is the disease of four channels: Liver, Kidney, Lung and Stomach'. According to this theory, the symptoms of the disease are in the lower limb, but the cause is maladjustment of the organic fluids. Treatment should regulate the circulation of Qi, Blood and Body Fluids, Yin and Yang, especially in Du Mai, the Sea of all the Yang. Points on the Liver, Kidney , Stomach and Spleen should be selected, nourishing Yin to restore Yang, as well as points on the Lung and Du channels to reinforce and warm Qi. It is also important to encourage the patient to take an active part in the recovery process.

> Case treated by Zhang Taoqing, case study by Liu Fu, HUANGFU
> MI INSTITUTE OF ACUPUNCTURE AND MOXIBUSTION, GANSU PROVINCE.

SPASMS

46. Involuntary clenching of the fist

Zhang, female, age 36, peasant

Case registered: May 1983

History: The patient had had an emotional upset. After an outburst of anger her right hand had suddenly clenched into a fist, and she was unable to open it again. Friends had forced her hand open for her, but it had sprung back into a fist the moment it was released. She was unable to work as a result. Before she was referred here she had been in hospital for 50 days, where the problem was diagnosed as hysteria or arthralgia syndrome.

Examination: The patient's right hand was tightly clenched and the fingers were stiff. Two walnuts had been pushed into the fist as deodorizers. Her speech was normal. Appetite poor. She had a feeling of fullness in the upper abdomen. She was extremely anxious that she might be crippled for life. *Tongue coating:* yellow and greasy. *Pulse:* wiry.

Diagnosis: Contracture: Liver Wind, Liver Qi Stagnation.

Treatment: Promote the circulation of Qi and dispel Wind.

Principal Points: Hegu L.I. 4
   The point was needled on the affected side with strong stimulation. The patient gave a cry of pain and then her fist opened. Her hand was then massaged, shaking the joints of the fingers to activate Qi and Blood. After about 30 minutes her hand was moving freely. The patient is back at work and there has been no relapse.

Explanation: The *Nei Jing* says, 'Any sudden stiffness comes from Wind'. This disorder was caused by Stagnant Liver Qi failing to disperse and remove. The vessels and tendons became stiff, resulting in this Wind syndrome. Treatment was designed to 'dispel the Liver when it is Stagnant'.

Hegu L.I. 4, the Source point, lifts and disperses, activates Qi, dispels Wind, activates the collaterals and relieves pain. This condition was thus cured with one single point only.

> Ma Shaochu, SHANDONG PROVINCIAL TCM SCHOOL
> (see *Journal of Shandong Traditional Chinese Medicine, Issue 3, 1984*)

47. Spasm of the hand

Liu, female, age 43

History: The patient had had paroxysmal tremors in both hands for about 10 years. The problem started when she had become frightened during labour. At first her hands shook and felt numb, but they gradually became painful. As the pain became severe she was disabled, and could not get dressed without assistance. Injections of calglucon gave relief for a day, and if she ate eggs with the shell she would also get temporary relief. The spasm would recur when she was angry or anxious, or if the weather was cold.

Examination: The patient was emaciated. Appetite, bowels and urination normal. Menstruation normal. *Tongue coating:* white and greasy. *Pulse:* wiry and thin.

Diagnosis: Contracture.

Treatment: Nourish and invigorate Qi and Blood, using points from Yang Ming and Shao Yang channels.

Principal Points: Hegu L.I. 4, Zusanli ST 36, Yanglingquan GB 34.

Secondary Points: Houxi SI 3 (needled less frequently).

The points were stimulated gently, and the needles were retained for 20 minutes. Moxibustion was given for 3–5 minutes whilst the needles were retained, until the patient felt relaxed and her skin had turned red. Treatment was given once a day.

After the first treatment there was no tremor for the rest of the day but it did return, less frequently than before. The prescription seemed effective, so it was repeated. Warm needle treatment was given at the principal points, and moxibustion on ginger at Qihai Ren 6 and Shenque Ren 8. After three treatments the patient showed great improvement, with no spasm for a week. If a treatment is effective, there is no need to change it, and the prescription was repeated for a month. During this time there were no more spasms. The case was followed up for a month and there was no relapse.

Explanation: Western medicine attributes spasm to deficiency of calcium in the blood. In TCM it is due to Deficiency of Qi and Blood, and malnutrition of the tendons and vessels. The disorder was so severe in this case that doses of calcium were only effective temporarily. It is remarkable that acupuncture and moxibustion were able to turn the condition around in so short a time.

Hegu L.I. 4 and Zusanli ST 36 are points of Yang Ming, which reinforces Qi and Blood. Yanglingquan GB 34, the Gathering (Hui) point of tendons relaxes the tendons and relieves pain. Houxi SI 3, the Shu-stream point and one of the eight Confluent points of the Extraordinary Vessels, opens Du Mai and is good for spasm in the hands. Moxibustion at Qihai Ren 6 and Shenque Ren 8 reinforces Kidney Qi and strengthens the body's resistance.

Zhang Fengrun, SHENXI PROVINCIAL INSTITUTE OF TRADITIONAL CHINESE MEDICINE
(see Journal of Traditional Chinese Medicine, Issue 10, 1980)

48. Spasm of the arm

He, male, age 36, cadre

Case registered: 8 September 1981

History: 10 days previously the patient caught a chill, with fever and headache. The symptoms cleared after 3 days, but on the 4th day he woke up to find that movement in his right elbow was restricted and very painful. Medication did not help, and the pain affected his sleep.

Examination: The patient's right elbow was flexed at an angle of 60°. The tendons of extensor carpi radialis longus and biceps brachii muscles were very taut. Flexion and extension of the forearm were restricted and the elbow was painful when palpated. His appetite, bowels and urination were normal. *Tongue body:* red. *Tongue coating:* white, yellowish and greasy. *Pulse:* wiry and slippery.

Diagnosis: Contracture: Stagnation of Damp Heat.

Principal Points: Quchi L.I. 11, Quze P 3, Shousanli L.I. 10, Waiguan TB 5, Yanglao SI 6, Neiguan P 6, Hegu L.I. 4.
Treatment for 3 days produced no improvement.

Scalp acupuncture: Sensory area.

A 28 gauge 2.5 cun needle was inserted deep at the centre of the area, to the aponeurosis. The needle was manipulated for 1 minute until sensation was referred from the top of the head through the neck to the right shoulder, elbow, wrist and fingertips. The patient immediately felt a sensation of lightness in the affected areas, and after a further 3 minutes was able to move his arm normally and without pain.

Explanation: The signs and symptoms indicate that this is Ju syndrome (contracture). The *Su Wen* says (Sheng Qi Tong Tian Lun chapter, Adaptation of the Human Body to the Environment) the disease 'is caused by Damp, the head feels like it is covered, Damp and Heat cannot be expelled. The large tendons contract, the smaller tendons relax'.

Contracture is Ju and relaxing is *Wei* (flaccidity). The disease is caused by Damp turning into Heat which obstructs the tendons and vessels, leading to contracture. In this case scalp acupuncture was indicated. Stimulation of the sensory area treated the affected parts directly, activating Qi and Blood, invigorating the tendons and channels to relieve the contracture and pain.

Dong Zibin, GANYU COUNTY PEOPLE'S HOSPITAL, JIANGSU PROVINCE
(see Journalof Traditional Chinese Medicine, Issue 6, 1983)

49. Spasm of the quadriceps

Yang, female, age 14, school student

Case registered: 14 August 1987

History: 5 days previously the patient suddenly developed tremors and pain in her left thigh. Each episode lasted about 5 minutes, and the pain was very severe. She did not respond to medication at the local clinic.

Examination: It was obvious the patient was in great pain. The tremor in her left quadriceps was clearly visible, and it was very tender on palpation. There were no other positive pathogenic signs. Blood tests were normal.

Diagnosis: Cold Bi syndrome.

Treatment: Activate Qi and Blood, dredge the collaterals and resolve stagnation to relieve pain.

Principal Points: Biguan ST 31, Fengshi GB 31, Xuehai SP 10, Liangqiu ST 34.

Electro-acupuncture was applied with a G6805 unit using continuous wave current: voltage 1.5 mV, frequency 60 per minute, duration 20 minutes. Cupping was administered for 5 minutes afterwards. After the first treatment there was considerable improvement in the pain, and after the second the disorder was completely cured. The case was followed up for 2 months and there was no relapse.

Explanation: In TCM spasm of the quadriceps is classified as arthralgia aggravated by Cold or Cold Bi syndrome. This was clear from the localization of the pain and the severe tenderness on palpation. Aetiology includes incorrect posture or application of force, e.g. lifting too much, moving suddenly, or trauma after physical impact, all of which result in disorders of Qi and Blood and spasm of the tendons and vessels. Zhang Jingyue says, 'When Cold and Damp rest between the muscle, tendon and bone, they stagnate and obstruct the Yang causing severe pain'. Electro-acupuncture and cupping at the above points activate Qi and Blood, dredge the collaterals and resolve stagnation to relieve pain.

He Jingui, ACUPUNCTURE AND MOXIBUSTION SECTION, JIAOZUO MUNICIPAL PEOPLE'S HOSPITAL, HENAN PROVINCE

50. Torticollis

CASE 1

Zhang, female, age 36, peasant

Case registered: Autumn 1956

History: The patient had previously been healthy and strong, but after washing one day her head suddenly tilted back and up. She was incapacitated and unable to move it. She was treated for 2 months in one hospital for 'nervous wryneck', and in another she was given local injections of procaine, but her condition remained unchanged.

Examination: The patient's neck felt hard on the left and flaccid on the right. Her head was tilted obliquely back and to the left. She had large and fearful eyes set in a very thin face. Examination of the channels revealed a hard lump in the right Juegu GB 39 area. *Tongue body:* pale. *Tongue coating:* thin and white. *Pulse:* wiry, and the artery extended at an angle into the thenar eminence.

Diagnosis: Wind stroke involving the neck.

Treatment: Expel pathogenic Wind, dredge the channels and collaterals.

Principal Points: Juegu GB 39 (right).
　　Electro-acupuncture was used, and the patient's head moved back

into position the moment the current was turned on. The case was followed up for 30 years, and there was no relapse.

Explanation: Torticollis and similar disorders are not uncommon, but cases of such severity are extremely rare. Juegu GB 39, the Gathering (Hui) point of Marrow, is an important point on the Gall Bladder channel. The hard lump on the skin at the right Juegu GB 39 area indicated Wind stroke involving the neck, a diagnosis borne out by the miraculous effect of the treatment.

Li Quanzhi, HEZE MUNICIPAL TCM HOSPITAL, SHANDONG PROVINCE

CASE 2

Yang, male, age 22

Case registered: 20 August 1980

History: The patient had previously been healthy and had no history of physical trauma. He had fallen asleep at his desk one night, and for the last 20 days the left side of his neck had been stiff and painful. His head tilted to the right and would nod involuntarily. The nodding was aggravated by stress. Electro-acupuncture, procaine, acupuncture and moxibustion, Western and traditional Chinese medication had so far been ineffective.

Examination: The patient's neck was stiff, tense, painful and very hot to the touch. It was immobile and inclined forward and to the right. The left sternocleidomastoid muscle was extended, stiff and slightly tender, and the right sternocleidomastoid was hard. The nodding was aggravated with spasm by stimulation of the head and left sternocleidomastoid muscle, but relieved or arrested completely by gentle stroking of the head. The left side of his face was contracted while the right side was flaccid. His left shoulder was raised. Temperature, pulse rate and BP normal. *Tongue body:* red. *Pulse:* wiry and rapid.

Diagnosis: Wind stroke involving the neck: Wind Phlegm obstructing the collaterals and vessels, accumulated Heat inducing Wind.

Treatment: Expel Wind, Heat and Phlegm to dredge the channels and vessels.

Principal Points: Houxi SI 3 (bilateral), Shenmai BL 62 (bilateral), Tianzong SI 11 (bilateral), Fenglong ST 40 (bilateral).
　　The patient lay on his back and Houxi SI 3 and Shenmai BL 62 were needled. The needles were rotated forcefully with a large amplitude till

Qi sensation was felt in the shoulders, and along the outside of the leg through the knee joint. The patient was advised to move his head during the manipulation, and the needles were retained for 10 minutes. After this the patient was able to hold and move his head normally.

He then sat up and Tianzong SI 11 on the left was reduced with Qi sensation referred to the shoulders. Tianzong SI 11 on the left was needled with gentle rotation and small amplitude to cause local numbness and distension. During these manipulations the patient was asked to move his shoulders. The shoulders became level after this.

Fenglong ST 40 was needled next, reinforcing and reducing evenly till Qi sensation reached the ankles. The condition recurred after the session, but it was much less severe. The treatment was repeated seven times, and the disorder was cured.

Explanation: The disease was in the Yang channels, caused by Wind and Cold invading the channels and collaterals of the neck and back. The True Qi was maladjusted locally, Wind Phlegm obstructed the channels and vessels, and accumulated Heat had induced Liver Wind. Reducing Houxi SI 3 and Shenmai BL 62 dredges Qi and Blood in the Taiyang channels, Du Mai and Yang Heel Vessel, clears Heat and subdues Wind. Tianzong SI 11 dredges and regulates the Qi of the shoulders. Fenglong ST 40 resolves Phlegm and clears the collaterals.

Xu Defeng, JINXIAN COUNTY TCM HOSPITAL, LIAONING PROVINCE

CASE 3

Zhang, female, age 40

Case registered: 26 August 1982

History: In 1979 the patient had developed a tremor in her right hand after losing her temper. Later a tremor developed in her neck, and her head tilted to one side. Over the last year her stools had become loose, her appetite had diminished, she felt faint and lost weight. She had malar flush, blurred vision, insomnia and dreamed frequently. She was diagnosed with 'nervous wryneck' and 'neurosis' and given medication, which did not help.

Examination: Tongue body: dark red. *Tongue coating:* thin and yellow. *Pulse:* deep and wiry.

Diagnosis: Liver Wind.

Treatment: Reinforce the Spleen, soften the Liver to expel Wind and control spasm.

Principal Points: Fengchi GB 20, Taichong LIV 3, Sanyinjiao SP 6, Quchi L.I. 11, Shousanli L.I. 10, Hegu L.I. 4.

Fengchi GB 20 expels Wind, Taichong LIV 3 dredges the Liver, Sanyinjiao SP 6 regulates and nourishes the Liver, Spleen and Kidney channels, Quchi L.I. 11, Shousanli L.I. 10 and Hegu L.I. 4 regulate the Yang Ming channels.

After 18 treatments there was no change in the patient's condition, so the Zi Wu Liu Zhu (Open Hourly Points) method was now adopted. Laogong P 8 and Taichong LIV 3 were opened on 20 September (date Stem 3, time Stem 2, Branch 8) to expel the Fire and soften the Liver. On 21 September (date Stem 4, time Stem 5, Branch 9) there was no specific point to open so Jiexi ST 41, the point for date Stem 9, was 'borrowed', to strengthen the Spleen and Stomach. On 23 September (date Stem 8, time Stem 2, Branch 8) Taichong LIV 3, Taiyuan LU 9 and Laogong P 8 were opened. On 26 September (date Stem 9, time Stem 5, Branch 9) the time's principal point, Jiexi ST 41, was opened. Yang points were therefore opened on Yang dates at Yang times, and Yin points were opened on Yin dates at Yin times. After five such treatments the tremor and spasm in the neck were cured and there was substantial improvement in the tremor of the hands.

Explanation: The disorder was caused by Deficient Spleen Yang leading to Deficient Liver Blood. When the Yin is deficient the Yang is not controlled and rises up. The patient's original outburst of anger aggravated the rising Liver Yang to create Fire and Wind. The Liver is in charge of tendons and the Spleen controls muscles. If the Liver is not properly nourished there will be spasm, and Liver Wind causes muscle tremor. The *Nei Jing* says, 'All Wind syndromes, stiffness in the body and faintness are related to the Liver'.

This case also demonstrates how effective the Zi Wu Liu Zhu method can be.

Yu Guangsheng, ACUPUNCTURE AND MOXIBUSTION SECTION, JILIN NO. 3 PEOPLE'S HOSPITAL
(see Shanghai Journal of Traditional Chinese Medicine, Issue 2, 1984)

51. Trismus (lockjaw)

CASE 1

Su, female, age 54, cadre

History: The patient had a previous history of hypertension. At present she found it hard to open her mouth and was having difficulty eating and talking. She also felt faint and her legs were weak. She found it hard to stand still or walk steadily and was distressed and sleeping badly. Her stools and urine were normal.

Examination: BP: 25.3/14.1 kPa (190/106 mmHg). No pathological reflexes. *Tongue coating:* thick and greasy. *Pulse:* wiry and rapid.

Diagnosis: Internal Wind.

Treatment: Clear Liver Wind, induce Blood to flow downwards, dredge and activate channels and tendons.

Principal Points: Tiaokou ST 38 through to Chengshan BL 57, Taichong LIV 3, Jiache ST 6, Dicang ST 4.

All these points were used bilaterally. Tiaokou ST 38 was needled to a depth of 3 cun with reinforcing technique. The needle was retained for 20 minutes and manipulated strongly once during this time. Taichong LIV 3 was reduced. After the needles were withdrawn, the sensation at the feet remained. This phenomenon is described in the *Ling Shu*: 'Sometimes the sensation continues to travel after the needle is withdrawn' (*Miraculous Pivot*, Xing Zhen, Manipulation chapter).

After treatment, the lockjaw and all signs of Exuberance in the upper part of the body and Deficiency in the lower part disappeared, although the sensation of heaviness in the legs persisted. The next day the patient's blood pressure measured 22.7/13.3 kPa (170/100 mmHg). Five more treatments were given and the disorder was cured. The case was followed up 6 months later and there was no relapse.

Explanation: The patient had a previous history of high blood pressure, and now had lockjaw and muscle tension. This pointed clearly to Internal Wind rising up with disturbance of Blood and Qi. The Stomach channel pathway 'goes up to the neck, controls the mouth and joins at the cheeks', so Stomach points were reinforced to strengthen the source of Qi and Blood. If Qi and Blood are full, the Wind will be subdued. This follows the principle of 'Treat Wind by treating the Blood first. When the Blood is activated the Wind subsides'.

Jiache ST 6 and Dicang ST 4 remove pathogens in the upper part of the Stomach channel. Reducing Taichong LIV 3 pulls Rebellious Qi back down.

Mang Xianxi, PEOPLE'S BANK OF CHINA CLINIC, KAIFENG MUNICIPAL BRANCH
(see *Journal of Traditional Chinese Medicine, Issue 8, 1984*)

CASE 2

Liu, male, age 20

History: The patient had had lockjaw for 142 days. It had started when he fell ill with high fever and coma, and spastic stiffness of the whole body. He was not given a formal diagnosis in his local hospital. After 3 days of treatment he recovered consciousness, and after 7 days the fever was relieved. After a month the spasm of the muscles was better, but the lockjaw remained unchanged and he was surviving on fluid infusion and glucose injections.

Examination: He was very weak. His jaw was tightly closed. The masseter and temporal muscles were stiff to the touch, as were the muscles of the floor of the mouth. He had great difficulty speaking and eating.

Treatment: Activate the channels and collaterals.

Principal Points: Xiaguan ST 7, Jiache ST 6, Lianquan Ren 23, Hegu L.I. 4. The points were reduced strongly, and the needles were not retained. After 1 minute he was able to move his jaw slightly. After 2 minutes he was able to open his jaw 2 cm. After 3 minutes he could open it 3.5. cm. Two more treatments were given, and the lockjaw was completely cured.

Ma Dingxiang, STOMATOLOGY DEPARTMENT, ARMY UNIVERSITY NO. 4

Editor's Note: This was a very difficult and chronic case of lockjaw following fever and systemic spasm. It responded so quickly because the treatment was designed to activate the channels and collaterals which relate to the mouth opening. Xiaguan ST 7, Jiache ST 6, Lianquan Ren 23 and Hegu L.I. 4 are all important points for difficulty in opening the mouth. It is important to note that all the points were reduced.

52. Spasm, facial

Luo, male, age 32, accountant

Case Registered: 17 April 1964

History: 2 months previously the patient began to have paroxysmal tremor affecting his left eyelid, left cheek and the left side of his mouth. He would have 5–6 attacks a day, and each one would last for 5–6 minutes. During an attack he felt sensations of heaviness in the eyeballs, contraction and pulling to the left of the facial muscles. There was no numbness or pain. The tremors only came during the day, not at night.

Examination: Apart from the spasm, he seemed to be generally in good health. Tongue and pulse normal.

Diagnosis: Invasion of the Yang Ming channels by Wind Cold.

Treatment: Activate the channels and collaterals, soothe Wind and stop spasm.

Principal Points:
1. Yangbai GB 14, Chengqi ST 1, Dicang ST 4, Hegu L.I. 4.
2. Sizhukong TB 23, Quanliao SI 18, Renzhong Du 26, Yizhong (Extra).

The two groups of points were alternated, and treatment was given daily. The points were strongly reduced and the needles were retained for an hour. The spasm stopped during the first session after the needles were inserted. When he came the next day his spirits were much improved. He had only had two minor twitches early that morning, and no sensations of heaviness. When he came for his third visit he had had no spasm at all. He was discharged as cured. A month later he had had no relapse.

Explanation: The cause of this disease was invasion of Wind and Cold into the Yang Ming channels. Pathogenic Wind is Yang and active in nature, and usually assaults the upper parts of the body. Pathogenic Cold is Yin and contracting in nature. When they combine they usually cause contraction and spasm of the tendons and vessels, and in this case caused facial tremor. The treatment was designed to dredge the channels and vessels, soothe Wind and relieve spasm. This conforms with the principle: 'When treating Wind, treat the Blood first. When Blood is activated the Wind calms down spontaneously'.

The Large Intestine and Stomach channels are rich in Blood and Qi. They go to the face, encircle the mouth and meet at Renzhong Du 26, so Chengqi ST 1, Dicang ST 4 and Hegu L.I. 4 were selected to regulate the Qi of Yang Ming. The Triple Burner and Gallbladder channels go to the face and the muscles around the eyes. Yangbai GB 14 and Sizhukong TB 23 were selected to relieve Wind and stop spasm, because the Gallbladder channel is Wood and corresponds to Wind. Renzhong Du 26 is also connected to Ren Mai. It readjusts Functional Yin and Yang Qi. Yizhong (Extra) is an empirical point for activating the Blood and the collaterals. The success of the treatment was also because the points were reduced and the needles were retained for a long time.

Yang Jiebin, CHENGDU TCM COLLEGE
(see Correspondence, Journal of Acupuncture and Moxibustion, Issue 1, 1987)

TREMORS

53. Shaking head

Zhong, male, age 25, peasant

Case registered: 6 April 1981

History: 2 months previously the patient got into a heated argument. Afterwards he drank some wine before going to sleep. The next morning he was constipated, restless, and his vision was blurred. His head started to shake intermittently. The tremor would stop if he slept. He was treated with Shu Gan Wan (Liver Comforting Pills), but his symptoms got worse and more frequent, interfering with his work. Neurological examinations in another hospital found nothing unusual, and Western medication also had no effect.

Examination: The patient was thin, with a red complexion. His head shook constantly. *Tongue coating:* yellow and greasy. *Pulse:* wiry and rapid.

Diagnosis: Liver Wind Agitating Within.

Treatment: Relieve Liver Wind, purge Fire and Heat.

Principal Points: Fengchi GB 20 (bilateral), Hegu L.I. 4 (bilateral), Xingjian LIV 2 (bilateral), Dazhui Du 14.
   After five treatments there was a big improvement in the shaking, but the patient's vision was still blurred and he was still distressed. After a course of 10 treatments the shaking would only occur about 10 times during the daytime, and the length of each episode would now vary. His other symptoms also improved. The shaking stopped after the next course, and a further course was given to consolidate the result. The case was followed up for 3 years and there was no relapse.

Explanation: Shaking of the head can arise from Excess or Deficiency conditions. Accumulated Heat in the Liver and Gall Bladder causing Agitated Liver Wind, or Heat in the Yang Ming channels, may cause shaking of the head, blurred vision, deafness, stiff and painful neck accompanied by high fever, distress, abdominal pain and constipation. Liver and Kidney Deficiency from old age, weakness after illness or Deficiency Wind Moving Within may cause shaking of the head and other symptoms of Deficiency.
   This was an Excess condition, so the treatment aims were to subdue Liver Wind and purge Fire and Heat. Fengchi GB 20 and Baihui Du 14 clear Heat and suppress Liver Yang. Hegu L.I. 4 and Xingjian LIV 2

relieve Liver Wind. Dazhui Du 14 regulates the functional Qi of the Yang channels.

Kong Lingju, JILIN FARM PRODUCE SCHOOL
(see Shengxi Traditional Chinese Medicine, Issue 4, 1978)

54. Tremor of the chin

Pan, female, age 18, peasant

Case registered: 17 March 1987

History: The patient had tremor of the chin for 5 days, which was worse over the last 2 days. She also had a bitter taste in the mouth, oppression in the chest and belching, which would stop when she was asleep.

Examination: Tongue body: pale. *Tongue coating:* thin and white. *Pulse:* wiry and thin.

Diagnosis: Stagnation of Liver Qi, Liver Wind rising upwards.

Treatment: Soothe the Liver Qi and calm Liver Wind.

Principal Points: Taichong LIV 3 (bilateral), Fengchi GB 20 (bilateral), Hegu L.I. 4 (bilateral), Xiaguan ST 7, Shanglianquan (Extra).
    The needles were retained for 80 minutes, and manipulated at 10 minute intervals. The tremor improved after 30 minutes, and disappeared altogether after 50 minutes.
    The tremor had returned more mildly by next day, but she had no bitter taste or oppression in the chest. The treatment was repeated.
    On the 3rd day all her symptoms had gone. She was given another consolidating treatment. The case was followed up for 6 years and there was no relapse.

Explanation: According to TCM these symptoms are caused by Liver Wind agitating within. The Liver and Gallbladder are a Yin–Yang pair. Taichong LIV 3, the Yuan-Source point, is used in combination with Fengchi GB 20, an important point of the Gallbladder channel, to calm the Liver Wind. Shanglianquan (Extra), although a new point, is by virtue of its location on Ren Mai, which passes through the chin. Hegu L.I. 4 and Xiaguan ST 7 are also on channels which pass through the chin. These three points were chosen because they are on vessels and channels which pass through the affected area.

Li Mengzhi, ACUPUNCTURE AND MOXIBUSTION SECTION, GANGYANG COMMUNE CLINIC, TAIXIAN COUNTY, JIANGSU PROVINCE
(see Shanghai Journal of Acupuncture and Moxibustion, Issue 3, 1982)

55. Nocturnal tremor of the back of the knee

Li, male, age 59, cadre

Case registered: 20 June 1977

History: For the last 2 years the patient had suffered from tremors in the back of the knee at night. They started in the left knee and then affected the right. Later his elbows tingled and itched as well. At first the symptoms had occurred every few months, but recently they had become more and more frequent. At present his knees trembled every few seconds and disturbed his sleep, sometimes all night long. He was tired and depressed. He had been to several hospitals for consultation and treatment but none had provided a cure or an accurate diagnosis. Finally he came here for acupuncture and moxibustion.

Examination: The patient looked depressed. He was of average stature with a dry yellow complexion. Skin, mucosa and lymph nodes negative. All the organs in the head, face and neck areas negative. Thyroid, carotid, heart, lungs, liver and spleen were normal. The popliteal and cubital fossae were normal in colour and temperature, but slightly tender. Muscle tone, strength and leg reflex were all normal. *BP:* 13.1/8.00 kPa (98/60 mmHg). *Laboratory examination:* cholesterol 7.02 mmol/1 (270 mg/dl). *Tongue body:* pale. *Pulse:* thin, slightly rapid.

Diagnosis: Deficiency of Liver and Kidney Yin.

Treatment: Nourish Liver and Kidney Yin.

Principal Points: Taixi KID 3, Taichong LIV 3, Weizhong BL 40.
  Medium strength manipulation was used, the needles were retained for 20 minutes and manipulated twice during this period.
  After the first treatment the tremor was less frequent and the patient was able to sleep for 4 hours. After five treatments the tremor had completely disappeared. The patient was able to sleep well. A persistent disease of 2 years' chronicity was cured.
  3 weeks later the patient relapsed. Further treatment to dredge and regulate the Qi in the channels was given.
  Chize LU 5 and Weizhong BL 40 were needled with the same stimulation as before. Treatment was given daily and the condition was cured after 4 days.
  The patient relapsed again 6 weeks later. Although mild, the twitching was disturbing his sleep.

Examination: Tongue body: swollen and pale. *Tongue coating:* yellow and white. *Pulse:* thin and rapid.

Diagnosis: Deficiency of Liver and Kidney Yin with Liver invading Spleen.

Treatment: Nourish the Yin and dredge the Liver to activate the channel Qi.

Principal Points: Taixi KID 3, Ganshu BL 18, Weizhong BL 40.
   The symptoms went after two treatments. The case was followed up for a further 2 years and there was no relapse.

Explanation: This is a difficult disease as no cause has been found and no accurate diagnosis can be made. From the pulse, tongue and symptoms it was clear that it could be attributed to Deficiency of the Kidney and Liver Yin, and points were selected accordingly.
   The *Ling Shu* says, 'When there is disease in the Five Organs treat the Twelve Source points' (Jiu Zhen Shi Er Yuan, *Nine Needlings*, Twelve Source points chapter). Taixi KID 3 is the Yuan-Source point, Taichong LIV 3 clears Heat in the Liver, Weizhong BL 54 activates the channel Qi and Body Fluids, Ganshu BL 18 relieves the Liver. The disease is extremely rare but was cured after only eight treatments, which shows the importance of clinical differentiation.

Guo Chengjie, SHENXI TRADITIONAL CHINESE MEDICINE COLLEGE
(see Shenxi Traditional Chinese Medicine, Issue 1, 1981)

56. Ataxia

CASE 1, POST-TRAUMATIC

Fu, female, age 28

Case registered: November 1975

History: The patient had an operation for hyperthyroidism in a London hospital in July 1968. She was under a general anaesthetic for 11 hours, and when she regained consciousness she felt faint and uneasy. A few hours later she was suffering from chills and dyspnoea from blood clots blocking the trachea. Her heart stopped for several minutes on the way back to surgery, and she was given emergency treatment and a tracheotomy. She went into coma for several weeks, during which time she had another cardiac arrest, accompanied by persistent high fever, spasm and clenched fists. 7 days later she recovered consciousness, but her field of vision was blurred and reduced, she was paralysed in her legs and arms and unable to speak. After over a year she regained some movement in her limbs, and a year after that she began slowly to speak again, but walking was still very difficult.

Examination: The patient was unable to walk steadily by herself, her speech was indistinct and she had tremor of the head and limbs. She felt faint and her mouth and eyes were dry. Her stools were dry and difficult to pass and she urinated frequently. *Tongue body:* red. *Tongue coating:* greasy. *Pulse:* deep and thin.

Diagnosis: Ataxia (sequela of cerebral ischaemia and anoxia): Deficiency of Blood and Qi in the brain, and Liver Wind.

Treatment: Activate Qi and Blood, nourish and refresh the brain.

Principal Points: Dazhui Du 14, Fengfu Du 16, Fengchi GB 20, Shousanli L.I. 10, Zusanli ST 36, Yanglingquan GB 34, Gaohuangshu BL 43.

Treatment was given once every 2 days and the needles were retained for 20 minutes.

Dazhui Du 14, Fengfu Du 16 and Fengchi GB 20 were reinforced with lifting, thrusting and twirling method and the needles were retained. When the patient came for her third treatment her symptoms had improved and the tremor in her limbs was reduced.

Secondary Points: Jingming BL 1, Tongziliao GB 1, Zhongji Ren 3, Hegu L.I. 4, Taichong LIV 3.

These points were added from the fourth treatment onwards. The needles were withdrawn immediately after insertion at Jingming BL 1 and Tongziliao GB 1, and retained for 30 minutes at the other points. Gaohuangshu BL 43 was cupped after needling.

After 30 treatments most of the patient's symptoms had gone, and she was able to stand and walk steadily without a stick. Her speech was clear, she was able to move her eyes easily, and the tremor in her head and limbs had gone. She was much stronger in her limbs and was able to hold a pen. After she got better she moved back to China permanently. The case was followed up after 5 years, and she was still healthy and stable.

Chen Weicang, ACUPUNCTURE AND MOXIBUSTION SECTION, SHANGHAI MEDICAL COLLEGE NO. 2, REIJIN HOSPITAL
(see Shanghai Journal of Traditional Chinese Medicine, Issue 4, 1980)

Editor's note: This was a very difficult case to treat, as there had been cerebral ischaemia and anoxia. From the symptoms and pulse,it arose from Deficiency of Blood and Qi in the brain, and Liver Wind. This was a result of Deficiency in Du Mai, the Liver, Spleen and Kidney, which could not supply the brain with Qi and Blood, or nourish the tendons and vessels. Dazhui Du 14, Fengfu Du 16, Fengchi GB 20, Gaohuangshu BL 43 and Zhongji Ren 3 nourish Kidney Qi and Blood and reinforce the brain. Zusanli ST 36 and Shousanli L.I. 10 strengthen the Qi and Blood of Yang Ming and tonify the source of Qi and Blood. Yanglingquan GB 34, Hegu L.I. 4 and Taichong LIV 3 relax the tendons and relieve spasm caused by Liver Wind. Jingming BL 1 and Tongziliao GB 1 relieve Wind and clear the eyes.

This prescription primarily nourishes and reinforces the Qi, Blood and Marrow of the whole body, and at the same time aids local recovery of the affected organs and tissues.

CASE 2, CEREBELLAR

Huang, male, age 30

Case registered: 18 April 1981

History: Early in 1976 the patient began to have difficulty moving his legs. This gradually got worse, and he became unable to walk without stopping frequently, and developed a tremor in his arms. He started to cough and choke at meals and his vision became blurred. If he looked to one side he would get double vision. If he saw striped patterns they would sway like a curtain moving in the wind. He also had headaches, muscular tension in his cheeks and a tremor in his right index finger.

Examination: Hoffmann's test positive. Extensor plantar response. Finger-nose test positive. Heel–shin test positive. Romberg's test positive. Dysdiadokokinesis.

Treatment: Nourish the brain and Marrow, balance Yin and Yang.

Scalp Acupuncture: Balance area (bilateral), Optic area (bilateral).
The needles were retained for 30 minutes and twirled rapidly for 2 minutes (150–200 times/min) every 10 minutes.

Principal Points: Shousanli L.I. 10, Houxi SI 3, Zusanli ST 36, Xuanzhong GB 39.
Treatment was given once every 2 days and a course consisted of 20 sessions. A 10-day interval was allowed between courses. After four treatments the heaviness and headache went, and the blurred vision and tremor improved. After nine treatments the tremor in the index finger improved. After 10 treatments the patient's vision improved some more. He no longer choked and coughed at meals, and could walk more steadily. The therapeutic effects of the scalp acupuncture endured. From the end of December up to the present time the patient's vision has been good. There has been no relapse in his coughing and choking. His speech is still not very clear, but he can walk steadily, going up and

down stairs without using the bannister, and has only a slight tremor in his arms.

> Dai Yi Jun, ACUPUNCTURE AND MOXIBUSTION SECTION, YUE YANG
> HOSPITAL, SHANGHAI TCM COLLEGE
> *(see Shanghai Journal of Acupuncture and Moxibustion, Issue 1, 1985)*

Editor's Note: Good results were obtained by using scalp acupuncture in combination with body acupuncture. The Balance area and Optic area are on the back of the head and are closely related to the balancing and visual centres in the brain. Shousanli L.I. 10 and Zusanli ST 36 reinforce Qi and activate Blood. Houxi SI 3, the Confluent point of Du Mai and Xuanzhong GB 39, the Hui-Converging point of Marrow, were used to nourish the Marrow and the brain, and balance Yin and Yang.

57. Parkinson's disease

CASE 1

Fan, female, age 70

Case registered: 4 December 1982

History: Recently the patient had begun to feel a heavy sensation in her head. She had become distressed, and clumsy with her right arm. Over the last 4 days it had begun to shake involuntarily, getting worse if she was agitated. The shaking would stop when she slept.

Examination: The patient was generally in good condition. Her arm was shaking involuntarily, and the muscle tone was poor. There was no sensory disturbance, but the tendon reflex was weak. *Tongue body:* red and a little dry. *Tongue coating:* thin, white and yellow. *Pulse:* wiry and rapid.

Diagnosis: Clonus.

Treatment: Reinforce Qi, calm the mind, soften the Liver Qi to relieve spasm.

Principal Points: Dazhui Du 14, Quchi L.I. 11, Jianshi P 5, Shenmen HT 7, Hegu L.I. 4.
   The needles were inserted quickly, retained for 30 minutes and manipulated with reducing method every 10 minutes. The patient's arm stopped shaking immediately the points were needled. Four more treatments were given to consolidate the effect, and there was no relapse.

Explanation: Parkinson's disease is mostly caused by aging and cerebrovascular disease. In TCM it is classified as clonus, arising from impairment of Qi, Blood and Body Fluids leading to malnourishment of the tendons and vessels. In addition, emotional upset can turn into Fire which, together with Wind, can disturb the extremities and cause spasm.

Dazhui Du 14 is the meeting of the Yang channels and dredges the Yang of the whole body. Shenmen HT 7 and Jianshi P 5 dredge Qi in the Heart and Pericardium channels, calming the mind. Quchi L.I. 11 and Hegu L.I. 4 nourish the major tendons. The combined effect of these points is to regulate Yin and Yang, clear the Heart and Liver, invigorate Qi and stop spasm.

Guan Xiaoxian, LONGTAN DISTRICT HOSPITAL, JILIN MUNICIPALITY, JILIN PROVINCE

CASE 2

Zhang, male, age 71, retired worker

Case registered: 26 November 1979

History: The patient had been diagnosed with Parkinson's disease 10 years previously. At first his left arm and leg had started to shake. He became weak and was unable to move them quickly. He did not respond to Western or traditional Chinese medicine, and by 1974 his legs were paralysed and he was bedbound.

Examination: The patient was conscious but he looked dull, as if wearing a mask. He was unable to stand and had pitting oedema on his legs. He found it hard to speak or swallow, and was producing a lot of saliva. *Tongue body:* wet. *Tongue coating:* thin and white. *Pulse:* wiry and slippery.

Diagnosis: Liver and Kidney Deficiency, with Liver Wind invading the collaterals. Consumption of Du Mai, weakness in the Yang Ming channels.

Principal Points: Baihui Du 20, Quchi L.I. 11, Hegu L.I. 4, Zusanli ST 36, Yanglingquan GB 34, Yinlingquan SP 9, Sanyinjiao SP 6.
  The points were needled every other day, and a course consisted of 10 treatments. After two courses the oedema had improved and the patient's legs were shaking less.

Secondary Points: Sishencong (Extra), Fengchi GB 20, Fengfu Du 16.
  These points were added to the principal points, and Baihui Du 20 was now omitted. Reinforcing and reducing evenly method was used.
  After the first of these modified treatments the patient's speech improved, and his legs felt more comfortable. After three more treatments the shaking stopped and he produced less saliva. He could walk around

his room with a walking stick. After the fourth course (4 months after his initial consultation) he was able to walk to a small park some 300 metres from his home.

Over the past 2 years the case has been followed up; there has been some relapse in the patient's symptoms, but he is still able to walk around the house with a walking stick.

Explanation: This is a severe and chronic case, but remarkable effects were achieved with acupuncture. At first, major points on the Stomach and Large Intestine channels were used to regulate and invigorate the Yang Ming channels. Sishencong (Extra) and Fengfu Du 16 strengthen Du Mai, dredge and regulate the three arm and leg Yang channels, circulate Qi and Blood smoothly and balance Yin and Yang. Fengchi GB 20 relieves Wind and controls spasm. The treatments addressed both the symptoms and the causes of the disease.

Zhang Jianqiu, ARMY MEDICAL UNIVERSITY 2, LONG MARCH HOSPITAL (*see Shanghai Journal of Acupuncture and Moxibustion, Issue 1, 1983.*

RHEUMATOLOGICAL AND ORTHOPAEDIC DISORDERS

58. Erythromelalgia

CASE 1

Zhang, male, age 24

Case registered: 18 May 1977

History: The patient suddenly began to experience burning pain in his left ring finger. The middle joint was red and swollen for more than a month. The pain was burning and throbbing, and most severe at night or on exposure to heat. Tests revealed normal blood indices and ESR. After unsuccessful treatment with salicylic acid he came here for treatment.

Examination: The patient's left ring finger was noticeably swollen at the middle joint. Flexion and extension were difficult, and he felt burning pain when the joint was touched.

Diagnosis: Arthralgia: Stagnation of Qi and Blood.

Treatment: Activate the channels and collaterals, stimulate the flow of Qi to relieve pain.

Principal Points: Waiguan TB 5, Zhongzhu TB 3.

The points were needled on the left with medium stimulation, and the needles were retained for 15 minutes. Treatment was given daily.

During the first treatment the patient felt an improvement in the pain and mobility in the joint. After seven treatments the problem was completely cured. The case was followed up for 2 months and there was no relapse.

Explanation: Western medicine attributes this condition to abnormal dilation of the vessels in the extremities from an imbalance in the autonomic nervous system. This is quite similar to the explanation in the *Sheng Ji Zhong Lu* (General Collection for Holy Relief) which says, 'Severe and migratory arthralgia is rooted in Deficiency of Qi and Blood. When attacked by Wind and Cold, Qi and Blood become stagnant and cannot circulate to the joints. The tendons are not nourished. The body resistance fights the pathogenic factors at the joints, and severe pain occurs, especially at night. The illness is called Lie Jie Feng (Wind through the joints, or severe and migratory arthralgia)'.

The pain was in the ring finger, which relates to the Triple Burner channel. The selection of the Shu-Stream and Luo-Connecting points of the channel cured the disorder quickly.

> Chen Keqin, SHENXI TRADITIONAL CHINESE MEDICINE INSTITUTE
> *(see Shenxi Modern Medicine, Issue 6, 1977)*

CASE 2

Sun, female, age 19, worker

Case registered: January 1982

History: The patient had had paroxysmal pains in the soles of her feet for 3 months. The pain was worse at night, and lasted 3–4 hours. 20 days previously she developed erythema on her toes and soles. These were red and tender, and gave her difficulty walking. She had a previous history of epilepsy.

She was treated at her local hospital with medication and point blocking therapy with 0.25% procaine, with no effect. When she was referred here, the Department of Dermatology at this hospital diagnosed her condition as erythromelalgia and she was prescribed luminal (pheno-barbitone), Dolantin (pethidine), wintermin, ephedrine, indomethacin, phenergan (dromethazine), diazepam, aspirin, root of Tripterygium and Carbamazepinum, but without effect.

Diagnosis: Arthralgia.

Treatment: Remove Heat and Damp, expel Wind and activate the channels.

Principal Points: Taichong LIV 3, Xiaxi GB 43, Shangqiu SP 5 and Qiuxu GB 40.

The points were needled bilaterally, reduced with light twirling and the needles retained for 15 minutes. By the 3rd day the heat and pain had improved.

Secondary Points: Fengfu Du 16.

This point was added to the prescription and reduced with lifting, thrusting and twirling manipulation. The needle was also retained for 15 minutes. On the 5th day the patient returned for her third treatment to report that she no longer had any severe pain, and that the red spots were less noticeable. Treatment was given once every 3 days. After 10 sessions all her symptoms had cleared. The case was followed up a year later and there was no relapse.

Chen Weicang, ACUPUNCTURE AND MOXIBUSTION SECTION, RUIJIN HOSPITAL, SHANGHAI NO. 2 COLLEGE,
(see Journal of Chinese Medicine, Issue 6, 1985)

CASE 3

Liu, male, 19, student

Case registered: 8 April 1984

History: For the last 2 weeks the patient had tingling, numbness and pain in his feet and was unable to walk. He had been in the habit of staying up late in a cold room to study. The disease had started some time before with tingling and numbness in his feet, which improved after exercise. He was not particularly concerned about this and had not considered it worth seeking medical advice. After a while he developed paroxysmal tingling pain in his feet, and his toes and soles would go red. An attack would last about 20 minutes and would only be eased by dipping them in cold water. He was prescribed piminodine, indomethacin and short-wave electrotherapy, but with no effect. He then came for acupuncture.

Examination: Temperature normal. Muscle power in the legs normal. Knee reflex normal, no pathological reflex. Scattered congestive erythema on the toes and feet, with obvious tenderness on palpation. *Blood test:* ESR 2 mm in 1 hour, O – antibody less than 300 units. Rheumatoid factor negative. WBC and differentiation normal. X-rays of the feet revealed no abnormality.

Diagnosis: Erythromelalgia.

Principal Points: Xingjian LIV 2 (bilateral), Xiaxi GB 43 (bilateral) and Baihui Du 20.

The points were reduced with 'Dragon and Tiger come to Blows' method. Then continuous wave electro-acupuncture was given for 20 minutes with a G6805 unit. The patient felt comfortable during the treatment, with a feeling of coolness in his feet, and was asleep by the end. When the needles were removed the pain had improved. Treatment was given daily for 4 days, and the condition was cured. The patient was able to walk several miles to college every day without relapse.

Explanation: The diagnosis of this disease was clear from the pain and erythema, but the cause is not yet clear and there is no sure cure. It is possible it arose from Cold and poor diet. The red spots receded when pressed, indicating congestion. This was due to excessive dilation of the capillaries, which meant that the congestion and pain would have been aggravated by the application of a poultice. Instead, the needle manipulation 'Dragon and Tiger Come to Blows' was used to reduce the points, adjusting Ying-Nutritive and Wei-Defensive Qi, dredging the channel Qi and promoting capillary contraction.

Qian Jifeng, ZHENJIANG MUNICIPAL MENTAL HOSPITAL, JIANGSU PROVINCE
(see Jiangsu Journal of Traditional Chinese Medicine, Issue 8, 1985)

59. Raynaud's disease

History: 2 years previously the patient noticed that the skin on his hands and feet would sometimes turn pale. After a while they would change to a dark red colour, and go numb. He began to get stomach ache, pass loose stools and he lost his appetite. The symptoms worsened and he went to a hospital in Shanghai, where his condition was diagnosed as Raynaud's disease. He did not respond to treatment there, so he turned to acupuncture and moxibustion.

Examination: The patient was thin. The skin on his hands and feet was pale. *Tongue body:* pale. *Pulse:* thin and slow.

Diagnosis: Deficiency of Spleen and Kidney Yang.

Treatment: Reinforce the Spleen and Kidney, regulate Qi and Blood.

Principal Points:
1. Hegu L.I. 4, Baxie (Extra), Shousanli L.I. 10, Waiguan TB 5; Bafeng (Extra), Sanyinjiao SP 6, Zusanli ST 36, Juegu GB 39.
2. Zhongwan Ren 12, Guanyuan Ren 4, Pishu BL 20, Shenshu BL 23.

Treatment was given once every other day, alternating the two prescriptions. A course consisted of 30 sessions. The needles were heated with moxa.

Secondary Points:
1. Dazhui Du 14, Zhiyang Du 9, Mingmen Du 4, Shangwan Ren 13, Zhongwan Ren 12.
2. Zusanli ST 36, Geshu BL 17, Pishu BL 20, Weishu BL 21, Shenshu BL 23.

After two courses of acupuncture and moxibustion, treatment was reduced to moxibustion alone, using 7–9 cones directly on the skin without blistering or scarring. One point was selected from each group during a session. Treatment continued for about 3 years and the disorder was largely cured. The case has been followed up and there has been no relapse to date.

> Case treated by Zhu Rugong et al, case history by Ju Xianshui and Lu Yanyao, SHANGHAI TCM COLLEGE
> *(see Shanghai Journal of Traditional Chinese Medicine, Issue 3, 1980)*

Editor's Note: The signs and symptoms pointed to Deficiency of Spleen and Kidney Yang. When the Kidney is Deficient it cannot transport Water. Invasion of the channels and collaterals by external pathogens caused Stagnation of Qi and Blood, leading to this disease. Thus treatment aims were to disperse Cold, activate the circulation of Blood and invigorate the collaterals. The moxibustion enhanced the effect of the acupuncture. The points selected for acupuncture activate Qi and Blood and invigorate the collaterals. Once this was achieved, the points selected for moxibustion , mainly on Du Mai, Ren Mai, the Spleen and Kidney channels and the Back-Shu points, coordinated Qi and Blood to effect a cure.

60. Rheumatoid arthritis

Zhu, female, age 34, worker

Case registered: 16 January 1985

History: The patient had had symmetrical pain in the joints of all her limbs for more than 4 years, especially in the knees and shoulders. Her joints were stiff in the mornings, and her movement was impaired. The pain was worse for cold. All her joints were tender when pressed. She had been taking 750 mg of DXM per day for 3½ years.

Examination: Blood test: rheumatoid factor positive, ESR 26mm. in 1 hour. Mucin 6.2 mg%. Immunoglobulins: IgG 12g/l (1200 mg%), IgA 2.1g/l

(210 mg%) and IgM 1.8 mg/l (180 mg%). The patient's knees were swollen and she had marked tenderness of the shoulders, restricted movement, and pain and swelling in the wrist, ankle and finger joints. *Tongue coating:* thin and white. *Pulse:* weak and floating.

Diagnosis: Cold Damp Bi syndrome.

Treatment: Strengthen the body's resistance whilst treating localized disease, expel pathogens and invigorate Stagnation of Blood.

Principal Points: Dazhui Du 14, Shendao Du 11, Shenzhu Du 12, Zhiyang Du 9, Jinsuo Du 8, Pishu BL 20, Shenshu BL 23, Xiaochangshu BL 27, Weizhong BL 40, Yanglingquan GB 34, Zusanli ST 36, Taixi KID 3, Qiuxu GB 40, Shangqiu SP 5.

Secondary Points: Tianzong SI 11 was added when the upper limb was affected, and Zhibian BL 54 when the lower limb was affected. Ashi points were used locally. Sifeng (Extras).

The principal points were needled superficially and reinforced with gentle twirling. The Ashi points were needled with relaxing needling method, trigger method, articular method and bleeding method, as outlined in the *Ling Shu* (*Miraculous Pivot*). The joints were moved passively at the same time.

The swellings at the wrist, ankle and knees, i.e. where the collateral branches of the main channels were stagnant, were bled with a triangular needle and then cupped.

When the patient had difficulty flexing and extending her fingers they were pricked at the Sifeng point with a triangular needle and a little mucus was squeezed out.

Auricular Therapy: Auricular points corresponding to the affected areas.

Two or three points were selected at a time. Each point was located by probing for a tender spot, then a vacarria seed (Wang Bu Liu Xing) was taped tightly in place.

This therapy was given twice a week for 5 weeks, with a 2-week rest between courses. The patient was given a general examination every 6 months or year. After one course of treatment her symptoms were much improved, and she had halved her dose of DXM. During the first break between courses tests showed: rheumatoid factor negative, ESR 18 mm in 1 hour, mucin 2.5 mg%, Immunoglobulins: IgG 1g/l (100 mg%). The case was followed up for another year and her condition remained steady and blood tests were normal.

Explanation: In TCM rheumatoid arthritis is classified as Bi syndrome. It starts from Deficiency of Nutritive and Defensive Qi, which allow penetration of Wind, Cold and Damp into the body. These pathogens stagnate the Defensive Qi, resulting in Stagnation of Qi and Blood, which eventually leads to Bi syndrome.

The treatment aims were to strengthen the body's resistance whilst treating the localized disease, and this approach gave good results. Clinical experience has shown that patients on steroids are able to come off them gradually and remain stable, indicating that acupuncture is able to regulate the immune system.

Bleeding and cupping local points and squeezing out a little mucus at the Sifeng (Extra) points promotes the circulation of Blood by removing Blood Stasis and alleviates local inflammation.

> Case treated by Xi Yongjiang, case study by Pu Yunxing and Xi Depei, ACUPUNCTURE AND MOXIBUSTION SECTION, SHANGHAI TCM COLLEGE HOSPITAL, YUEYANG
> (see Correspondence, Journal of Acupuncture and Moxibustion, Issue 1, 1987)

61. Lupus erythematosus, systemic

CASE 1

Han, female, age 37

History: The patient had low-grade fever and fatigue for 4 years. Her limbs were painful for 2 years, and worse over the last 4 months. She had symmetrical erythema in the face. She was admitted to the Dermatology Section of this hospital with 'lupus sebaceous' on 29 January 1985. Her limbs were very painful, especially at the knees and at night. Her cheeks were dark, with bright red capillaries. She experienced photosensitivity and Raynaud's syndrome. Urine protein (+++). Alopecia.

She was given prednisolone (40 mg per day), Dicentrinum (3 tablets per day) and intramuscular injections of diazepam to help her sleep through the pain (10 mg per day). More prednisolone or AP-237 was administered between 12.00 and 2.00 a.m. in an attempt to give her 2–4 extra hours sleep. After a month it was decided to try acupuncture and moxibustion as a temporary measure to ease the pain in the knees.

Examination: The patient's complexion was dark, and she was very thin. She was clearly in pain and restless, lying curled up in fetal position. *Tongue body:* dark red. *Tongue coating:* white and greasy. *Pulse:* slippery, and weak in the chi position.

Diagnosis: Severe Wind Bi syndrome.

Treatment: Activate Qi and Blood, strengthen body resistance to stop pain.

Principal Points: Xuehai SP 10, Liangqiu ST 34, Xiyan (Extra, medial and lateral), all bilaterally.

The day after this treatment there were no outbreaks of pain in the night and the patient slept well without sedatives or painkillers. Unfortunately continued acupuncture treatment of this patient was not requested. The pain recurred 3 days later, so the prescription was now repeated, with the addition of Open Hourly Point therapy (Zi Wu Liu Zhu).

Supplementary Points: Waiguan TB 5, Zulinqi GB 41, Zusanli ST 36.

Waiguan TB 5 and Zulinqi GB 41 were opened. 10 daily treatments were administered, with the addition of Zusanli ST 36 for the last five. No more sedatives were required by this stage as the patient was sleeping peacefully and no longer in pain. Her spirits and appetite improved, she began to put on weight and the colour returned to her face.

Secondary Points: Qihaishu BL 24, Guanyuanshu BL 26, Shenshu BL 23, Weizhong BL 40.

Acupuncture and moxibustion were given at these points to readjust Qi and Blood and the channels and collaterals of the whole body. Five treatments were given over a 10 day period. The patient's dosage of steroids was reduced, and when she was discharged some months later she was only on a maintenance dose.

Explanation: In this case the treatment principle was 'In emergencies treat the symptoms'. Initially local points were chosen, and the relapse occurred because acupuncture therapy was withdrawn. Waiguan TB 5 and Zulinqi GB 41 were chosen because the pain was most severe at night (Branch 1). This relieved the pain which did not occur again. Zusanli ST 36 was added to strengthen the body resistance and reinforce the Stomach. The effects were thus consolidated. The remaining five treatments were to regulate the whole body by activating Qi and Blood, and the channels and collaterals.

> Liang Yiqiang, ACUPUNCTURE AND MOXIBUSTION SECTION, BEIJING SINO-JAPANESE FRIENDSHIP HOSPITAL

CASE 2, CEREBRAL

Yu, male, age 31

Case registered: 3 May 1983

History: The patient had had lupus erythematosus for more than 2 years. He often suffered fevers with migratory arthralgia and red spots, which would appear one after the other. This was originally diagnosed as rheumatoid arthritis, and he was prescribed various drugs, including indomethacin, which did not help. Later he developed pain in the liver area, with urine containing albumen and red and white blood cells. This was diagnosed as chronic hepatitis and nephritis, and standard treatments were given. It was not until this spring that his doctors became alarmed at butterfly shaped spots on his face. Lupus cells were found in his blood and he was hospitalized on 20 March . His symptoms responded to treatment until 30 April, when his condition suddenly deteriorated. He developed a severe headache, with vomiting and diarrhoea, then went into spasm, later becoming rigid and comatose.

Socket pressing reaction disappeared. Pupils not equal. Diminished reaction to light. *Temperature:* 39°–40°C. *BP:* 20.0–22.7/12.0–14.7 kPa (150–170/90–110 mmHg). *WBC:* 13.8×10^9/l (13.8×10^3/mm³), neutrophils 89%. Urinary protein (+++), urinary red blood cell (++++), urinary white blood cell (++). Creatinine 353.6 mmol/l (sic). Urea nitrogen 20.8 micromol (sic). CO_2 combining power 29.12 mmol/l. Albumin 60g/l. Globulin 35g/l. Thymol turbidity test 14 units. Zinc sulphate turbidity test 18 units. Hepatic ultrasound: turning dense, dense, minute, low and small, medium small, dentate. Ascites 1.5m. Spleen negative. Rales could be heard all over both lungs.

The disease was diagnosed as cerebral lesion caused by lupus erythmatosus, cerebral hernia, hypertension, metabolic acidosis, severe destruction of liver and kidney functions with secondary lung infection. Emergency treatment was given for 4 days with mannitol, DXM, furosemide (frusemide), lobeline, Cormelaine (dilazap), sodium bicarbonate, phenytoin sodium, gentamicin, penicillin, chloramphenicol, reserpine, Xing Nao Jing (Brain Refresher), San Shen Zhen (adrenaline, noradrenaline, isoprenaline), as well as fluid infusion and oxygen. The patient did not regain consciousness, and was referred for acupuncture and moxibustion.

Examination I (3 May): The patient was comatose. His face was flushed and dotted with erythema and his eyes were filled with exudate. Phlegm could be heard in his throat. *Tongue body:* dark red with prickles. *Tongue coating:* thick, yellow and dry. *Pulse:* wiry, slippery and rapid.

Diagnosis: Wind Phlegm Heat.

Treatment: Resolve Phlegm, calm Wind, purge Heat and resuscitate the Mind.

Principal Points: Renzhong Du 26, Fengchi GB 20, Fengfu Du 16, Fenglong ST 40, Shixuan (Extras).

All the points were reduced, except the Shixuan (Extras), which were bled. When Renzhong Du 26 was needled the patient flinched. By the time the Shixuan (Extras) were bled he had opened his eyes and looked around, and was even able to move his hands and feet when asked. His family were watching and were overjoyed.

Explanation: The Du Mai goes through the brain, so needling Renzhong Du 26 resuscitates the Mind. Fengchi GB 20 and Fengfu Du 16 purge Wind Fire. Reducing Fenglong ST 40 resolves Phlegm and removes the Turbid. Bleeding the Shixuan (Extras) removes Heat toxins in the Ying stage.

This treatment was given once a day for 3 days.

Examination II (6 May): The patient reacted to his name and could open his mouth and put out his tongue. There were some signs of his spirits improving. He was still unable to speak, however, and did not seem very aware. There were still red stripes on his face. *Tongue body:* dark red. *Tongue coating:* dark and dry. *Pulse:* slippery and rapid.

Diagnosis: The Wind Phlegm Heat was still Exuberant, and his recovery was only tentative.

Treatment: Purge Fire and resolve Phlegm to refresh the Mind. Clear Heat in the collaterals to prevent Heat Toxins from transforming into Dryness and impairing the Body Fluids.

Principal Points: Renzhong Du 26, Fengchi GB 20, Fengfu Du 16, Erjian L.I. 2, Daling P 7, Fenglong ST 40, Lidui ST 45, Shixuan (Extras).

All the points were reduced, except the Shixuan (Extras), which were bled.

Explanation: Erjian L.I. 2, the Yong-Spring point, and Lidui ST 45, the Jing-Well point, are used together to clear the Yang Ming channels and remove Heat toxins. Daling P 7, the Yuan-Source point, refreshes the Mind and cools the Blood.

Examination III (7 May): The patient's condition improved after this treatment. He was more aware and could sometimes answer questions, but he was constipated. *Tongue coating:* dry stripes. *Pulse:* rapid, wiry and thin.

Diagnosis: Exuberant Yang consuming the Yin fluids.

Treatment: Purge Heat to preserve Yin.

Principal Points: Fujie SP 14, Erjian L.I. 2, Fengchi GB 20, Fengfu Du 16, Daling P 7, Fenglong ST 40, Lidui ST 45, Fuliu KID 7.

All the points were reduced except Fuliu KID 7, which was reinforced.

Explanation: It was important to waste no time and put Zhang Zhongjing's principle of 'Purge quickly to preserve Yin' into practice. Fujie SP 14 activates the Qi of the Fu and promotes intestinal peristalsis. When reduced it is effective for cases where Pathogenic Heat has impaired the Yin. Fuliu KID 7 is both the Jing-River point and the Mother (tonification) point of the Kidney channel, and nourishes Kidney Yin when reinforced.

Examination IV (8 May): The next day the patient passed some dry stools. After this he seemed in better spirits, and wanted to drink more. He could only speak a little, but was articulate and able to move his limbs.

Treatment: Clear Heat, resolve Phlegm, nourish Yin fluids.

Principal Points: Erjian L.I. 2, Fengchi GB 20, Daling P 7, Fenglong ST 40, Lidui ST 45, Fuliu KID 7.
  All the points were reduced except Fuliu KID 7, which was reinforced.

Examination V (10 May): The patient's appetite returned and he asked for food. He was still weak. *Tongue body:* red and dry. *Tongue coating:* striped. *Pulse:* thin and weak.

Diagnosis: Deficiency of Qi and Yin after severe disease.

Treatment: Nourish and readjust Qi and Yin.

Principal Points: Guanyuan Ren 4, Zusanli ST 36, Taixi KID 3.

Explanation: Guanyuan Ren 4 reinforces the Vital Qi of the Kidney. Zusanli ST 36 supports the Qi of the Stomach. Taixi KID 3, the Yuan-Source point, nourishes Yin fluids.

Examination VI (13 May): The patient was becoming thinner, and hiccupped frequently. Although the pathogens had been removed, the Spleen and Stomach Qi was impaired and deficient. *Tongue body:* pale red and dry. *Tongue coating:* patchy. *Pulse:* thin and weak.

Diagnosis: Weakness and Deficiency of the Shao Yin and Tai Yin channels. Irregularity of the Middle and Lower Burners, which fail to raise Qi and descend Qi.

Treatment: Nourish the Spleen and Stomach to reinforce the Qi of the Middle Burner.

Principal Points: Guanyuan Ren 4, Zusanli ST 36, Taixi KID 3, Zhongwan Ren 12, Gongsun SP 4.
  All the points were reinforced.

Explanation: Stomach Qi is generated in the Stomach, but it has its root in the Kidney. Zusanli ST 36, Zhongwan Ren 12 and Gongsun SP 4 regulate the Spleen and Stomach and reinforce the Qi of the Middle

Burner. At the same time Taixi KID 3 and Guanyuan Ren 4 were used to strengthen Kidney Qi so it could receive the Qi of the Middle Burner.

Examination VII (15 May): The patient's appetite was better and he hiccupped less frequently, but he now felt a sensation of fullness in the abdomen.

Principal Points: Guanyuan Ren 4, Fuliu KID 7, Gongsun SP 4, Zusanli ST 36, Jianli Ren 11, Futonggu KID 20.
All the points were reinforced.

Explanation: In accordance with the principle of 'reinforcing the Mother point when the related organ is deficient', Fuliu KID 7 was substituted for Taixi KID 3 in the previous prescription. Zusanli ST 36 and Jianli Ren 11 used together reinforce the Qi of the Middle Burner. Gongsun SP 4 opens into Chong Mai, and Futonggu KID 20 is the place of origin for the Qi of Chong Mai. Used together these two points suppress Rebellious Qi in Chong Mai.

Examination VIII (18 May): The Rebellious Qi in Chong Mai was suppressed and the patient no longer hiccupped, but the sensation of fullness in the abdomen remained and was aggravated by eating. *Tongue body:* pale. *Tongue coating:* patchy. *Pulse:* thin and weak.

Treatment: Support and activate the Spleen (Earth), reinforcing the Qi of the Middle Burner to promote astringency.

Principal Points: Pishu BL 20, Taibai SP 3, Zusanli ST 36, Guanyuan Ren 4, Jianli Ren 11.

Explanation: This approach is known as 'treating obstructive disease by tonification'. The first three points reinforce and activate the digestion, and the last two consolidate Qi to promote astringency.

Examination IX (21 May): The patient's abdominal fullness was relieved and his appetite improved further. He looked better and was getting stronger.

Treatment: Continue to reinforce Spleen and Stomach and nourish Kidney Qi.

Principal Points: Zhongwan Ren 12, Qihai Ren 6, Zusanli ST 36 Taibai SP 3.
After a week of this treatment all his symptoms were relieved and the disease was cured.

Sun Jishan, SHANGHAI MUNICIPAL INSTITUTE OF ACUPUNCTURE, MOXIBUSTION, CHANNELS AND COLLATERALS
(see Shanghai Journal of Acupuncture and Moxibustion, Issue 3, 1983)

Editor's Note: This was a very serious and difficult case. The doctor's first approach was to remove Phlegm, calm Wind, purge Heat and resuscitate the Mind. Once the patient regained consciousness he shifted the focus of treatment to remove Phlegm, open the clear orifices and clear Heat in the collaterals. When the patient was fully conscious and able to speak, treatment was changed immediately to purgation to protect Yin. When the Qi of the Fu organs was activated and the patient's spirits had improved, treatment was modified to support Prenatal and Postnatal Qi, nourishing the Kidney at the same time to consolidate the result. Correct differentiation of the disease and accurate and skilful selection of points turned the tide and brought final success.

CASE 3

Zhao, female, age 28, school teacher

Case registered: July 1970

History: The patient had suffered from systemic lupus erythematosus since 1964. She had been treated for 5 years, but her symptoms had got steadily worse. She presented here with symmetrical red facial erythema, oedema of the limbs and body, pain in the joints, the sides of the body and the liver area. Her lips were livid, and the whites of her eyes were red. She also had low fever and blurred vision.

Examination: Her face was as described above. There were also bilateral round tubercles at Shenshu BL 23 and Ganshu BL 18. Each tubercle was the size of a broad bean and tender on palpation. *Tongue body:* dark red with purple spots. *Pulse:* thin and wiry.

Diagnosis: Butterfly spots.

Principal Points: Danzhong Ren 17, Qihai Ren 6, Hegu L.I. 4 (bilateral), Taichong LIV 3 (bilateral), Zhangmen LIV 13 (bilateral), Neiguan P 6 (bilateral), Yintang (Extra, bilateral).
  The points were needled with reinforcing and reducing evenly method, and the needles were retained for 30 minutes. Treatment was given once every other day.

Point Injection: Ganshu BL 18, Pangguangshu BL 28, Xuehai SP 10, Sanyinjiao SP 6, and the related Back-Shu points.
  A solution of Hong Hua and Dang Gui was prepared (*Flos carthami* and *Radix angelicae sinensis*). The syringe was inserted and manipulated with birdpecking method until there was sensation, then 0.3–0.5 ml of the solution was injected into the point.

Point injection therapy was given once every other day, alternating with the moxibustion. The patient was advised to cut down on her intake of hormones.

After 3 months the erythema on her face and body began to recede. The pain in her joints and liver area improved. The whole condition was clearly under control and her spirits improved.

Secondary Points: Yingxiang L.I. 20, Tai Yang (Extra), Fuliu KID 7.

These points were added to the previous prescription. The patient was advised to stop her hormones completely and to take up Tai Chi. After continuous treatment for a further year and a half, the erythema was gone, her period started again and she gained 3 kg in weight. All her tests proved normal. She gave birth to a baby boy a year later. The case has been followed up for many years, and there has been no relapse. She has been in full-time employment.

Explanation: This is an autoimmune disease. It can be divided into two types: discoid and systemic. The causes of the disease are not yet clear. The symptoms are similar to what is called 'red butterfly', 'solar dermatitis' and 'ghost face' in TCM, and can be differentiated in the same way as Bi syndrome.

The disease is located in the channels and collaterals, and is mostly related to the Ren, Du, Bladder and Stomach channels. Treating the Front-Mu and Back-Shu points readjusts Yin and Yang. The tubercles are usually found on the back on the Bladder channel, and the erythema is usually on the face around Chengqi ST 1 and Sibai ST 2. In this case tender tubercles were found on the back. They may have been due to Stagnation of Qi and Blood. Injection of medication at these points softens and may eventually cure them. As the tubercles improve the other symptoms will also improve. The best results are achieved with the combination of moxibustion, point injection therapy and exercise.

Chang Mingqi, DONGDAJIE HOSPITAL, XI'AN
(see Shenxi Traditional Chinese Medicine, Issue 2, 1987)

62. Lupus erythematosus, discoid

Fang, female, age 30

Case registered: 30 May 1974

History: The patient had red patches on both cheeks level with the bridge of the nose. She did not feel the symptoms were severe, and came for acupuncture and moxibustion.

Examination: The patches resembled frostbite. On each patch there were inflammatory papules, with scaling and symmetrically distributed pigmentation.

Diagnosis: Butterfly spots.

Auricular Points: Ear, Lung, Cheek, Adrenal, Endocrine.

Treatment was given once every other day. The needles were retained for 30 minutes. After 12 treatments the margins of the areas of pigmentation showed improvement. The inflammatory papules shrank and became flat, and the scaling disappeared. After 30 treatments the skin rash was mostly resorbed.

The patient also had gynaecological problems. When probed Uterus, Pelvic Cavity and Tip of Tragus points were very tender, so these were added to the prescription. After 40 sessions the skin lesions were completely resorbed, and the papules were reduced to areas of slight pigmentation. Her gynaecological disease had also greatly improved. The patient was re-examined 10 years later in April 1984: her skin was completely normal and there were no traces whatsoever of the disease.

Explanation: Auricular therapy is effective for discoid lupus erythematosus. The author of this article has treated 10 cases successfully with this method. It is important for the patient to have faith in the doctor, so that treatment is not cut short or irregular.

If the patient has marked itching it will generally be relieved by 2–5 treatments. On the other hand if the patient has little or no itching, the first treatment might aggravate it, and the itching might not be relieved until the skin lesions were healed.

The healing process can be divided into several stages. At first the lesions become less red, and are less prominent. Then the lesions begin to be absorbed, and there is less and less scaling. Finally the lesions disappear, leaving behind only a few areas of pigmentation. Continued treatment can lighten this pigmentation or even cure it altogether. Moreover, auricular therapy treats the whole body, so other systemic symptoms such as poor appetite or sleep may also improve. This in turn will promote the healing of the lesions.

Chen Yusheng and Hu Xiu'e, DERMATOLOGY DEPARTMENT, XI'AN
MEDICAL COLLEGE HOSPITAL NO. 2
(see Journal of Traditional Chinese Medicine, Issue 12, 1984)

63. Prepatellar bursitis

Sun, male, age 24, member of staff

History: 3 months previously the patient had developed pain and swelling in his right knee, accompanied by feelings of heaviness. He had no recollection of any previous injury. It was diagnosed as prepatellar bursitis and he was treated with herbs and acupuncture but without success. He then came here for treatment.

Examination: The knee was swollen and painful, and felt heavy. The problem was worse in damp weather. The upper left margin of the patella was tender on palpation. Floating patella test positive. Body temperature 36.2°C.

Diagnosis: Damp Bi syndrome.

Treatment: Warm the channels and disperse Cold, remove Damp and dredge the collaterals.

Principal Points: Liangqiu ST 34, Yanglingquan GB 34 through to Yinlingquan SP 9, Zusanli ST 36, Sanyinjiao SP 6.

Treatment was given for a month without any improvement in the condition. Then the same prescription was given with the addition of moxibustion on the ends of the needles. Reinforcing and reducing evenly method was used. The needles were removed when the moxa was completely burned. Treatment was given daily. After the first session there was a noticeable improvement in the pain and swelling. After the third all the symptoms had gone and the patient was discharged as cured. The case was followed up a year later: there had been no relapse and the patient was able to do some light work.

Explanation: This problem had lasted for months and had failed to respond to herbal medicine and acupuncture. The patient had been exposed to Cold and Damp pathogens. Cold is a Yin pathogen which impairs the Yang. When the Yang is Deficient for a long time, diseases of Cold and Stagnation will arise. The *Nei Jing* says, 'Qi and Blood prefer warmth and abhor cold. If it is cold then Qi and Blood will stop flowing; when it is warm Qi and Blood flow and the disease is removed'. In this case warm needle therapy was used to obtain a cure.

Han Youdong, ACUPUNCTURE AND MOXIBUSTION SECTION, SHANDONG TCM COLLEGE HOSPITAL

64. Chondromalacia patellae

Wang, female, age 49

Case registered: December 1982

History: In 1973 the patient had dislocated her left patella in an accident, and X-rays confirmed a diagnosis of chondromalacia patellae. She had had pain in her left knee for 9 years, and severe pain in both knees over the last 3 months. The pain in her left knee was there all the time, and if she lifted anything heavy the right one became painful.

Examination: Both knees were swollen: the circumference at the midpoint of the patella was 41.5 cm on the left knee and 43 cm on the right knee. Movement was restricted, with crepitus. Floating patella test positive.

Diagnosis: Damp Bi syndrome.

Principal Points: Heding (Extra), Xiyan (Extra), Renying ST 9, Yinmen BL 37, Sidu TB 9.

All the points were needled bilaterally, using warming and invigorating manipulation. After 21 treatments there were noticeable improvements in the swelling and pain. Floating patella test was now negative. Functional movement of the knee was normal. The knees now measured 38 cm on the left and 37 cm on the right.

> Guo Xiaozong, XUE LIGONG ET AL, ACUPUNCTURE AND MOXIBUSTION INSTITUTE, CHINA ACADEMY OF TCM
> *(see Correspondence, Journal of Acupuncture and Moxibustion, Issue 1, 1987)*

65. Tumour of the knee

Qu, male, age 50, peasant

Case registered: Autumn 1975

History: 1 year previously the patient started to feel pain in his right knee after a period of overwork. It became red, swollen and painful and his movement was restricted. He was hospitalized for 4 months but things got worse until finally he was unable to move. The disease was diagnosed as 'malignant bone tumour', and his doctors recommended amputation. The patient and his family did not accept this, and brought him home where he could be treated with acupuncture and moxibustion.

Examination: The patient had severe pain in his right knee, especially at night, fever all over, thirst, dry stool and reddish urine.

He looked emaciated and depressed. The circumference of his right knee was 1.5 times larger than the left, and his thigh and lower leg were noticeably thinner. His knee was very bright and shiny like the skin of an eggplant, and was hot and very tender on pressure. *Tongue body:* dark red. *Tongue coating:* yellow and greasy. *Pulse:* rapid and slippery.

Diagnosis: Wind Cold and Damp transforming to Heat.

Treatment: Remove Damp Heat, resolve obstruction, activate Blood and collaterals and relieve pain.

Principal Points: Liangqiu ST 34, Xuehai SP 10, Zusanli ST 36, Yinlingquan SP 9, Kunlun BL 60, Xixia (Extra).

The points were reduced and the needles retained for 30 minutes. A course consisted of 10 daily treatments, and a 3-day interval was allowed between courses. After the first course the patient reported that the pain was better and his sleep had improved. After the fourth course the swelling subsided and he was able to walk with a stick, although it was painful. There was oedema below the knee and ankle, which were signs of Qi and Blood beginning to circulate freely. After six courses all his symptoms had gone and the disease was cured. The patient was recommended functional exercises. The case was followed up for 7 years and there was no relapse.

Explanation: In TCM the joints of the body are said to be in charge of movement. They can be impaired by overwork and External Pathogens. The knee joint in particular carries a great load and is one of the joints most easily affected by exposure to Wind, Cold and Damp. In clinic, most cases of joint pain are caused by these pathogens or by overwork, and acupuncture and moxibustion are especially effective in these cases.

In this case Western doctors had diagnosed the disease as a malignant bone tumour, and had been unable to help. The analysis of the disease process in TCM is very different:

The problem had lasted for a year. The redness, swelling, heat, pain and restricted movement in the knee were caused by overwork which impaired the body's resistance. This resulted in Deficiency of the Qi and channels which left the body open to invasion by External Pathogens. Wind, Cold and Damp battled at the knee joint and transformed into Stasis and Heat. When Heat and Damp stagnate in the joint, the Blood and collaterals are obstructed. When Heat is Exuberant it forms swellings, and when there is obstruction there is pain. The treatment principle is to clear and activate.

Points on the Stomach and Spleen channels were selected to remove Heat and Damp. If the pathogen has a way out and Qi can circulate through the channels, the Stasis and obstruction will resolve spontaneously. Liangqiu ST 34, Xuehai SP 10, Zusanli ST 36, Yinlingquan SP 9 and Xixia (Extra) are all local points to dredge the obstruction of Qi and Blood in the channels and collaterals and activate the circulation of Blood. Yinlingquan SP 9 removes Damp and strengthens the Spleen. Zusanli ST 36 clears Heat and is especially effective to nourish Qi. Using both together strengthens the body's resistance and expels pathogens. Xuehai

SP 10 activates the Blood and resolves Stasis. Liangqiu ST 34 activates Qi and removes Stasis. Kunlun BL 60 relaxes the tendons, activates Blood and eases the movements of the joints.

Xie Linyuan, WENDEN BONE SETTING HOSPITAL, SHANDONG PROVINCE

66. Prolapsed lumbar disc

CASE 1

Qin, male, age 31, cadre

History: The patient had had lumbar pain for 6 months, especially on the right. He was unable to stand straight. Movement in his right hip was impaired and as a result he had a lot of pain in his right leg and was unable to sit still for long. He had dull pain in his right knee and ankle. The severity of the pain prevented him from sleeping, and was aggravated by cold and damp. Treatment with Western and Chinese medication in the prefectural hospital had not helped. A provincial hospital advised surgery after X-ray examination revealed a prolapsed lumbar disc, but the patient was reluctant to take this option and decided to try acupuncture and moxibustion.

Examination: The patient was obviously in great pain and had difficulty walking. The lumbar vertebrae projected posteriorly. Straight leg raising test positive at 30°. *Tongue coating*: white. *Pulse:* deep and thin.

Diagnosis: Cold Bi syndrome.

Treatment: Reinforce the Kidney and waist, promote flow of Blood to relieve pain, expel pathogenic factor and relax the tendons.

Principal Points: Shenshu BL 23, Qihaishu BL 24, Zhibian BL 54, Huantiao GB 30, Yanglingquan GB 34, Feiyang BL 58.

Secondary Points: Juliao ST 3, Juegu GB 39, Zusanli St 36, Chengfu BL 36.
Treatment was given once every 2 days. The needles were manipulated with medium stimulation with reinforcing and reducing equally method and retained for 20–30 minutes, with manipulation every 10 minutes.

After the first two treatments there was some improvement in the level of pain, and the patient's mobility. After five treatments he could almost stand up straight. After 12 treatments he could walk unaided, and after 30 he had almost no pain. The straight leg raising test was negative, and the case was discharged as cured. The case was followed up for 2 years and there was no relapse.

Explanation: Lumbar disc prolapse is classified in TCM as arthralgia or Bi syndrome. The *Su Wen* says, 'Arthralgia is caused by the combination of Wind, Damp and Cold. If Wind is predominant the arthralgia migrates, if Cold is predominant the arthralgia is worse for cold, if Damp is predominant the arthralgia is worse for damp' (Bi Lun, *Familiar Conversations*, Arthralgia Syndrome chapter). The *Nei Jing* says, 'Arthralgia is aggravated by cold and relieved by warmth'. Zhang Jingyue of the Ming dynasty said, 'Arthralgia is caused by external pathogenic factors which cause Stasis of Qi and Blood'. According to these theories the disease is caused by obstruction of Qi and Blood resulting from invasion of the channels and collaterals by Wind, Cold or Damp.

From the signs and symptoms, this was a case of arthralgia aggravated by Cold. Shenshu BL 23 and Qihaishu BL 24 strengthen the waist, back and Kidney. If the Kidney Yang is sufficient and the flow of Qi and Blood is normal then the external pathogenic factor will be expelled. Zhibian BL 54, Huantiao GB 30, Yanglingquan GB 34 and Feiyang BL 58 relax the tendons and relieve pain by invigorating Blood and activating the channel. Regular treatment produced satisfactory results.

Sun Xianbao, ACUPUNCTURE AND MOXIBUSTION SECTION, JINAN TCM MUNICIPAL HOSPITAL, SHANDONG PROVINCE

CASE 2

Jiang, male, age 39, worker

Case registered: 3 June 1975

History: The patient had had a lumbar sprain 1 year ago. The pain was so severe he required local injections to block the sensations. It improved, but did not completely disappear, and was aggravated by fatigue. In the previous month he had tired himself out, and as a result had developed pain in his right hip which spread down his right leg. The outside of the leg also felt dull. The pain was more severe at night and disturbed his sleep, but was relieved if he bent his leg. He also noticed the muscles on the back of his right leg were slightly atrophied. He was treated with Western and Chinese medication, but without effect.

Examination: The patient was obviously in pain, leaning to the left and limping. He was tender on palpation on the right of vertebrae L3 and L4, and the sensation radiated down his right leg. Straight leg raising test positive on the right at 45°. Dorsal bending test positive. Heel–hip test positive. Ankle reflex absent on the right. Diminished sensation on the lateral side of the right leg and slight muscular atrophy. Diminished muscle power. X-rays showed narrowing between L3 and L4.

Diagnosis: Cold Bi syndrome.

Treatment: Reinforce the Kidney and waist, relax the tendons, promote the Blood circulation to relieve pain.

Principal Points: Siyao (Extra), Wuyao (Extra)[1], Ciliao BL 32, Zhibian BL 54, Chengfu BL 36, Yanglingquan GB 34, Tiaokou ST 38 through to Chengshan BL 57.

At Siyao (Extra) and Ciliao BL 32, 2.5–3 cun needles were inserted at 80°–90° angles to a depth of 1.5–2 cun, then manipulated with twirling method until electric shock sensations passed from the lumbar area to the foot. Electro-acupuncture was administered for 20–30 minutes, one pole at Zhibian BL 54, the other at Yanglingquan GB 34, using high frequency pulse current at a level tolerable to the patient. Treatment was given daily and a course lasted 6 days, with 1–3 days in between courses.

After 10 treatments the pain had improved dramatically, and the straight leg raising test on the right was now negative.

Secondary Points: Ciliao BL 32, Huantiao GB 30, Yinmen BL 37, Yanglingquan GB 34, Tiaokou ST 38 , Yangfu GB 38.

The points were needled on the affected side and stimulated with electro-acupuncture for 30 minutes, once a day. After another 12 treatments most of the symptoms had disappeared, but the sensations of dullness and heaviness in the right leg remained. To treat this, Dubi ST 35, Zusanli ST 36 and Fenglong ST 40 were selected on the right, retaining the needles for 20 minutes. This new prescription was given daily. After 5 days all the symptoms had gone and the patient was discharged. The case was followed up for a year and there was no relapse.

Explanation: Acupuncture and moxibustion are frequently used in TCM to treat pains in the leg and lumbar area and there are many different techniques. The *Zhen Jiu Da Cheng* (Great Compendium of Acupuncture and Moxibustion) recommends treatment with Huantiao GB 30, Fengshi GB 31, Yinshi ST 33, Weizhong BL 40, Chengshan BL 57 and Kunlun BL 60. The *Zhen Jiu Jia Yi Jing* (Rudiments of Acupuncture and Moxibustion Classic) recommends similar points for these symptoms, e.g. Ciliao BL 32 for cold and pain in the lumbar area and back, Chengfu BL 36 for pains in the waist, back, hip and thigh aggravated by cold, Yinmen BL 37 for lumbar pain from injury, Tiaokou ST 38 for leg pains and difficulty raising the leg, and Yanglingquan GB 34 for pains in the hip, leg and knee with dullness and spasm.

---

[1]Siyao and Wuyao are on the back, 2 cun lateral to the spinous processes of vertebrae L4 and L5, respectively.

In this case the two groups of points were selected from points recommended in the classics and those which in the author's experience have proved effective. Siyao (Extra) and Wuyao (Extra) were discovered by the author of this article. After many years of observation they have been found to relieve pain promptly, shorten the duration of treatment and consolidate its therapeutic effects. The key to using them is skilful manipulation of the needles, correct angle and depth of insertion. Qi sensation must be propagated from the lumbar area to the foot. Excessive needling of these two points may damage the nerve. If the needle scrapes the bone, it should be lifted and reinserted at a slightly different angle. Both points used together get better results. Electro-acupuncture is effective for mild cases and migratory pain. It is less effective for chronic cases.

When these two points are needled with strong sensations, the patient will feel a sudden tremor in the waist and affected limb. This tremor may realign the joints and increase the space between the vertebrae, repositioning the nucleus pulposus, or relieve the pressure of the disc on the nerve roots.

> Zhang Dengbu, ACUPUNCTURE AND MOXIBUSTION SECTION, SHANDONG TCM COLLEGE
> (*see Shandong Journal of Chinese Medicine, Issue 1, 1977*)

67. Pains in the buttock when coughing

Zhang, male, age 28, worker

Case registered: 15 December 1984

History: The patient had sprained his back when doing some heavy lifting 2 days previously. He had restricted movement when bending, stretching and turning at the waist. The pain in the lumbar area was worse when he coughed.

Examination: The pain was in the buttock area. There was no redness, swelling or marked tenderness. Tongue and pulse were normal.

Diagnosis: Localized Stagnation of Qi.

Treatment: Regulate Qi and remove Stagnation.

Principal Points: Yuji LU 10 (bilateral).

The points were reduced with lifting thrusting and twirling method. After 5 minutes the patient was asked to cough, and reported that he could feel no pain. The needles were retained for 20 minutes and manipulated at 5-minute intervals. The patient was asked to move his waist during the session. The treatment was repeated the next day and all the pain and symptoms disappeared.

Explanation: The only recorded use of Yuji LU 10 for pain in the buttocks when coughing is in the *Zhen Jiu Da Cheng* (Great Compendium of Acupuncture and Moxibustion) by Yang Jizhou of the Ming dynasty, but other books, both ancient and modern, make no mention of this. The author of this article has found the point to be very effective in cases of severe pain which is aggravated by coughing, when there is no localized redness, swelling or tenderness. It is important for the patient to move his waist during the treatment.

Xiao Xianggao, ACUPUNCTURE AND MOXIBUSTION SECTION OF MIANXIAN COUNTY TCM HOSPITAL, SHENXI PROVINCE
(see Shenxi Traditional Chinese Medicine, Issue 12, 1985)

68. Sequelae of infected Achilles tendon rupture

Gao, male, age 35, school teacher

Case registered: June 1984

History: A year previously the patient ruptured his Achilles tendon playing ball games. He was given an operation to restore the tendon but the ankle became infected, resulting in restricted movement.

Examination: The right ankle joint was stiff. There was swelling on both sides of the Achilles tendon and a 10 cm scar on the tendon. Dorsiflexion 15°. Plantar flexion about 15°. There was atrophy of tibialis anterior and soleus muscles. Grade 4 muscle power. No pathological reflex. *Tongue coating:* thin, with purpura on the sides. *Pulse:* thin and wiry.
Diagnosis: Stasis of Qi and Blood after injury.

Treatment: Regulate Ying-Nutritive Qi and Wei-Defensive Qi, nourish the muscles and tendons, increase mobility. Electro-acupuncture and standard acupuncture were alternated. Treatment was given every day.

Electro-acupuncture: Chengshan BL 57 (+), Kunlun BL 60 (–), Zusanli ST 36 (+), Jiexi ST 41 (–), Sanyinjiao SP 6 (+), Taixi KID 3 (–).
The points were needled on the right. After sensation was obtained the needles were twirled to reduce, then twirled to reinforce. After sensation had radiated from around the needles, current was applied for 10 minutes with a G6805 unit before the needles were removed.

Principal Points: Shenmai BL 62, Xuanzhong GB 39, Yanglingquan GB 34, Taichong LIV 3.

The points were needled on the right. Qi was propagated to the affected area and the needles were retained for 15 minutes.

Massage was given after acupuncture, and the patient was taught functional exercises. The injury was cured after 50 treatments and the patient was discharged.

Explanation: The *Su Wen* says, 'For flaccidity use the points of Yang Ming only' (Wei Syndrome chapter). The first prescription follows this principle. Zusanli ST 36, the He-Sea point, and Jiexi ST 41 regulate the Qi of the Middle Burner and the function of Ying-Nutritive and Wei-Defensive Qi. This treats the cause of the disorder. Chengshan BL 57 and Kunlun BL 60 remove the Stasis and promote new growth.

In the second prescription, Shenmai BL 62 is the place where the channel Qi of the Yang Heel is generated. The Yang and Yin Heel Vessels control healthy walking. Xuanzhong GB 39. the Hui-Converging point of Marrow and Yanglingquan GB 34, the Hui-Converging point of tendons, strengthen the tendons and the bone. Taichong LIV 3, the Yuan-Source point, also strengthens tendons. Good results were achieved by alternating the two prescriptions and supplementing the therapy with massage and functional exercises.

Yang Yongnian, SHANGHAI RAILWAY BUREAU, QIANJIANG SANATORIUM
(see Shanghai Journal of Acupuncture and Moxibustion, Issue 3, 1986)

69. Pain in the sole of the foot

Sun, male, age 48

History: For the last week the patient had pain in the sole of his right foot. He had no history of injury.

Examination: The sole of the patient's right foot was red, swollen and very tender. *Tongue body:* red. *Tongue coating:* dry. *Pulse:* rapid.

Diagnosis: Deficiency of Kidney Yang and Damp.

Treatment: Raise sinking Yang.

Principal Point: Baihui Du 20.

The point was reduced. The needle was inserted against the flow of the channel, and manipulated with advancing and withdrawing technique (jin tui): the needle was first inserted 1.2–1.5 cun deep, then pulled out slowly in three stages. At each stage lifting and thrusting method to reduce was used. The needle was retained for 60 minutes, then the hole was enlarged with shaking technique when it was withdrawn.

After treatment the pain improved and the patient was able to stand up and walk. He returned the next day, however: the redness and swelling had gone but there was a 2 cm round lump under the 5th metatarsal, which was tender on palpation. The treatment was repeated and the lump disappeared by the next day. The case was followed up for 6 months and there was no relapse.

Explanation: The *Ling Shu* says, 'The Kidney channel originates from the tip of the fifth toe, and ascends at an angle through the middle of the sole to the navicular bone, the medial malleolus, the inside of the ankle to the heel, and continues along the inside of the lower leg up along the inside of the thigh'.

The author of this article believes that this disorder usually affects women after childbirth and people who are overweight. It is due to Deficiency of Kidney Yang. Of the channels which pass through the sole, only the Kidney channel goes through the whole sole. It is closely related to the Du Mai, the governor of all the Yang and the Sea of Yang. Du Mai leads from the sacrum and coccyx up along the spine to Luo Nao (around the brain). Externally Du Mai governs the Yang channels, and internally it connects the channel Qi of all the organs. Baihui Du 20 is the meeting point of Du Mai with the six Yang channels. It raises depressed Yang Qi, regulates and nourishes Kidney Qi, dredges the Triple Burner, strengthens the waist and knee and activates the Functional Qi.

Wang Jiyuan, SHANGU COAL MINE HOSPITAL, YANBEI PREFECTURE, SHANXI PROVINCE
(see Shanxi Traditional Chinese Medicine, Issue 2, 1986)

SWEATING DISORDERS

70. Profuse generalized sweating

CASE 1

Hao, female, age 50, worker

Case registered: 6 May 1980

History: 2 years previously the patient had been exposed to wind. She had sweated profusely ever since. Her current symptoms included flushing, continual sweating and feeling hot. This would happen 5–6 times a day, even in a cold room. She also felt faint, tired, weak and had palpitations.

Examination: The patient had a red face and was sweating all over. *Tongue body:* pale. *Tongue coating:* white. *Pulse:* weak and thin.

Diagnosis: Deficiency of Qi and Blood.

Treatment: Regulate and nourish Qi and Blood.

Principal Points: Tai Yang (Extra) (bilateral), Fengchi GB 20 (bilateral), Dazhui Du 14, Jiaji (Extra).
 Electro-acupuncture was given daily. Low frequency faradic current was applied to these points at the following voltages: 2V, 10V, 15V, and 15V respectively, for 30 seconds at each point. The patient's condition improved straight away, and she was cured after 10 treatments. Six more consolidating treatments were given. The case was followed up for 2 months and there was no relapse.

Explanation: Abnormal sweating is usually caused by Deficiency, for example spontaneous sweating from Deficient Yang and nightsweats from Deficient Yin. In this case the patient had been exposed to wind after working. Wind is a Yang pathogenic factor and its property is to make things open. When it lodges in the skin the pores open, causing the person to sweat. In this case both Yin and Yang were Deficient.
 Dazhui Du 14 is the meeting point of Du Mai with the six Yang channels, and treats Exterior syndromes. The Jiaji points activate the Yang. Fengchi GB 20 and Tai Yang (Extra) are important head points and meet with all the Yang channels; they are therefore used to activate Yang in the channels.

Miao Xiaowei and Zhang Shubin, ZHANGJIAKOU PROSPECTING MACHINES FACTORY HOSPITAL, MINISTRY OF GEOLOGY
(see Journal of Traditional Chinese Medicine, Issue 1 1981)

CASE 2

Shen, male, age 46, school teacher

Case registered: 15 June 1981

History: The patient had been in hospital with bronchitis and bronchiectasis for 50 days. His symptoms had improved after treatment with penicillin, streptomycin and kanamycin, but he now sweated profusely all over, especially on his forehead. Chinese herbs had not helped.

Examination: The patient was sweating profusely on his forehead and all over. The sweating was worse on exertion. His complexion was yellow and he looked fatigued. His voice was weak and quiet, he spoke little and was short of breath, with sensations of fullness in the chest. *Tongue body:* pale red and dry. *Pulse:* slow floating and weak on pressure.

Diagnosis: Deficient Qi and weak Defensive Qi.

Treatment: Reinforce Qi and Defensive Qi to stop sweating.

Principal Points: Hegu L.I. 4 (bilateral), Fuliu KID 7 (bilateral), Zusanli ST 36, Neiguan P 6.

Hegu L.I. 4 was reduced with gentle twirling, Fuliu KID 7 was gently reinforced. Zusanli ST 36 and Neiguan P 6 were also gently reinforced, and needled on alternating sides with each treatment. Treatment was given daily for 10 days. After the 3rd day the symptoms began to improve. After 10 days the patient was in good spirits and the profuse sweating had stopped.

Explanation: Both spontaneous sweating from Yang Deficiency and nightsweats from Yin Deficiency are symptoms of low body resistance. Treatment should regulate and reinforce Yin and Yang to tonify the weak body resistance. The *Ling Shu* says, 'When the five Zang are diseased, use the 12 Source points' (Jiu Zhen Shi Er Yuan, 9 Needlings and 12 Source Points chapter). Hegu L.I. 4, the Source point, directly reflects the condition of the Large Intestine and treats diseases of that organ. Fuliu KID 7 is the Jing-River point, where the Qi of the channel passes through. Reducing the former and reinforcing the latter activates the True Qi, benefits the circulation of all the Body Fluids and regulates and strengthens both the Exterior and the Interior. When Yin and Yang are harmonized and Water circulates evenly throughout the body, there will be normal perspiration.

Wang Kan, SHANDAN COUNTY TCM HOSPITAL, GANSU PROVINCE
(see Journal of Traditional Chinese Medicine, Issue 3, 1985)

71. Profuse sweating of the hands and feet

CASE 1

Ding, male, age 23, cadre

History: The patient had suffered from profuse sweating on the limbs for about 9 years, especially in the centre of his palms and soles, and on the tips of his fingers and toes. He was also short of breath and felt weak.

Examination: Tongue coating: thin and white. *Pulse:* wiry and thin.

Diagnosis: Spleen and Kidney Yang Deficiency, Deficiency of Defensive Qi.

Treatment: Nourish the Yang and strengthen Defensive Qi to reduce sweating.

Auricular Points: Lung, Kidney, Sympathetic, Endocrine.

Four treatments were given, but with little effect. Channel points were then selected.

Principal Points: Pishu BL 20, Shenshu BL 23, Zhigou TB 6, Hegu L.I. 4, Houxi SI 3.

The points were reinforced, and moxibustion added at Pishu BL 20 and Shenshu BL 23. The treatment was repeated nine times, and the condition was cured.

Explanation: The Spleen governs the four limbs and digestion. Deficiency of Spleen Yang causes weakness in the interstices of the skin leading to profuse sweating. If the Kidney Yang is weak the Defensive Qi will be weak.

Reinforcing technique followed by moxibustion at Pishu BL 20 and Shenshu BL 23 strengthens the Spleen and Kidney functions, and so strengthens Defensive Qi and builds Original Qi.

Reinforcing Zhigou TB 6, Hegu L.I. 4 and Houxi SI 3 regulates the three Yang channels and collaterals, and tightens the interstices to stop perspiration.

XIA LINGQING, YIXING COUNTY PEOPLE'S HOSPITAL, JIANGSU PROVINCE
(see Journal of Traditional Chinese Medicine, Issue 12, 1983)

CASE 2

Zhou, male, age 28, peasant

Case registered: 27 November 1980

History: 6 months previously the patient discovered a snake when working in the fields. He was very frightened and broke out in a sweat all over. Ever since he sweated profusely on his palms and soles, and this had got worse over the last month. The sweating was worse if he was anxious, and his arms would tremble. He had a dry mouth, was sleeping badly, his bowels were sluggish and he passed yellow urine.

For the last 2–3 months he had received diverse treatments. Western doctors diagnosed his condition as a functional disturbance of the autonomic nervous system and gave him oryzanol, vitamins and luminal (phenobarbitone). TCM doctors prescribed him Zhu Sha An Shen Wan (Sedative Bolus), Mu Li San (Oyster Shell Powder) and Bu Zhong Tang (Reinforce the Middle Burner Decoction), but none of these had helped.

Examination: The patient was well-built and healthy looking. His palms and soles were normal in colour, but were sweating profusely. If he closed his hands for a short while sweat would collect in his palm, and his shoes and socks were wet. He was also sweating on his forehead. *Tongue body:* red. *Tongue coating:* white and slightly moist. *Pulse:* deep and slightly rapid.

Diagnosis: Yin and Yang disharmony from shock.

Treatment: Regulate Yin and Yang, clear Heat to stop sweating.

Principal Points: Hegu L.I. 4, Fuliu KID 7, Neiguan P 6.

All the points were needled bilaterally. Fuliu KID 7 was reinforced, producing sensations of warmth, and the others were reduced, producing sensations of coolness. Treatment was given once a day. After 10 days there was a noticeable improvement in all his symptoms, and after another 15 sessions the disease was cured. The case was followed up 2 years later and there was no relapse.

Explanation: The profuse sweating in this case was due to shock, causing Yin and Yang disharmony in the organs and collaterals.

Reducing Hegu L.I. 4 activates Qi in the channels, strengthens resistance to External attack and regulates the functions of the pores. Reinforcing Fuliu KID 7 regulates and nourishes the Kidney Yin, reinforces Qi, builds Body Fluids and strengthens the Defensive Qi. When the pathogenic Qi is expelled, the Body Fluids circulate, the Defensive Qi is strong, the pores close and the profuse sweating will stop. In the *Yu Long Ge* (Jade Dragon Songs), Wang Guorei says, 'For Cold without sweat, reduce Fuliu: for profuse sweating, reduce Hegu'. The *Zhen Jiu Da Cheng* (Great Compendium of Acupuncture and Moxibustion) says, 'For profuse sweating first reduce Hegu, then reinforce Fuliu'. These theories have been borne out by clinical practice.

Neiguan P 6, the Luo-Connecting point of the Pericardium channel and Confluent point of Yin Wei Mai connects and clears the External and Internal channels, helping the main points disperse the Stagnant Internal Heat.

Wang Kan, SHANDAN COUNTY TCM HOSPITAL, GANSU PROVINCE
(see Journal of Traditional Chinese Medicine, Issue 3, 1985)

72. Profuse sweating in brother and sister

CASE 1

M, female, age 25, foreigner

Case registered: 5 April 1982

History: The patient had sweated profusely since childhood, especially on her hands and feet. The problem was worse when she was anxious or tired, or during her period. Her hands and feet constantly dripped with sweat, and as a result she often had to wear sandals rather than shoes. She occasionally had palpitations, shortness of breath, cold limbs and felt weak. Her period was regular but a little heavy, and the blood was pale. Her appetite, bowels and urination were normal.

Examination: The patient looked big but not very strong. Temperature, BP, heart and lungs normal. Liver and spleen not enlarged. Movement of spine and limbs normal. Her palms and soles were dripping with sweat. *Tongue body:* pale red. *Tongue coating:* thin and white. *Pulse:* weak.

Diagnosis: Deficiency of Heart and Kidney Yang, Deficiency of Defensive Qi.

Treatment: Nourish the Heart and Kidney, tighten the interstices to stop sweating.

Principal Points: Hegu L.I. 4 (bilateral), Fuliu KID 7 (bilateral), Qihai Ren 6.
Hegu L.I. 4 was reduced, the other points were reinforced, and the needles were retained for 15 minutes. Treatment was given daily. After eight sessions the symptoms improved, and after a further six treatments there was much less sweating. After a total of 24 treatments the disorder was completely cured. The case was followed up for 4 months and there was no relapse.

CASE 2

M, male, age 28, foreigner, brother of Case 1

Case registered: 6 May 1982

History: The patient had sweated profusely since childhood, especially on his hands and feet. The problem was worse if he was anxious. The sweating had gradually got worse and, like his sister, he too was compelled to wear sandals rather than shoes. Change of weather had no effect on the problem. He had occasional palpitations, insomnia, and dreamed excessively. His waist ached, and he had spermatorrhoea. Appetite, bowels and urination were normal.

Examination: The patient looked thin and delicate. Temperature, BP, heart and lungs normal. Liver and spleen not enlarged. Movement of spine and limbs normal. Hands and feet were normal in colouring and temperature, but dripping with sweat from the palms and soles. *Tongue body:* red. *Tongue coating:* thin. *Pulse:* thin and rapid.

Diagnosis: Heart and Kidney Yin Deficiency.

Treatment: Nourish the Heart and Kidney Yin, regulate Nutritive and Defensive Qi to tighten the interstices and stop sweating.

Principal Points: Hegu L.I. 4, Fuliu KID 7, Yinxi HT 6.

  The points were needled bilaterally and the needles retained for 15 minutes. Treatment was given daily. After 6 days the symptoms had markedly improved. Six more treatments were given and the disorder was cured. The case was followed up for 3 months and there was no relapse.

Explanation: It is not unusual to encounter cases of profuse sweating in clinic, but it is quite rare to see it in brother and sister, especially with such severity and chronicity.

  Sweating can be healthy or pathological. Healthy sweating is a sign of harmony between Yin and Yang, Qi and Blood, Nutritive and Defensive Qi and Exterior and Interior; pathological sweating indicates these things are in disharmony. Spontaneous sweating may arise from Deficiency of the Lung or Kidney, Deficiency of Liver Yin, Liver Yang rising, Deficient Yang, or Deficient Defensive Qi. Nightsweats arise when the Yin is Deficient and unable to anchor the Yang, or if the Yang is Deficient, causing weak Defensive Qi.

  In the first case the Heart and Kidney Yang were Deficient and the Defensive Qi was weak and unable to regulate sweating. In the second case the signs and symptoms indicated the Heart and Kidney Yin were Deficient, with Deficiency Fire pushing out the sweat. Lan Jiang Fu said, 'When there is no sweat reinforce Hegu and reduce Fuliu: if the sweating is unchecked reinforce Fuliu and you will see the miracle' (Songs of Halting the Flow of the River). In the first case Fuliu KID 7 and Qihai Ren 6 were reinforced, strengthening the Heart and Kidney Yang to help the Defensive Qi. The sweating stopped when the Defensive Qi functioned properly and was tight. In the second case Fuliu KID 7 and Yinxi HT 6 were reinforced, nourishing the Yin to anchor the Yang. The sweating stopped when the Heart and Kidney Yin were strong and could control the Yang.

  The Lung and the Large Intestine are an Interior/Exterior pair. The Lung controls the skin. Reducing Hegu L.I. 4, the Source point, regulates the Nutritive and Defensive Qi and closes the pores.

Zhang Dengbu, ACUPUNCTURE AND MOXIBUSTION SECTION, SHANDONG TCM COLLEGE HOSPITAL
(see New Chinese Medicine, Issue 11, 1984)

73. Nightsweats

CASE 1

Han, female, age 43, peasant

History: The patient had malaria in autumn 1966 and suffered from nightsweats ever since. She became concerned in 1971 when the problem became worse; she would sweat as soon as she closed her eyes, and in such quantities that her clothes were always wet. Her face would feel flushed and she felt hot in her palms and soles. She was faint and dreamed a lot. The problem was always worse a few days before her period.

She was treated unsuccessfully with Chinese herbs and Western drugs, including Dang Gui Liu Huang Tang (Angelica and Six Yellow Decoction), Liu Wei Di Huang Wan (Six Ingredients Pill with Rehmannia), Zhi Bai Di Huang Wan (Anamarrhena, Phellodendron and Rehmannia Pill), diazepam, oryzanol and placental tissue fluid.

Examination: The patient looked thin and frail. *Tongue body:* pale. *Tongue coating:* white. *Pulse:* weak and thin.

Diagnosis: Kidney Yin Deficiency.

Treatment: Tonify Yin to arrest sweating.

Principal Points: Fuliu KID 7, Yinxi HT 6, Sanyinjiao SP 6.

Seven treatments were given, but there was no improvement. Further enquiries revealed that although the patient had feverish sensations in her face, palms and soles, she also felt chills and had cold limbs. The sweating was worst when she had a feeling of cold in her back.

Revised treatment: Reinforce Yang to strengthen the interstices.

Principal Points: Dazhui Du 14, Xinshu BL 15.

The points were needled strongly with reinforcing by obtaining sensations of heat method, then warmed with moxibustion to strengthen the effect. That night the patient sweated much less, and did not soak her clothes. The next day her back felt less cold, and her hands and feet were slightly warm.

Treatment continued, and after five sessions her nightsweats were markedly reduced. After 14 treatments the problem was cured. Six more consolidating treatments were given. After 8 years this persistent condition responded very quickly to acupuncture, and there has been no relapse up to this time.

Zhang Naiqing, RUGAO COUNTY TCM HOSPITAL, JIANGSU PROVINCE
(see Shanghai Journal of Acupuncture and Moxibustion, Issue 4, 1986)

CASE 2

He, male, age 45, cadre

Case registered: 12 July 1983

History: During the past 2 months the patient had sweated profusely during his afternoon naps and at night. His clothes and bedding would be soaked. The problem had become worse in the last 3 weeks. His palms and soles felt hot, his eyes were dry and his cheeks were flushed. Chest X-ray and blood sedimentation tests were normal. Medication had not helped.

Examination: Temperature: 37.8°C. Slight malar flush. *Tongue body:* slightly red and dry. *Pulse:* thin and rapid.

Diagnosis: Deficiency Heat.
    Treatment: Nourish the Yin to cool Heat, regulate the channels and vessels to stop sweating.

Principal Points: Hegu L.I. 4, Fuliu KID 7, Sanyinjiao SP 6.
    All points were needled bilaterally and retained for 20 minutes, with manipulation at 5-minute intervals. Hegu L.I. 4 and Sanyinjiao SP 6 were gently reduced, and Fuliu KID 7 was gently reinforced. Treatment was given daily.
    After 7 days the nightsweats improved, and after 20 sessions the disorder was completely cured.

Wang Kan, SHANDAN TCM COUNTY HOSPITAL, GANSU PROVINCE
(see Journal of Traditional Chinese Medicine, Issue 3, 1985)

Editor's Note: This case of nightsweats was caused by Deficiency of Yin. The Yin was unable to control and anchor the Yang, which escaped with the Yin fluids. Reducing Hegu L.I. 4 and reinforcing Fuliu KID 7 clears and regulates the Exterior and Interior, regulating and invigorating Yin and Yang. Reducing Sanyinjiao SP 6 gently nourishes the Yin and pulls down Heat. The sweating stopped when Yin and Yang were harmonized.

74. One-sided facial sweating

Wang, male, age 28, peasant

Case Registered: 3 July 1976

History: The patient had sweated on one side of his face and neck for over 6 years. The difference between the two sides was more marked in summer. The right side sweated a lot, and was very sensitive to cold.

The left side was warm and flushed. The condition was diagnosed as a functional disturbance of the autonomic nervous system, but after various treatments it was no better.

Diagnosis: Yin–Yang face.

Auricular Points: Lung, Sympathetic, Endocrine.

The points were needled on the right. He stopped sweating immediately and the needles were withdrawn. The next day he still had some sweating on the right, so needle embedding therapy was used at the same points. The needles were removed after 7 days. He sweated little during this period. After 5 days' observation he was discharged. He relapsed some time later, but was cured with 10 courses of the above treatment. The case was followed up for 6 years, and there was no further relapse.

Explanation: This disease is quite rare. In Western medicine it is regarded as a functional disturbance of the autonomic nervous system. In TCM it is held to be due to maladjustment of the channels and vessels, Stagnation of Qi and Blood, obstruction of the vessels by Pathogenic Wind, Cold or Phlegm leading to a breach between Yin and Yang. In this case auricular therapy gave long-lasting effects.

Case treated by Xia Lianqing, case study by Huang Shifu,
ACUPUNCTURE AND MOXIBUSTION SECTION, YIXING COUNTY PEOPLE'S
HOSPITAL, JIANGSU PROVINCE
(see Journal of Traditional Chinese Medicine, Issue 12, 1983)

75. Anhidrosis

Yang, female, age 39, worker

Case registered: 3 June 1980

History: The patient had terminated a pregnancy in August 1977. At the time she had been exposed to wind when the weather had been going through dramatic changes, with the temperature during the day varying from 40°C to –20°C. She now felt cold and was unable to sweat, even when it was very hot and other people were. She also felt faint, with palpitations, headache and a feeling of oppression in the chest. She had taken 48 doses of Chinese herbs when in Jianxi Province, but these had no effect. Her symptoms had got worse since she started work here. By the time she came for treatment she still had all of the above symptoms, but also felt restless, with a headache which radiated into her neck. She had an aversion to cold, and was still wearing her autumn clothes in summer. At night she would feel cold even with two quilts. She would take a nap at midday and wake up feeling faint with a bitter taste in her mouth and a dry throat.

Examination: Tongue body: pale. *Tongue coating:* white. *Pulse:* wiry and tight.

Diagnosis: Exterior Wind Cold, Nutritive and Defensive Qi disharmony.

Treatment: Relieve Exterior syndrome, raise Yang, regulate Nutritive and Defensive Qi.

Principal Points: Tai Yang (Extra) (bilateral), Fengchi GB 20 (bilateral), Dazhui Du 14, Jiaji (Extra).

Low frequency electro-acupuncture was used, 2V at Tai Yang and Fengchi, 10V at Dazhui and 15V at the Jiaji (Extra) points. Current was applied for 30 seconds to each point, once a day. After three treatments the patient felt comfortable and the palpitations, feeling of distress in the chest and faintness had improved. She sweated a little on her forehead when it was hot. After five treatments her aversion to cold was less pronounced and she was sweating more on her head. After 10 treatments the palpitations, distress in the chest, bitter taste and faintness had gone. She was cured after 13 treatments.

Explanation: The patient was exposed to severe cold when she was very weak after her abortion. External Wind penetrated the body, closing the pores, blocking the Defensive Qi and causing Stagnation of Defensive and Nutritive Qi. This gave rise to her aversion to cold, stiff neck, headache and inability to sweat. After the disease became chronic, the damaged Yang began to affect the Yin, causing restlessness, distress in the chest and faintness, so this case is a good example of disharmony between Nutritive and Defensive Qi, Yin and Yang.

Dazhui Du 14 reinforces all the Yang and expels External attack. Fengchi GB 20 and Tai Yang (Extra) relieve Exterior syndromes. The Jiaji (Extra) points are on the back of the body, its Yang surface, so they were used to reinforce Yang and relieve Exterior syndrome.

Miao Xiaowei and Shang Shublin, ZHANGJIAKOU PROSPECTING MACHINES FACTORY HOSPITAL, MINISTRY OF GEOLOGY, *(see Journal of Traditional Chinese Medicine, Issue 1, 1981)*

76. Anhidrosis, left side of body

Zeng, female, age 28, member of staff

Case registered: 4 September 1986

History: 3 months previously the patient had been injected with gentamicin and penicillin after admission to hospital with pain in the right kidney and abdomen. The pain stopped and she was discharged after 10 days. Following this she stopped sweating on the left side of her body from head to toe. Some mild pain returned in the right kidney area.

Examination: The patient was well developed and well nourished. Complexion light brown. Heart, lungs, appetite, bowels and urination normal. Five sense organs normal. *Tongue body:* pale red. *Pulse:* wiry and thin.

Diagnosis: Obstruction of the channels and collaterals, imbalance of Yin and Yang.

Treatment: Regulate Yin and Yang and clear the channels and collaterals. Principal Points: Shenshu BL 23, Fuliu KID 7. Hegu L.I. 4.

Secondary Points: Tapping with a plum blossom needle over the Bladder channel from the neck to the waist, and over the Jiaji (Extra) points.

Both sets of points were used once daily, reducing the principal points then reinforcing afterwards, and retaining the needles for 30 minutes. The day after the first treatment the patient noticed some sweating on her left lumbar area, and on her head and body. After 5 days she was sweating normally and the disorder was cured.

Explanation: The original right-sided abdominal and lumbar pain was caused by Heat obstructing the channels and collaterals. The pain was relieved after treatment, but the imbalance of Yin and Yang was not addressed.

Shenshu BL 23 reinforces Kidney Qi, and Fuliu KID 7 and Hegu L.I. 4 are empirical points for controlling sweating. The Jing-River points have a dual regulating function: they reinforce Deficiency and reduce Excess, regulate the channel Qi and harmonize Yin and Yang.

Case treated by Lin Wenyang, case study by Lin Pengzhi,
ACUPUNCTURE AND MOXIBUSTION SECTION, GUANGDONG PROVINCIAL TCM HOSPITAL.

77. Anhidrosis, migrainous, right side of the face

Gong, male, age 32, member of staff

Case Registered: 24 February 1982

History: For the last 2 years the patient had migraines on the right, together with an inability to sweat on the right side of his face. He tried various treatments without success.

Examination: The skin on the right side of his face was dry and did not sweat. The left side was red and moist. His right eyelids were slightly more closed than on the healthy side. The dividing line between the two sides was exactly down the middle of his face.

Principal Points: Tai Yang (Extra) through to Jiache ST 6.

The point was needled on the right, down through Xiaguan ST 7, under the zygomatic bone to Jiache ST 6. Strong stimulation was given with large amplitude lifting and thrusting. Treatment was given once every other day. After three treatments he was sweating on the right almost as much as on the left. His migraines were also cured simultaneously. The case was followed up for 6 months and there was no relapse.

Explanation: This disease is mentioned in some books, but there are no detailed records of its aetiology, pathology or treatment.

Han Weipeng, FUSHUNCHENG CLINIC, XINFU DISTRICT, FUSHUN
(see Journal of Traditional Chinese Medicine, Issue 6, 1983)

SKIN DISORDERS

78. Pruritus

CASE 1, GENERALIZED

Na, female, age 8

Case registered: August 1980

History: For the last 6 months the patient had been itching all over. Her appetite was poor and she was losing weight. However, she liked snacks but would defaecate immediately after eating. Her stools were loose and contained undigested food. She was treated with Chlor-trimeton (chlorpheniramine), Benadryl (diphenhydramine), hydrocortisone and Gastrozepine (pirenzepine) but these did not help. Recently her skin had got worse, affecting her sleep and schoolwork.

Examination: The patient was pale, emaciated and lacklustre. Her stomach felt full. Heart and lungs were normal. RBC and WBC within normal ranges. Haemoglobin 100 g/l (10 g%). *Tongue coating:* slightly greasy. *Pulse:* soft and weak.

Diagnosis: Infantile malnutrition.

Treatment: Treat malnutrition and indigestion.

Principal Points: Sifeng (Extras).

The points were needled on both hands and squeezed to let out some yellow and white mucus. After the first treatment there was less itching and the patient's stools became more firm. Her appetite improved. Treatment was given once every 5 days. After three sessions the itching disappeared. Her stools became normal and her appetite was good. The case was followed up a year later and there was no relapse.

Explanation: In TCM these symptoms are believed to be due to irregular diet impairing the Stomach and Spleen. There are some old sayings in TCM: 'When the Blood is deficient there will be Wind' and 'All itching belongs to Wind'. Itching is therefore caused by Stomach and Spleen Deficiency. The Sifeng (Extras) address the root cause, as they are empirical points for infantile malnutrition and indigestion.

Zhang Juru, ACUPUNCTURE AND MOXIBUSTION SECTION, LIAONING TCM COLLEGE HOSPITAL
(see Journal of Traditional Chinese Medicine, Issue 5, 1982)

CASE 2, EPISODIC, FOLLOWING HEPATITIS

Zhu, male, age 21, technician

Case registered: 25 October 1987

History: The patient was recovering from hepatitis with jaundice. In the previous week he suffered bouts of unbearable itching whenever he ate hot porridge. Each attack lasted half an hour. Medication did not help. He was also distressed, with poor, dream disturbed sleep. His urine was dark, his stools were loose and irregular and he had a bitter taste in his mouth.

Examination: The patient had a rosy complexion and looked healthy. The skin on his hands and feet was normal.

Diagnosis: Itching due to Liver Heat and Wind.

Treatment: Soothe Liver Wind, regulate Qi and Blood.

Principal Points: Quchi L.I. 11, Hegu L.I. 4, Waiguan TB 5, Xuehai SP 10, Yanglingquan GB 34, Taichong LIV 3.
    The points were needled bilaterally, and the needles were retained for 20 minutes. Quchi L.I. 11 and Waiguan TB 5 were needled superficially. Hegu L.I. 4 and Taichong LIV 3 were reduced, and then stimulated with electric current. Xuehai SP 10 and Yanglingquan GB 34 were needled with reinforcing and reducing evenly method.
    After the first session the patient went home and ate some porridge to test the efficacy of the treatment. There was no reaction straight away,

but after half an hour he had a mild attack. The treatment was repeated 2 days later, and the disorder did not recur. The case was observed for a month and there was no relapse.

Explanation: The patient had had acute liver disease for a month. There was Heat and Wind in the Liver channel which had not yet been purged. The accumulated Heat in the channel became Wind, and the Heat and Wind battled in the extremities, causing the intense itching. It was aggravated by the hot porridge because Wind is more severe with Fire.

Quchi L.I. 11 and Hegu L.I. 4 are part of Yang Ming, which is rich in Qi and Blood. They remove external Wind and pathogens, and regulate Qi and Blood. Xuehai SP 10, also known as Bai Chong Ke (Nest of 100 Worms), is used for Blood diseases, regulates Qi and Blood, and purges accumulated Heat in the Blood to relieve itching. This follows the principle of 'Treat Wind by treating Blood first. When the Blood is tonified the Wind dies down'.

Waiguan TB 5 and Yanglingquan GB 34, the He-Sea point, regulate the Functional Qi of the Triple Burner, soothe Liver Wind, normalize the function of the Gall Bladder and purge Damp Heat. Together with Taichong LIV 3, the Yuan-Source point, they soothe and relieve Liver Heat, and activate the Blood and channels. When Hegu L.I. 4 is used together with Taichong LIV 3 it is called the 'Four Gates'. This combination readjusts the functions of the organs. The entire treatment was effective because it took into account both Exterior and Interior, treating both Qi and Blood.

Xu Futian, BAOCHANG TOWNSHIP CLINIC, HAIMEN COUNTY, JIANGSU PROVINCE

CASE 3, CHRONIC PERIANAL

Huang, male, age 45, cadre

History: 5 years previously the patient began to suffer from unbearable paroxysmal itching around the anus. This gradually became worse and the episodes, which had originally lasted a few minutes, would now last hours. He had been to both the dermatology and proctology departments, where the condition was diagnosed as perianal pruritus, but both oral and topical medication had made no difference. The problem continued to get worse, affecting his sleep. He was now tired and thin, and his appetite was poor. The affected area was bleeding and painful from scratching. Surgery was suggested as an option.

Examination: The skin around the patient's anus was lichenified. The skin was damaged: there were scratch marks, fissures and bloody scabs. Tests ruled out mycotic infection, enterobiasis, and related anorectal disease.

Diagnosis: Anal itching: Stasis and accumulation of Damp Heat in the channels and collaterals.

Treatment: Root amputation: dredge the channels and collaterals to relieve itching.

Principal Points: Dachangshu BL 25 (bilateral), Changqiang Du 1, Chengshan BL 57 (bilateral), Yaoshu Du 2, Guanyuanshu BL 26 (bilateral).

The patient lay on his side. Dachangshu BL 25 (bilateral) and Changqiang Du 1 were sterilized and 0.1 mg of 0.5% procaine solution was injected into each one, until a raised lump had appeared. A scalpel was used to make a superficial incision 5 mm long, just deep enough to cause a little bleeding. A suture needle was inserted into the opening to hook up the white fibres inside and break them. 5–8 fibres were broken at each point. The incisions were then swabbed with 75% alcohol and covered with sterile gauze. For the second treatment Chengshan BL 57 and Changqiang Du 1 were selected. Treatment was given every 5–7 days. 2–3 points were used each time.

After the first session there was almost no itching, and the patient's skin became less lichenified. After 1 month his skin was normal. The case was followed up for a year and there was no relapse.

Explanation: Perianal pruritus is a localized paroxysmal and persistent disease with complicated aetiology. In TCM it is called anal itching. There are many therapies for this disease, but none of them is ideal. Root amputation has a long history in TCM, and combines point blocking with procaine, stone needling and acupuncture. Used alone these therapies are not as effective. All the points mentioned above are effective for anal disease, which in this case was caused by Stagnation and accumulation of Damp Heat in the channels and collaterals. Strict asepsis is recommended. This therapy is contraindicated in pregnancy, heart disease, and for patients who are very weak or allergic to procaine. Irritating foods, e.g. hot peppers, should not be eaten after treatment.

Xuan Guowei, GUANGDONG PROVINCIAL TCM HOSPITAL
(see New Chinese Medicine, Issue 12, 1982)

79. Molluscum contagiosum

Fan, female, age 16, student

Case registered: 7 July 1919

History: The patient's skin broke out in pea-sized lumps 4 months previously. These were on her chest, back and the upper part of her limbs. They were very itchy and affected her sleep and schoolwork. She tried oral and topical medications without success and the problem grew worse.

Examination: The patient had about 80 hemispherical lumps on her chest, back, shoulders and the upper parts of the limbs. Each lump was smooth on the surface with a depression in the middle.

Diagnosis: Warts.

Treatment: Purge Heat in the Liver, Spleen and Lung.

Principal Points: Yinbai SP 1, Dadun LIV 1, Shaoshang LU 11.
   The points were pricked with a three-edged needle and a few drops of blood were drawn. The blood was cleaned off after 5 to 10 minutes. Treatment was given twice every 3 days. After the first treatment the itching was markedly better and the base of each wart had become red and was easily removed with scratching. Six treatments were given in total, and all the warts came off.

> Li Liang'an, DERMATOLOGY DEPARTMENT, LUOYANG RAILWAY HOSPITAL, HENAN PROVINCE
> *(see New Chinese Medicine, Issue 11, 1983)*

Editor's Note: This disease is mentioned very early. When discussing the Small Intestine Luo-Connecting channel symptoms, the *Nei Jing* says, 'When Zhizheng SI 7 is excessive the joints are flaccid, and the elbow is paralysed. When it is deficient there are warts'. Chao Yuanfang of the Sui Dynasty stated that warts are caused by a battle with Pathogenic Wind in the muscles (*Zhu Bing Yuan Hou Lun*, Chao's General Treatise on the Causes and Symptoms of Diseases). Chen Shigong of the Ming dynasty said they were caused by emotional factors impairing the Liver, which becomes malnourished, so that the tendon Qi comes out (*Wai Ke Zhen Zong*, Orthodox Manual of External Disease). The *Xue Shi Yi An* (Xue's Case Studies) says that warts are a disease of the Liver and Gall Bladder channels, caused by Wind and Heat drying up the Blood, or anger agitating Liver Fire, or Pathogenic Qi invading the Liver.
   In conclusion, the disease is due to Ying-Nutritive and Wei-Defensive Qi imbalance, and Liver and Gall Bladder disharmony. In this case the Jing-Well points of the Liver, Spleen and Lung channels were bled. This purges Heat in the Liver, Spleen and Lung, regulates the Liver and Gall Bladder, soothes Wind and moistens dryness.

80. Psoriasis

Wang, male, age 58, peasant

Case registered: November 1973

History: The patient had had psoriasis for 20 years. It started with pale red eruptions dotted over the lateral parts of his limbs. The eruptions were in clusters, with white scales which came off when scratched. The psoriasis spread to his back and head and became very itchy, especially when dressing and undressing. He would scratch until he was bleeding. The disease was better in summer, and became severe with the onset of winter. He had been to many hospitals, but treatment had not helped. Now the eruptions were all over his body.

Examination: The patient's skin was damaged all over. There were many scaly pale red eruptions dotted all over his body. The scales came off if scratched, and the skin underneath would bleed.

Diagnosis: Bai Bi: Pathogenic Wind invading the skin, Dryness from Deficiency of Blood.

Treatment: Embedding therapy: Tonify Qi and Blood in the skin.

Principal Points: Feishu BL 13 (bilateral).
    The area 1 cun below the point was sterilized with gentian violet, then 1 ml of 2% procaine solution was injected into each point. The middle of a piece of sterilized catgut was slowly inserted with a thread embedding needle into a point 1 cun below Feishu BL 13 until no ends were visible above the skin and the thread had reached Feishu. Sterile gauze was taped over the point to prevent infection. The patient was advised not to bathe for the first 2 days, and to avoid foods that might cause infection and Wind, such as seafood, mutton and garlic.
    Generally catgut takes 2–3 weeks to be absorbed by the tissues. The night after the treatment the patient's itching was much better. After a week there was no new skin damage. The treatment was re-administered after 2 weeks. There was a steady improvement. By the fourth treatment the skin damage had nearly disappeared, and there were only a few areas of pigmentation. Two consolidating treatments were given. The case was followed up for 2 years and there was no relapse.

Explanation: Psoriasis is a chronic recurrent skin disease. In TCM it is called 'Bai Bi'. The Yi Zong Jin Jian says, 'The disease is usually called Snake Wind. It is a skin disease which resembles scabies, and white scales form after scratching' (Wai Ke Xin Fa Yao Jue, External Disease).

The *Wai Ke Zheng Zhi Quan Shu* says, 'Bai Bi can also be called Bi Feng. The skin is dry and itchy. The condition resembles scabies and white scales form with scratching. The skin becomes dry and bleeds. This is a very painful problem' (The Complete Book of Symptoms and Treatments of External Diseases).

The disease is usually due to emotional factors which cause Stagnation of Qi. This then accumulates and becomes Fire. The Fire becomes Exuberant and the Fire toxin stays in the Blood. It can also be caused by irregular diet or ingestion of seafood or other foods which engender Wind and infection, causing disharmony between Spleen and Stomach.

Repeated onsets consume the Blood and cause an imbalance of Qi and Blood, leading to Dryness and Wind or Stagnation in the channels and collaterals. This causes the scaling and eruptions on the skin.

'The Lung dominates the skin', so thread embedding therapy at Feishu BL 13 gives long lasting stimulation to activate Qi and Blood in the skin and nourish it. If the skin damage is on the head, Lingtai Du 10 could also be treated in this way.

Xia Lianqing, ACUPUNCTURE AND MOXIBUSTION SECTION, YIXING COUNTY PEOPLE'S HOSPITAL, JIANGSU PROVINCE

81. Alopecia areata

Wan, male, age 42, cadre

Case registered: 29 June 1979

History: The patient had alopecia areata at the back of his head for many years. He also suffered from insomnia and dream-disturbed sleep. Medication did not really help, so he decided to try acupuncture and moxibustion.

Examination: There was a 2×3 cm bald patch at the back of the patient's head. *Tongue body:* pale. *Pulse:* thin and rapid.

Diagnosis: You Feng: Deficiency of Lung and Kidney Yin.

Treatment: Point injection therapy: Nourish Lung and Kidney Yin.

Principal Points: Feishu BL 13, Shenshu BL 23, Geshu BL 17.

1 microgram of vitamin B_{12} and 1 mg of strychnine nitrate were injected into one pair of Bladder points per day. The points were rotated with each treatment. After seven sessions thin, light coloured hairs began to grow in the bald area. Later the hairs became darker. After 17 sessions the bald patch was completely covered in new healthy hair.

Explanation: Alopecia areata is called 'You Feng'. It is characterized by hair loss over a short period of time which leaves a shiny area of skin. The hair may be lost over one area or all over the head. Usually this disease is due to Blood Deficiency or Dryness causing malnutrition of the hair. Modern medicine calls this condition neural alopecia. Treatment should aim to nourish the Lung and Kidney. In TCM the Lung is in charge of the skin and hair, and the Kidney stores the essential substances of the body.

Feishu BL 13 and Shenshu BL 23 nourish the Heart and Kidney. Geshu BL 17 generates Blood to nourish hair. The medication reinforces the effect of nourishing the Lung and Kidney, activating the channels and tonifying Qi and Blood.

> Case treated by Zhang Heyuan, case study by Liu Mingyi and Sunhao, GUIYANG TCM COLLEGE

82. Erysipelas

Fan, male, age 45, school teacher

Case registered: 6 May 1979

History: The patient had erysipelas on his left leg for more than 5 years. It would break out two or three times a year. Antibiotics were prescribed during acute attacks, but the disease was never cured. His present symptoms were redness, swelling, heat and pain on the inside of his left leg, accompanied by fever, poor appetite and aversion to cold.

Examination: Temperature: 38.5°C. *WBC:* $14 \times 10^9/1$ ($14 \times 10^3/\text{mm}^3$), neutrophils 84%. *Tongue coating:* yellow. *Pulse:* rapid and wiry.

Diagnosis: Tui You Feng: Toxic Heat retained in the muscle and skin.

Treatment: Cool the Blood by clearing Heat, resolve Toxin and remove Damp.

Principal Points: Diji SP 8, Xuehai SP 10, Sanyinjiao SP 6, Fenglong ST 40, Taichong LIV 3, all on the left side.

The points were reduced with slow and fast, twirling, lifting and thrusting method. The needles were retained for 20 minutes and manipulated once during this time. Dispersed needling (San Ci) with a three edged needle was used over the red and swollen areas after the other needles were withdrawn. These points were bled and then cupped. Treatment was given once a day.

Treatment III: After two treatments the redness and swelling on the patient's medial thigh were much improved. *Temperature:* 37.1°C. *WBC:* $9.1 \times 10^9/1$ ($9.1 \times 10^3/\text{mm}^3$), neutrophils 74%.

Principal Points: Diji SP 8, Xuehai SP 10, Shangqiu SP 5, all on the left, Zusanli ST 36 on the right.

The points were manipulated as before.

Treatment V: The redness, swelling and pain in the leg had almost completely gone. Temperature normal. *WBC:* $7.5 \times 10^9/1$ (7.5×10^3 mm^3) Neutrophils 68%.

Principal Points: Yinlingquan SP 9, Zusanli ST 36, Sanyinjiao SP 6.

The points were all needled on the left with reinforcing and reducing evenly method. The needles were retained for 20 minutes.

From this time on treatment was given twice a week, and after a month it was reduced to once a week. Three months later consolidating treatment was given once a fortnight. The case was followed up for a year, and there was no relapse.

Explanation: Erysipelas is called Liu Huo (Flowing Fire), Tui You Feng (Travelling Wind of the Leg), Bao Tou Huo Dan (Head Holding Fire Redness) and Da Tou Wen (Big Head Plague). It usually affects the head and the leg, and has a high rate of recurrence.

In 1979 this ward treated 20 cases of acute erysipelas and achieved clear short term effects with acupuncture. The treatments followed the principles of 'reducing Excess' and 'removing Stasis'. Points on the Spleen channel were selected, in combination with the Stomach Back-Shu points.

Modifications: This principle was modified according to the presentation.

Principal Points: Diji SP 8, Xuehai SP 10, Sanyinjiao SP 6, Fenglong ST 40, Taichong LIV 3, all on the affected side.

Secondary Points: Yinlingquan SP 9, Shangqiu SP 5, Zusanli ST 36, Ligou LIV 5.

Severe Heat in the Blood: points on the Liver channel were added to cool Blood and clear Heat.

Symptoms on the head and face: Yifeng TB 17, Touwei ST 8, Hegu L.I. 4, Sibai ST 2.

Severe cases: If the patient is quite strong and the damage is severe, use a long needle to puncture the affected area obliquely.

Pronounced redness and swelling: Use a three-edged needle to bleed or tap with a cutaneous needle to bleed. Cupping may be added. Stop the bleeding when the redness and swelling subside.

Clinical observation has found that acupuncture can alleviate the symptoms in the acute phase of erysipelas, normalizing white blood cell indices within 2 to 3 days. Oblique puncture with a long needle or bleeding and cupping over the affected area can relieve pain and swelling, and clear Heat.

> Case treated by Xi Yongjiang, case study by Pu Yunxing and Xi Depei, SHANGHAI TCM COLLEGE HOSPITAL, YUEYANG
> (see Correspondence, Journal of Acupuncture and Moxibustion, Issue 1, 1987)

PSYCHIATRIC DISORDERS

83. Insomnia

Chen, female, age 52, worker

Case registered: 13 October 1984

History: The patient had become unable to sleep after a period of feeling exhausted. She slept intermittently, and sometimes stayed awake for 3 months at a time. With sleeping pills she might sleep for 2 or 3 hours. Her limbs felt heavy, her appetite was poor, she was a little thirsty and she felt faint and distressed.

Examination: The patient looked weary and fatigued. *Tongue body:* pale. *Tongue coating:* white. *Pulse:* weak.

Diagnosis: Deficiency of Qi and Blood.

Treatment: Invigorate the Qi and calm the mind.

Principal Points: Baihui Du 20.
　　Direct moxa with pea-sized cones was given. After 10 cones the patient could feel local sensations of heat. After 32 cones the sensations spread along the channel to Yintang (Extra). After 40 cones her head felt heavy, as if there was a 10 cm square weight resting on it, her neck ached and she could hear ringing in her left ear. 30 minutes after moxibustion the sensations of heaviness and heat began to recede, and the patient began to feel refreshed. That night she slept quietly for 4 hours. After six treatments she could sleep for 6 hours, and her distress, faintness and thirst stopped. She became energized and regained her appetite.

Explanation: The *Huang Di Ming Tang Jiu Jing* (Ming Tang Moxibustion Book of the Yellow Emperor) says, 'Baihui (Du 20) controls feelings of heaviness in the head, nasal obstruction and absent-mindedness'. Baihui Du 20 is the meeting point of Du Mai with the hand and feet Yang channels, and is used to expel Heat, for resuscitation, to refresh the mind and calm the spirits. In clinical practice moxibustion at Baihui Du 20 is often used to treat faintness, insomnia and amnesia.

Hao Shaojie, ACUPUNCTURE AND MOXIBUSTION SECTION, SHENXI PROVINCIAL TCM INSTITUTE HOSPITAL
(see Shenxi Traditional Chinese Medicine, Issue 9, 1985)

84. Narcolepsy

CASE 1

Chen, female, age 46, school teacher

Case registered: 18 December 1980

History: In 1969 the patient began to suffer from narcolepsy, which had gradually got worse. At present she was suffering four or five attacks a day. During an attack she would collapse and fall asleep instantly, no matter what she was doing: eating, walking, attending a meeting or preparing a lecture. Usually these attacks would occur two or three times in the mornings and once or twice in the afternoons. An attack would generally last no more than 10 minutes. She was also afraid to laugh out loud. Whenever she did she would lose her balance and fall on the ground, although she would quickly recover.

She had been to several hospitals, which had all diagnosed her condition as 'paroxysmal lethargy'. She had taken stimulants like caffeine and Centrofenoxine (meclofenoxate) for about 6 months, but with little effect. She had previously been healthy and there was no family history of the same problem.

Examination: Temperature, pulse and BP normal. Skull, heart and lungs negative. Abdomen flat and soft. Liver and spleen not enlarged. Spine and limbs normal. Physiological reflex normal, no pathological reflex induced.

Diagnosis: Lethargy.

Treatment: Invigorate Heart Yang and regulate Qi and Blood.

Principal Points: Shenmen HT 7, Neiguan P 6.

The points were needled bilaterally. After Qi was obtained the needles were rotated, lifted and thrusted for 1 or 2 minutes before withdrawal. Treatment was given once a day. After 9 days the patient said she was able to control the sleepiness in the mornings, but that it would return once or twice in the afternoons. After 16 treatments the attacks would only occur occasionally at night. After a total of 24 treatments the condition was cured. The case was followed up for 6 months and there was no relapse.

Explanation: The *Su Wen* (Ch. 9) says, 'The Heart is the root of life and the source of spirit . . . the Tai Yang of all the Yang'. The *Ling Shu* says, 'The Heart is the king of all the organs, and houses the spirit' (Miraculous Pivot, Xie Ke chapter, Evil Visitors). These quotations show that the Heart controls consciousness and is the most important of all the organs. If the Heart Yang is activated, Qi and Blood circulate properly and a person will be active and rest appropriately. If they do not, the person will feel tired and rest inappropriately.

Both Neiguan P 6 and Shenmen HT 7 calm the mind and activate the channels and collaterals. Needling them invigorates Heart Yang, promotes the circulation of Qi and Blood, and harmonizes Yin and Yang.

> Xu Benren and Ge Shuhan, ACUPUNCTURE AND MOXIBUSTION
> SECTION, SHENYANG AIRFORCE HOSPITAL
> *(see Beijing Traditional Chinese Medicine, Issue 4, 1985)*

CASE 2

Dang, male, age 20
Case registered: 20 March 1985

History: The patient had suffered from narcolepsy for the last 3 years. The attacks would come after eating, usually around 9.00 a.m. Before an attack he would feel weak, restless and irritable. During a severe attack he would collapse and sleep for about an hour, but would wake up feeling normal. He also suffered from poor memory and was unable to concentrate in class. As a result his grades had been poor and he had had to leave school.

Examination: Skull, heart and lungs normal. Nervous system normal. *Tongue body:* red. *Tongue coating:* thin and white. *Pulse:* wiry and thin.

Diagnosis: Lethargy: imbalance of Yin and Yang.

Treatment: Regulate Yin and Yang Heel Vessels.

Principal Points: Baihui Du 20, Daling P 7 (bilateral), Taixi KID 3 (bilateral). These points were needled seven times, but with no effect.

Revised Points: Jiaoxin KID 8, Fuyang BL 59.

After two treatments the patient's symptoms improved and there were less frequent attacks. After 10 more treatments his symptoms were considerably improved and he was in much better spirits. He was given another course of treatment and the disorder was cured.

Explanation: In TCM narcolepsy is classified as 'lethargy', 'inclination to sleep' or 'oversleep'. The earliest record is in the *Su Wen* (Zhen Yao Jing Zhong Lun chapter, Diagnosis), which states that the disease is a sign of disharmony between Yin and Yang. In the theory of Root and Branch the root of the channels and vessels is located below the elbows and knees, and the branch is located in the head and trunk. The True Qi of the channels starts in the extremities and affects the head, face and trunk. In the *Qi Jing Ba Mai Kao* (Study of the Eight Extraordinary Vessels), Li Shizhen said, 'When the Yang enters the Yin, the person sleeps: when the Yin comes out from the Yang, the person wakes'.

The Yin Heel Vessel starts from the inside of the ankle and ascends along the Kidney channel. The Yang Heel Vessel starts from the outside of the ankle and ascends along the Bladder channel. Both Heel Vessels meet on the inside of the eyelid. They control the movements of the limbs as well as the opening and shutting of the eyelid. The Xi-Accummulation points are where Qi and Blood of the channels and vessels converge. Jiaoxin KID 8, the Xi-Accumulation point of the Yin Heel Vessel, and Fuyang BL 59, the Xi-Accummulation point of the Yang Heel Vessel regulate the two Vessels.

Yin Kejing, ACUPUNCTURE AND MOXIBUSTION SECTION, SHENXI TCM COLLEGE

CASE 3

Chen, female, 42, homemaker

Case registered: 2 November 1983

History: The patient had suffered from narcolepsy since the winter of 1976. The attacks would usually come after breakfast, and she would collapse asleep in the middle of what she was doing. Prescribed stimulants helped only temporarily. Over the last few years the attacks had become more frequent; she would suffer 10 a day, and they would last 10 to 15 minutes. She was diagnosed with 'paroxysmal lethargy', but neither Western nor traditional Chinese medication had proved effective.

Examination: The patient was emaciated. Her breathing was weak and shallow, and she was reluctant to speak. She was tired and her limbs felt heavy, with oedema on the back of both feet. Neurological and physiological tests normal. *Tongue body:* pale. *Tongue coating:* thin and greasy. *Pulse:* soft and weak.

Diagnosis: Lethargy: Deficient Spleen Yang.

Treatment: Warm and strengthen Spleen Yang.

Principal Points: Baihui Du 20, Sanyinjiao SP 6 (bilateral), Zusanli ST 36 (bilateral), Xinshu BL 15 (bilateral).

The needle was inserted to a depth of 1 cun at Xinshu BL 15, angled towards the bottom of the spinous process, and manipulated with rotation, lifting and thrusting until sensation spread to the front of the chest. Baihui Du 20 was needled obliquely. The needles at the other points were inserted deeply and manipulated until sensation spread to the feet. The needles were retained for 15–20 minutes, and manipulated once or twice over this period with reinforcing and reducing equally method.

After 15 treatments there was a big improvement and the attacks became less frequent, occurring only 2–5 times in the afternoons. After 26 treatments the attacks were less severe, of shorter duration and the patient was able to fight them more. After a further eight sessions the disorder was cured. The case was followed up for 3 years and there was no relapse.

Explanation: In TCM lethargy is caused by Deficiency of Yang and Internal Damp. Yang governs activity and Yin governs quietness. If Yang is Deficient and Yin is Excessive, the person will have to sleep.

Zusanli ST 36 strengthens the Qi of the Middle Burner, promotes digestion and Original Qi. Sanyinjiao SP 6, the meeting of the three leg Yin channels, generates Qi in the three Yin channels, reinforces the Spleen and clears Damp. Baihui Du 20, the meeting of the Yang channels with Du Mai, the Governor of Yang, tonifies Yang and calms the mind. Xinshu BL 15 calms the mind and opens the sense organs.

Kong Lingju and Guo Yihua, DA'AN COUNTY TCM HOSPITAL, JILIN PROVINCE
(see The New Chinese Medicine, Issue 11, 1986)

85. Somnambulism

CASE 1

Kang, male, age 63

Case registered: October 1975

History: The patient had had nightmares and talked in his sleep almost every night for 10 years. Whilst dreaming he would get out of bed and walk around, sometimes quarrelling and fighting with people, then return to his bed, remembering nothing when he woke up. He had tried many treatments without success, and was deeply distressed.

Examination: The patient was an articulate and cooperative old man.

Temperature, pulse and BP normal. Heart and lungs normal. Liver and spleen not enlarged. Physiological reflex normal, no pathological reflex induced.

Diagnosis: Somnambulism: Heart and Kidney Yin Deficiency.

Treatment: Calm the mind, regulate Yin and Yang.

Principal Points: Baihui Du 20, Qianding Du 21, Shangxing Du 23, Naohu Du 17, Naokong GB 19 (bilateral), Sishencong (Extra).

The needles were inserted deep to the aponeurosis, then sparse—dense electro-acupuncture was used. The needles were retained for 20 minutes, and treatment was given daily. A course consisted of 10 treatments.

The disorder was cured after two courses, and another two were given to consolidate the result. The case was followed up for 6 months and there was no relapse.

Explanation: In TCM somnambulism arises from malnourishment of the Heart and Mind, and Yin-Yang disharmony. Modern medicine explains the disease as an imbalance in the central nervous system between inhibitory and stimulative functions.

In this case there was a Deficiency of Heart and Kidney Yin causing the mind to be malnourished and an imbalance between Yin and Yang. For this reason points on the head were selected, and electro-acupuncture was used to enhance the effect.

Ma Dingxiang, STOMATOLOGY DEPT, NO. 4 ARMY MEDICAL UNIVERSITY
(see Shenxi Traditional Chinese Medicine, Issue 12,1987)

CASE 2

Liu, male, age 37, cadre

Case registered: 2 June 1963

History: The patient had a previous history of sleepwalking in his childhood. From 1950 the problem had become more frequent and each episode would last longer. Whilst asleep he would get out of bed, run around aimlessly, jump from high places, fire a gun or brandish his sword. He would then return to bed and wake up the next morning with no memory of having left it. At first this would only happen once a month, but it was now happening once a week. He had been treated in many different hospitals for nearly 10 years, but with no effect. He was forced to leave the army and return to his home town in Fujian province, where he received more herbs and acupuncture, but the problem became worse.

Examination: The patient was emaciated. No abnormal findings. *Tongue coating:* thin and white. *Pulse:* thin and weak.

Diagnosis: Deficient Yin failing to control Exuberant Yang, Yin-Yang disharmony.

Treatment: Readjust Yin and Yang.

Principal Points: Hunmen BL 47, Pohu BL 42, Shenmen HT 7, Taichong LIV 3.

The points were reinforced, and treatment given daily. The patient was given 43 treatments over a 2-month period. During this time there was only one episode of somnambulism, and this only lasted 2 minutes. Treatment was discontinued for 6 months at this point, as the patient had other commitments. In March 1964 he received another 15 treatments, and the disorder was cured. The case was followed up till November 1981 and there was no relapse.

Explanation: In TCM, 'the Liver houses the Ethereal Soul (Hun) and the Lung houses the Corporeal Soul (Po)'. Somnambulism occurs at night and is therefore Yin in nature. The *Su Wen* says (Yin Yang Ying Xiang Da Lun chapter, Concept of Yin and Yang), 'The master of the needle induces Yang from Yin and induces Yin from Yang'. This disease was caused by Deficient Yin failing to control Exuberant Yang, and the combination of points strengthened the mind, calmed the Spirit and regulated Yin and Yang.

Huang Zhiguang, FUZHOU MUNICIPAL PEOPLE'S HOSPITAL
(*see Journal of Traditional Chinese Medicine, Issue 3, 1982*)

86. Fear of women

CASE 1

Lin, male, age 28, fisherman

History: The patient had been unable to have sexual relations with his wife since they got married 2 years previously. Each time they tried, he would be so frightened that he would become impotent, with goose pimples and chills, faintness, distress in the chest and palpitations. These symptoms were much worse if she touched him. As the problem progressed he developed pain in the lumbar area and would be unable to sleep for the rest of the night.

Before getting married he had often felt sexual urges and had spermatorrhoea every 1 or 2 weeks. After marrying he was treated with pantocrine, testosterone propionate and chorionic gonadotrophin, as well as some Chinese herbs, but without any effect.

Examination: The patient was well developed. Liver and spleen not enlarged. No abnormalities were found in his head, heart, lungs, abdomen, limbs or exterior genitalia. *Tongue coating:* thin and white. *Pulse:* hollow.

Diagnosis: Deficiency of Kidney and Heart.

Principal Points: Guanyuan Ren 4, Shenmen HT 7, Sanyinjiao SP 6, Shenshu BL 23.

The points were needled with reinforcing and reducing evenly method, with moxibustion at Guanyuan Ren 4 after acupuncture. Needle sensation at Guanyuan was propagated to the tip of the penis. Treatment was given once a day, and the patient was advised to abstain from sex during the course. 2 days later, he reported that his libido was stronger, and that he could maintain an erection for longer periods of time. During sex with his wife the faintness, palpitations, distress in the chest and the chills had not appeared.

Secondary Points: Qihai Ren 6, Yaoyangguan Du 3, Yangwei (Extra)[1], Taixi KID 3, Baihui Du 20.

This group of points was alternated with the principal points to consolidate the treatment. The patient came for four more sessions and the disorder was cured. He wrote 3 months later to say his wife was pregnant, and they had a baby girl later the same year.

Explanation: In TCM this disorder is classified as alarm and anxiety impairing the Kidney and Heart, so treatment is aimed primarily at adjusting the functions of these two organs. Shenmen HT 7, the Shu-Stream point, tranquillizes the mind and calms the Spirit. Guanyuan Ren 4, the Front-Mu point of the Small Intestine and the meeting point of Ren Mai with the three leg Yin channels, is the place where the Qi of the Triple Burner is generated. It strengthens the Kidney and Vital Qi of the body. With moxibustion it strengthens Deficiency in the lower part of the body and warms it. Sanyinjiao SP 6 and Shenshu BL 23 reinforce Kidney Yin. Baihui Du 20 is the meeting of all the Yang and calms the mind. Qihai Ren 6 is the place where Vital Qi is generated, and regulates and reinforces the functional Qi of the Lower Burner as well as the Qi of the Kidneys. Yaoyangguan Du 3 and Taixi KID 3 reinforce Kidney Qi.

---

[1]Yangwei is located in the depression midway between Yaoshu Du 2 and Changqiang Du 1.

From the rapidity of the cure it is clear that the diagnosis and selection of points were correct.

Chen Yijiao and Fang Jinbang, FUJIAN TCM COLLEGE
(see Fujian Traditional Chinese Medicine, Issue 4, 1982)

CASE 2

Li, male, age 28, peasant

Case registered: 10 February 1982

History: The patient was married in October 1981. On his wedding night he and his wife had retired when some mischievous youths who were hiding under the bed leaped out from underneath, yelling and screaming and playing other practical jokes. Ever since, the patient had been unable to go to bed with his wife without feeling faintness, palpitations, distress in the chest, insomnia and impotence. This condition had not responded to Chinese herbs or modern tranquillizers and sedatives, and he was frightened that it might ruin his relationship.

He had a previous history of occasional spermatorrhoea.

Examination: External genitalia were normal. *Tongue coating:* thin. *Pulse:* slow and choppy.

Diagnosis: Heart and Kidney Deficiency disturbing the Shen.

Treatment: Calm the mind, combining acupuncture with psychotherapeutic training.

Principal Points: Xinshu BL 15, Shenmen HT 7, Sanyinjiao SP 6.
'Grain of wheat' shaped embedding needles were used. At Xinshu BL 15 the needles were inserted to a depth of 1 cm. Shenmen HT 7 was needled 0.5 cm above the point and at Sanyinjiao SP 6 the needle was inserted obliquely upwards under the skin.

Auricular Points: Shenmen, Heart, Kidney, Brain and Sympathetic.
Ear tacks were inserted and retained in the ear, alternating from left to right with each treatment. Treatment was given once a day.

The patient was advised to press and rub all the points several times a day, concentrating especially on Shenmen HT 7 and Sanyinjiao SP 6 for 5–10 minutes before going to bed. After 20 days the disorder was cured. In Spring 1985 the patient reported that his wife had given birth to a baby boy.

Zhang Weihua, ACUPUNCTURE AND MOXIBUSTION SECTION, SHENXI TCM COLLEGE
(see The New Chinese Medicine, Issue 7, 1985)

87. Fear of men

Song, female, age 24, peasant

Case registered: 5 August 1979

History: The patient came with her mother, who reported that her daughter had always been very healthy. In October 1978, however, she had begun to be frightened of her husband at night. This fear would intensify if he touched her, and she would develop distress in the chest, palpitations, faintness and her whole body would shudder. She had consulted many doctors but none had been able to help.

As the interview progressed the patient disclosed that she had had a normal sexual appetite before getting married, but the first time she and her husband had had intercourse it had been extremely painful. She had bled profusely afterwards and developed secondary infections, which were cured with treatment. The fear, however, was not.

Her periods were regular, with normal flow and colour.

Examination: Heart, lungs, liver and spleen all normal. Genitalia normal. *Pulse:* deep, thin.

Treatment: Calm the mind, combining acupuncture with psychotherapeutic training.

Principal Points: Xinshu BL 15, Shenmen HT 7, Sanyinjiao SP 6.
'Grain of wheat' shaped embedding needles were used. At Xinshu BL 15 the needles were inserted to a depth of 1 cm. Shenmen HT 7 was needled 0.5 cm above the point and at Sanyinjiao SP 6 the needle was inserted obliquely upwards under the skin.

Auricular Points: Shenmen, Heart, Kidney, Brain and Sympathetic.
Ear tacks were inserted and retained in the ear, alternating from left to right with each treatment. Treatment was given once a day.

The patient was advised to press and rub all the points several times a day, concentrating especially on Shenmen HT 7 and Sanyinjiao SP 6 for 5–10 minutes before going to bed. The patient's husband was asked not to touch her for the first 10 days of treatment and to refrain from sexual intercourse with her for a month. Instead he was advised to sit down and chat with her.

After as little as a week the patient was able to sit freely with her husband and chat without fear, but she would still get nervous if touched. Treatment continued for another 20 days, after which the couple were able to have sexual intercourse without any problem. After 6 months the patient reported that she was 3 months pregnant.

Explanation: Fear of men is a psychological maladaptation, usually due to a disturbance in the autonomic nervous system caused by psychological factors. In this case the cause was the severe pain and secondary infection of the vagina following intercourse for the first time. The doctor followed the principle of 'treating diseases of the Shen by treating the Heart'. Xinshu BL 15 calms the mind and relieves mental strain, Sanyinjiao SP 6 balances Yin and Yang. Shenmen HT 7 is at the wrist joint and is therefore not suitable for subcutaneous needle therapy, but if the needle is inserted 0.5 cm above the point it will reinforce the calming effect of Xinshu BL 15.

The auricular points were used to restore normal balance between the Heart and Kidney, nourish the Blood, calm the mind and enhance activity in the genitals. Embedding needles were used to give continuous stimulation. Psychotherapeutic training was given to help relieve the anxiety and at the same time desensitize the patient. In *Medical Psychology*[1] Shen Geng observes that psychotherapeutic training can reduce the activity of the sympathetic nervous system, reduce oxygen consumption and systolic blood pressure, slow down heart and respiration rates and alter brain waves. The relaxation induced by such training can therefore reduce stress and anxiety.

Zhang Weihua, ACUPUNCTURE AND MOXIBUSTION SECTION, SHENXI TCM COLLEGE
(see The New Chinese Medicine, Issue 7, 1985)

88. Mania

CASE 1

Wang, female, age 17, peasant

Case registered: 24 October 1980

History: The patient's parents reported that the illness had started 10 days previously, when she had got overexcited. She wept for no reason, was restless, unable to sleep and had no appetite. She was emotional and her speech was illogical. Sometimes she was offensive, even aggressive. She was given medication, acupuncture and moxibustion at local town and county hospitals, but did not respond, so her parents brought her here.

Examination: Tongue body: normal. *Tongue coating:* yellow and greasy. *Pulse:* wiry, tight, rapid and slippery.

---

[1]*Medical Psychology,* Renmin Weisheng Press, 1982, p. 117.

Diagnosis: Mania: Exuberant Phlegm Fire rising up to disturb the Mind.

Treatment: Clear Heat in the Heart, remove Phlegm, send down the Turbid Qi and calm the Mind.

Principal Points: Renzhong Du 26, Shaoshang LU 11, Yinbai SP 1, Daling P 7, Shenmai BL 62, Fengfu Du 16, Jiache ST 6, Chengjiang Ren 24, Laogong P 8, Shanxing Du 23, Quchi L.I. 11, Haiquan (Extra). *Needling method:* Renzhong Du 26, 0.3 cun deep; Shaoshang LU 11, 0.3 cun deep; Yinbai SP 1, 0.2 cun deep; Daling P 7, 0.5 cun deep; Shenmai BL 62, Fire needle; Fengfu Du 16, 0.5 cun deep, warm needle; Jiache ST 6, 0.2 cun deep; Chengjiang Ren 24, 0.3 cun deep; Laogong P 8, 0.5 cun deep; Shanxing Du 23, 1 cun deep, oblique insertion; Quchi L.I. 11, Fire needle, 2 cun deep; Haiquan (Extra), bleeding. Treatment was given on Yin dates, i.e. even numbered days, and the points were needled in the order given above. The points were reduced except Fengfu Du 16, and needles were not retained.

After the first two treatments the patient's sleep improved, and she wept and cried less. After the third treatment she was making normal conversation and eating. After the fourth she seemed fully aware and had stopped behaving offensively. Her appetite and sleep had improved but she seemed listless and withdrawn. *Tongue coating:* slightly greasy. *Pulse:* tight, slippery and wiry.

After the sixth treatment all her symptoms had gone and she was discharged as cured. She and her family were advised that she should avoid getting upset. The case was followed up for 3 years and there was no relapse.

Explanation: Mania is caused by disturbance of the Mind resulting in Turbid Phlegm obstructing Qi and impairing the Heart and Mind. The *Lin Zheng Zhi Nan* (A Guide to Clinical Practice with Case Histories) says, 'Mania is caused by excessive alarm or anger. The illness is in the Liver, Gall Bladder and Stomach channels'. Sun Simiao's *Qian Jin Yao Fang* (Important Prescriptions Worth A Thousand Gold Pieces) says, 'For diseases caused by the Hundred Evils treat the Thirteen Points'. The *Zhen Jiu Da Cheng* (Great Compendium of Acupuncture and Moxibustion) records the use of the Thirteen Ghost Points to treat mania.

Renzhong Du 26 is a meeting point of Du Mai with the Large Intestine and Stomach channels and dredges obstructed Yang. Shaoshang LU 11, the Jing-Well point, clears Heat in the Lung. Chengjiang Ren 24 is a meeting point of Ren Mai, Du Mai and the Large Intestine and Stomach channels. It regulates Yin and Yang, clears Heat and regulates Qi. Laogong P 8, the Yong-Spring point, clears the Heart and Mind and removes

Pathogenic Heat. Fengfu Du 16 is a meeting point of Du Mai with the Bladder channel, and a Sea of Marrow point. These five points together resolve Phlegm and refresh the Mind. Reinforcing and reducing evenly method should be used at Fengfu Du 16, and the rest of the points should be reduced.

Daling P 7, the Shu-Stream Yuan-Source point calms the Mind and clears Pathogenic Heat. Yinbai SP 1, the Jing-Well point, calms and refreshes the Mind, reinforces the Qi of the Middle Burner and resolves Phlegm. Haiquan (Extra) refreshes the Mind, removes Fire and soothes alarm. These three points in combination strengthen the body's resistance and calm the Mind. Yinbai SP 1 should be reinforced and the other points should be needled with reinforcing and reducing evenly method.

Shenmai BL 62 is one of the Eight Confluent points of the Extra channels and connects with Du Mai. It activates Qi and Blood and relieves Stasis. Shangxing Du 23 refreshes the sense organs and clears Heat. Jiache ST 6 clears Pathogenic Heat and regulates Stomach Qi. Quchi L.I. 11, the He-Sea point, activates Qi and Blood and readjusts the functions of Defensive and Nutritive Qi. These four points used in combination activate Qi, relieve Stasis, remove Phlegm and dredge obstruction. All four should be reduced.

Jianshi P 5 and Houxi SI 3 can be added as supplementary points to refresh the Mind and resolve Phlegm.

All these points used together reinforce and reduce, dredge and regulate, reinforce the body's resistance to expel pathogens, refresh the Mind, move Stasis and restore the normal flow of Qi, so Clear Qi and the Spirit come and go freely. It is clear from this that the ancient masters crafted their technique flawlessly and effectively. Needling the points on Yin days follows the principle of 'Dredging Yang from Yin'.

Li Shuxian, QINGYANG PREFECTURAL PEOPLE'S HOSPITAL, GANSU PROVINCE
(see *Yunnan Journal of Traditional Chinese Medicine,Issue 2, 1983*)

CASE 2

Yang, male, age 30, worker

Case registered: 21 February 1984

History: The patient's family reported that the patient had become disturbed after an argument: his language became illogical. At work he became very emotional and aggressive, and had to be taken home. He went to a mental institution twice, but his symptoms were not controlled. Gradually he became more restless, crying and singing for no reason. He was unable to sleep, and his language became more and more illogical, sometimes offensive. He would sometimes make an exhibition of himself, for example taking off his clothes in public.

Examination: The patient's face and eyes were red. He was constipated, and urinated little. His language was illogical and offensive, and he spat frequently. He was irritable and restless. *Tongue body:* red. *Tongue coating:* yellow. *Pulse:* wiry, slippery and rapid.

Diagnosis: Mania: Stagnation of Liver Qi, Phlegm disturbing the Mind.

Treatment: Resolve Stagnation of Liver Qi, refresh the Mind by clearing Phlegm.

Principal Points:
1. Jiaji (Extras) at T1, T5, T9, T11.
2. Jiaji (Extras) at T1, T5, T9, T10.

The points were reduced, and the needles were retained and manipulated every 5 minutes for 25 minutes. After the needles were withdrawn the Jiaji at T5 and T9 were cupped. The patient fell asleep during the treatment, and once he got home slept till 6.00 a.m. the next morning. The next day his mind was a little clearer, but his language was still offensive and he was restless.

The second group of points was needled next, reducing and cupping after needling.

After five treatments the patient was much more aware and much less restless. He was speaking normally but he still had heaviness and pain in the head.

Secondary Points: Jiaji (Extras) at T3 and T7.

These points were added to the others, and reduced. Treatment was given for another 3 months: most of his symptoms cleared and he regained his mental health. The case was followed up for 2 years and there was no relapse.

Meng Xianxi, INDUSTRIAL AND COMMERCIAL BANK OF CHINA CLINIC, KAIFENG BRANCH

Editor's Note: This is quite an original treatment for mania. The Jiaji at T1, T5, T9 and T10 refresh and tranquillize the Mind, regulate the functions of the Liver and Gall Bladder, resolve Phlegm and clear the chest. Cupping reinforces the clearing and dredging effects. The Jiaji at T3 and T7 clear accumulated Pathogenic Heat in the Upper Burner to relieve the ache and heaviness in the head.

89. Schizophrenia

CASE 1

Zhang, male, age 25, worker

Case registered: 20 November 1973

History: The patient's mother revealed that he had argued with his family 2 weeks previously and had become disturbed afterwards. He slept badly at night, sometimes not at all, was dizzy and absent-minded and did not want to move. He looked lacklustre and depressed, and had no appetite. He would hide in a corner and talk to himself, crying and smiling at the same time. His language was illogical, and he was pessimistic and suspicious. He had a previous history of mental illness.

Examination: The patient appeared depressed, and was reluctant to speak. His responses to questions were not to the point. Tongue body: pale red. *Tongue coating:* white and greasy. *Pulse:* deep and wiry.

Diagnosis: Depressive psychosis: Stagnation of Liver Qi and Stasis of Phlegm.

Treatment: Eliminate Phlegm, regulate the flow of Qi, relieve mental stress and refresh the Mind.

Principal Points: Renzhong Du 26, Baihui Du 20, Shenmen HT 7 (bilateral), Fenglong ST 40 (bilateral), Sanyinjiao (bilateral).

At Renzhong Du 26 the needle was inserted obliquely upwards and twirled with large amplitude to get strong sensations. The needles were retained for 15 minutes, and treatment was given daily.

After six treatments the heaviness and dull sensation in the head improved, and the patient was able to sleep at night. After six more sessions he was making normal conversation. 24 treatments were given altogether and the disease was cured. The case was followed up for 6 years and there was no relapse.

Explanation: Depressive psychosis is a disturbance of the Mind, and Yin in nature. It is usually caused by Stagnation of Liver Qi and Stasis of Phlegm. The patient's mind and sense organs became dulled, so he spoke little, and his speech was illogical. He wept and smiled unpredictably and his behaviour was very abnormal. Renzhong Du 26 was the key point of the prescription, because it is the intersection of Du Mai with the Large Intestine and Stomach channels, and an important point for mental disorders. The *Xi Hong Fu* (Songs of Xi Hong) says, 'Renzhong

Du 26 is the most effective point for depressive psychosis'. Baihui Du 20 and Shenmen HT 7 relieve mental stress and refresh the Mind. Fenglong ST 40 and Sanyinjiao SP 6 dissolve Phlegm, relieve depression and reinforce the Liver, Spleen and Stomach.

Zhang Dengbu, ACUPUNCTURE AND MOXIBUSTION SECTION, SHANDONG TCM COLLEGE HOSPITAL
(see Heilongjiang Traditional Chinese Medicine, Issue 4, 1983)

CASE 2

Wang, female, age 37, worker

Case registered: 2 April 1982

History: The patient had become mentally disturbed after a traumatic experience 10 years previously and had never fully recovered. She was depressed and pessimistic all the time, and would sit on her own criticizing herself. She also suffered from visual and auditory hallucinations. These symptoms became worse after her divorce. She had headaches and sensations of energy rising to the top of her head. Her stools were dry and towards the end of her period she would get dark blood with clots. She also felt as if something sticky was obstructing her throat. She dreamed a lot, and slept badly. Her EEG was abnormal, and she was diagnosed as a schizophrenic. For 10 years she had gone from one hospital to another looking for effective treatment, and at last came here for acupuncture and moxibustion.

Examination: The patient's complexion was dark, with ecchymosis, and she seemed absent-minded. *Tongue body:* normal. *Tongue coating:* greasy and yellow. *Pulse:* slippery and slightly rapid.

Diagnosis: Depressive psychosis: Phlegm rising up to disturb the Mind, Liver and Gall Bladder disharmony.

Treatment: Regulate the Liver and Gall Bladder, resolve Phlegm and send down the Turbid Qi, relieve mental stress.

Principal Points:
1. Jiaji (Extras) at T5, T10, T11, L2 (all bilateral).
2. Jiaji (Extras) at T5, T10, T12, L2, L3 (all bilateral).

The points in the first group were reduced and the needles retained for 20 minutes. After the needles were removed the points were cupped. For the second treatment all the points in the second group were reinforced except at L3. The needles were again retained for 20 minutes and the points were cupped afterwards.

After two treatments the patient's headache and the sensations of heaviness improved. Her sleep got better and she was a little less anxious. Treatment was continued, alternating the two groups of points. After two more treatments her visual and auditory hallucinations were considerably better. At this point she was advised to make her lifestyle more regular and to avoid emotional overstimulation. After two more treatments she was sleeping even better, the sensations of energy rising up had gone and she felt well and comfortable.

Treatment continued daily. After her 25th treatment she relapsed at the beginning of her period and became distressed. The Jiaji points at T7 were added, and the next day the Jiaji points at L5 were reduced. Treatment continued once every other day for another 5 months, by which time her condition was stable. Another week's consolidating treatment was given, and this chronic disease of 10 years' duration was cured. The case was followed up 2 years later: the patient was back at work and there had been no relapse. An EEG taken in June 1984 was normal.

Meng Xianxi, INDUSTRIAL AND COMMERCIAL BANK OF CHINA CLINIC, KAIFENG BRANCH

Editor's Note: This condition is classified in TCM as depressive psychosis. The doctor got good results by using the Jiaji (Extra) points. These points are located between Du Mai and the Bladder channel. The *Ling Shu* says, 'Depressive psychosis starts from dorsal spasm causing pains in the back. To treat it use the Bladder channel' (*Miraculous Pivot*, Dian Kuang, Manic Depressive Psychosis chapter). This technique is based on the principle of 'inducing Yin from Yang', i.e. treating diseases of Yin nature by selecting points on a Yang channel. In this case the Jiaji points were used to regulate Yin and Yang, refresh the Mind, resolve Phlegm and send down Rebellious Qi.

90. Hallucinations, auditory and visual

Zhang, male, age 15, middle school student

History: Over the last 2 years the patient had seemed to become very lazy. He was unable to concentrate and was doing worse and worse at school. He complained that he could hear people talking about him and could see things spinning around and changing shape. He had a violent temper and occasionally attacked people or property. His condition was diagnosed as adolescent schizophrenia, but he did not respond to treatment, and eventually came for acupuncture and moxibustion.

Diagnosis: Depressive psychosis.

Treatment: Calm the Mind.

Principal Points: Houding Du 19 through to Baihui Du 20, Zhengying GB 17 through to Muchuang GB 16, Luxi TB 19 through to Yifeng TB 17.
The needles were inserted obliquely under the skin and twirled and vibrated for 1–3 minutes to get strong sensation, then retained for 3 hours without manipulation. Treatment was given daily. After 10 treatments the hallucinations disappeared. The patient was able to live a normal and regular life, helping his family with housework, doing exercise and studying hard.

Explanation: Hallucinations are a manifestation of hysteria. In TCM they are classified as depressive psychosis. Generally they can be improved by 10 treatments with head acupuncture. The therapy is safe and has no side effects, acts quickly and gives long-lasting results.

Zhang Mingjiu, TCM DEPARTMENT, NANJING HOSPITAL OF NEUROLOGICAL AND MENTAL DISEASES
(see Journal of Traditional Chinese Medicine, Issue 6, 1987)

91. Hallucinations, olfactory

Xing, male, age 37, worker.

Case registered: 21 October 1986

History: On the morning of 12 August 1986 the patient woke up feeling headachy and sick. He could smell burning cotton but when he searched the house he could not find any. His condition was diagnosed as 'olfactory hallucination' and he was given vitamin B_1 and vitamin C orally. The symptoms did not improve, and he was referred for acupuncture and moxibustion. He had no previous history of mental illness, and there had been no incident which might have triggered the hallucinations.

Examination: The patient seemed fully aware. He spoke fluently and his answers were to the point. Examination of the head, neck, eyes, nose, mouth and ears revealed no abnormalities. Spine and limbs negative. Physiological reflexes normal, no pathological reflexes induced. *Tongue body:* pale red. *Tongue coating:* thin and white. *Pulse:* wiry.

Treatment: Tonify the Lung and Heart.

Principal Points: Lieque LU 7, Neiguan P 6, Yingxiang L.I. 20, Yintang (Extra), Hegu L.I. 4.
The points were reduced, and treatment was given once a day for 10 days. There was no improvement, so auricular points were added.

Auricular Points: Shenmen, Subcortex, Forehead, Internal Nose.
The points were reduced with twirling method once a day. After four

treatments the patient was cured. He no longer smelled burning cotton, and was able to distinguish the smell of alcohol from gas. The case was followed up for 6 months and there was no relapse.

Explanation: In TCM the nose is believed to be the 'opening of the Lung', and the Heart is said to be 'in charge of smelling'. According to the *Ling Shu* (*Miraculous Pivot*, Length of Channels chapter), 'The Qi of the Lung passes through the nose. When the Lung is in harmony, the nose can distinguish smells'. The *Nan Jing* (Book of Difficulties, Difficulty 40) says, 'The Heart is in charge of smelling, and tells the nose to know the smells'.

In Western medicine this disease is caused by a disturbance of the temporal lobe in the brain, or is seen in mentally disturbed patients.

In this case body acupuncture was not very effective, but the success of the auricular points shows that this therapy should not be overlooked. 'The ear is the convergence of the assembled meridians, and goes to the brain.'

Ear Shenmen, Subcortex and Forehead readjust levels of stimulation and inhibition in the cerebral cortex, and are used to treat diseases of the central nervous system. Internal Nose is used to treat nasal diseases.

Wang Fuchun, ACUPUNCTURE AND MOXIBUSTION SECTION, CHANGCHUN TCM COLLEGE HOSPITAL

GENITO-URINARY DISORDERS

92. Hypofunction following ureteroplasty

Feng, female, age 28, cadre

Case registered: December 1983

History: The patient had a congenital stricture of the right ureter, which resulted in hydronephrosis (accumulation of urine in the renal pelvis), renal calculus and renal dysfunction on the right. On 24 November she had ureteroplasty on the right renal pelvis. A week later there was leakage of urine from the incision. On 19 December contrast medium examination via the drainage tube showed marked pyelectasia and caliectasis (dilatation of the renal pelvis and calyx) but the ureter could not be visualized. On 22 December cystoscopic examination showed the bladder and right ureter to be normal but the patient still had low pressure in the right kidney and diminished discharge of urine from the renal pelvis to the ureter. At this point she was referred for acupuncture and moxibustion.

Examination: The patient's general condition was not too bad. Her complexion was pale and her voice was low and thin. She had a drainage tube in her right kidney area. Her urine was clear and light yellow. *Tongue body:* pale. *Tongue coating:* thin and white. *Pulse:* deep and thin.

Diagnosis: Deficiency of Kidney Qi.

Treatment: Nourish Kidney Qi, regulate Qi and Blood.

Principal Points: Sanyinjiao SP 6 (bilateral), Taixi KID 3 (bilateral).

The points were reinforced, then given sparse-dense wave electric stimulation for 20 minutes. After this treatment, for the first time since the operation, there was no leakage of urine around the incision. Treatment was given daily. There was no further leakage. After 12 days the drainage tube was clipped up, and the patient felt no discomfort for 24 hours. Six more treatments were given. Further X-rays of the operation site still showed marked pyelectasis and caliectasis, but the contrast medium now entered the bladder through the ureter. After comparison to the images taken on 19 December, it was clear that the function of the ureter had been restored and the acupuncture was stopped on 21 January 1984.

Explanation: In this case the symptoms were caused by Deficiency of Kidney Qi impairing the digestion. Treatment aims were to reinforce the Kidney Qi and tonify the body's resistance.

Taixi KID 3, the Yuan-Source point, is closely related to the Triple Burner. The *Ling Shu* says, 'When the Five organs are sick, needle the twelve Source points' (*Miraculous Pivot*, Jiu Zhen Shi Er Yuan, Nine Needlings and Twelve Source Points chapter). This point nourishes and reinforces the Kidney channel. When the Kidney is reinforced, renal and ureteric functions will improve.

Sanyinjiao SP 6 is a meeting point of the Kidney, Liver and Spleen channels. It is in charge of Blood. It regulates the Qi and Blood of the Yin channels, activates their physiological functions and benefits urination.

Wang Xianhua, ACUPUNCTURE AND MOXIBUSTION SECTION, SHANDONG PROVINCIAL HOSPITAL

93. Postoperative urinary incontinence

Huo, male, age 50

Case registered: 25 April 1962

History: In June 1960 the patient had two bladder stones removed. During the operation the right ureter was opened to check for obstruction. There were two stones, each 1.8×0.4 cm. Afterwards the site of the operation became swollen, and the patient developed anuria, high fever and headache. The incision was reopened, and it was found that the ureteric opening had not closed. There were problems at the incision: obstruction of urination, adhesion of the bladder wall to the muscle, posterior urethral stricture and extensive infection. These were given standard treatment, but for more than a year there was continuous leakage of urine from the incision, localized swelling and occasional discharge of pus. *Bacillus coli* positive; *Mycobacterium tuberculosis* negative. Later the patient underwent operations for phlegmon (suppurative inflammation of subcutaneous connective tissue) but there was no improvement in his symptoms, and he finally came here for acupuncture and moxibustion.

Examination: The patient was urinating frequently, sometimes as often as 20 times a night. He found urination uncomfortable, with a feeling of pressure. His clothes were often wet with urine. He felt weak and painful all over and was short of breath. His appetite was poor and he was irritable and restless. He looked lacklustre and exhausted.

His lower abdomen was crisscrossed with scars, and urine and a little pus leaked from the unhealed incision. There was swelling around the incision, and pitting oedema in the legs. *Tongue body:* pale. *Tongue coating:* thin and white. *Pulse:* deep, slow and weak.

Diagnosis: Deficiency of Qi and Blood, Spleen Deficiency with retention of Damp.

Treatment: Warm and nourish Qi and Blood, strengthen the Spleen and expel Damp.

Principal Points: Kunlun BL 60 (Extra), Qihai Ren 6, Guanyuan Ren 4.
    At Kunlun BL 60 the needles were inserted with a twist to a depth of 1.5 cun, then light and heavy birdpecking method was used. Needle sensation was propagated to the hips.
    At Qihai Ren 6 and Guanyuan Ren 4 the needles were inserted with finger pressing and twisting method, to a depth of 0.7–1.0 cun. At Qihai Ren 6 the patient felt sensation propagated around the front of the abdomen and the lumbar area along Dai Mai. This is rare, and according to the *Nei Jing* shows that the treatment is effective.
    The needles were retained for 30 minutes and manipulated during treatment to give sensations of soreness, heaviness, numbness and fullness.

Local Points: 3–4 points were needled around the site of the original operation. The needles were inserted 1–1.5 cun deep with finger pressing and twisting method.

After the first treatment the patient's symptoms improved slightly, and after two treatments there was less leaking of urine. After three treatments the leaking stopped and he urinated less often, perhaps seven or eight times a night. He also had more force, so he now produced a steady stream of urine, rather than a series of droplets. His lower abdomen became softer and the oedema subsided. After five treatments his urinary control and frequency were almost normal, except at night if he was tired. His upper abdominal pain disappeared, his abdominal circumference became less and his appetite improved. Some sutures emerged from the incision.

Secondary Points: Zusanli ST 36, Zulinqi GB 41.

These points were added to consolidate the treatment and strengthen the body's resistance. 10 more treatments were given. The oedema gradually subsided. The patient became stronger and stronger, and was able to work part time and do some household chores. He was discharged as cured and the case was followed up for 10 years. He continued to work part-time and had no relapses.

Explanation: Kunlun BL 60 is on the Bladder channel which passes through the bladder organ. Guanyuan Ren 4 is a meeting of the three leg Yin channels with Ren Mai, and Qihai Ren 6 regulates Functional Qi. Together these three points readjust and activate the Bladder, warm the Kidney, invigorate the Functional Qi and activate the circulation of fluids. The local points helped nourish the Kidney Qi and tighten the bladder.

> Xu Dexin, SHANDONG PROVINCIAL INSTITUTE OF MEDICINE AND SCIENTIFIC LABOURING
> *(see Shandong Journal of Traditional Chinese Medicine, Issue 5, 1983)*

94. Ureteric calculus and hydronephrosis

Wu, male, age 33, cadre

Case registered: 29 January 1983

History: The patient had pains in his sides and lumbar region. His hospital diagnosed ureteric calculus and hydronephrosis. He was advised to have surgery, but decided to try acupuncture and moxibustion.

Examination: There was marked pain on percussion of the kidney area.

Urinary red blood cell (+++), protein (+). Nephropyelography showed enlarged shadow of the right kidney: 11 × 7.5 cm.

Diagnosis: Lin syndrome: Damp Heat in the Lower Burner.

Treatment: Clear Damp Heat, expel stone and ease urination.

Principal Points: Jingmen GB 25, Shenshu BL 23, Zusanli ST 36.
    All the points were needled on the right. Jingmen GB 25 was needled to a depth of 1.5 cun, Shenshu BL 23 was needled through to Jingmen GB 25, 4 cun deep, and Zusanli ST 36 was needled 2.5 cun deep. The points were reduced and the needles were retained for 30 minutes and manipulated at 5-minute intervals.
    After 13 treatments the patient passed out a stone which was the same size as the one detected in the nephropyelography. The stone was pale grey and mostly made of calcium. Re-examination by X-ray confirmed that the stone was removed and the patient was discharged as cured. The case was followed up for 4 years and there was no relapse.

Yang Dinglin, SHANGAO MUNICIPAL TCM HOSPITAL, JIANXI PROVINCE.

Editor's Note: Renal and ureteric calculi are classified in TCM as Lin syndrome. The cause is often excessive intake of hot and spicy food, such as hot pepper, so that Damp Heat accumulates in the Lower Burner. The Damp Heat then heats the urine and substances in the urine condense into stones, obstructing the kidney or ureter and causing hydronephrosis.
    Acupuncture is quite effective for this disease. From the above it is clear that not only can it be used to expel the stones and ease urination, but it also relieves the hydronephrosis.
    Jingmen GB 25 is the Front-Mu point of the Kidney, and Shenshu BL 23 is the Back-Shu point of the Kidney. Using the Front-Mu and Back-Shu points together reinforces the Kidney, eases urination, helps to expel stones and relieves obstruction.
    Zusanli ST 36 activates the Middle Burner and helps remove stone obstruction and Damp.

95. Fainting on urination

Zhou, male, age 15

Case registered: 12 May 1983

History: The patient's father reported that since the previous September the boy would lose consciousness when he got up to urinate at night. He would come to after about 5 minutes, and would feel generally weak. His doctors diagnosed nycterine (nocturnal) epilepsy and prescribed him phenytoin sodium and oryzanol. These had no effect, and in the last week he had fainted three times, so he was brought to try acupuncture and moxibustion.

Examination: Blood tests normal. EEG normal. *Pulse and tongue:* normal.

Diagnosis: Retained Pathogen due to Deficiency of Qi, and failure of Clear Yang to rise.

Treatment: Tonify Qi, raise Clear Yang and eliminate Phlegm.

Principal Points: Baihui Du 20, Fengfu Du 16, Yaoqi (Extra), Shenmen HT 7 (bilateral), Zhaohai KID 6 (bilateral), Fenglong ST 40 (bilateral).
   Moxibustion was applied after needling at Baihui Du 20. After three treatments the patient did not faint for a month. Another three consolidating treatments were given. A year later the patient's father wrote to say there had been no relapse and to express his thanks.

Explanation: This illness is very rare. The major symptoms are sudden blackout and loss of consciousness when the patient passes water at night. In TCM this is believed to be due to a disturbance of Functional Yin Qi and Yang Qi, which fail to meet. The head is the uppermost part of the body, and is where the Yang channels meet. On the inside of the head is the Sea of Marrow, and on the outside are the clear orifices. When the Sea of Marrow is full, and the Clear Yang sufficient, the Blood and Qi of the body are in harmony and the orifices are clear. When the Yin is Deficient and the Sea of Marrow is not full, the Liver is malnourished, causing Qi to move about. When the Qi is Deficient it permits pathogenic obstruction and the Clear Yang cannot rise. At night Qi and Blood do not work at full capacity, so the fainting occurs at this time, when the person gets up to urinate. The *Nei Jing* says, 'When the Sea of Marrow is Deficient the brain spins and the ear rings'. Fainting is therefore closely linked to the functioning of the brain.
   Moxibustion after needling at Baihui Du 20 lifts the Clear Yang, as all Wind syndromes and faintness belong to the Liver channel, which connects with Baihui Du 20 at the top of the head. Baihui Du 20 is therefore used to remove Heat from the Liver and calm Internal Wind. 'To treat Wind with acupuncture the first points to use are Baihui and Fengfu.' These points in combination are used to calm Internal Wind and relieve faintness.
   Yaoqi (Extra) is at the lower end of Du Mai. It regulates Yin and Yang and the Functional Qi. Shenmen HT 7 tranquillizes and refreshes the

Mind. Zhaohai KID 6 reinforces Kidney Yin and the brain. Fenglong ST 40 removes Phlegm and clears the orifices to prevent fainting.

Xia Lianqing, ACUPUNCTURE AND MOXIBUSTION SECTION, YIXING COUNTY PEOPLE'S HOSPITAL, JIANGSU PROVINCE

96. Chronic enuresis

Han, female, age 19, worker

Case registered: 6 May 1983

History: The patient suffered from enuresis for 13 years. This happened once or twice a night. She was therefore unable to drink water or porridge at supper. She felt weak, with lumbar pain, weakness in the knees, occasional faintness, and she dreamed excessively. She had various treatments, including medication, acupuncture and moxibustion, but nothing helped.

Examination: The patient looked pale, thin and dispirited. Her hair was dry and withered. *Tongue body:* pale. *Tongue coating:* thin and white. *Pulse:* thin.

Diagnosis: Enuresis: Spleen and Kidney Deficiency.

Treatment: Warm the Kidney and regulate water.

Principal Points: Chengjiang Ren 24, Baihui Du 20, Guanyuan Ren 4.

Secondary Points: Zusanli ST 36 (bilateral), Sanyinjiao SP 6 (bilateral).
    At Chengjiang Ren 24 the needle was inserted obliquely upwards to a depth of 0.3–0.5 cun with reinforcing and reducing equally method. Guanyuan Ren 4 was reinforced, followed by moxibustion for 5–10 minutes. The needles were retained for 20 minutes. Treatment was given once a day, and a course consisted of 12 treatments. After one course the patient's enuresis was less frequent. After two courses there was no more enuresis, and the patient was able to wake up to go to the toilet. Another course of consolidating treatment was given and the disease was completely cured. The case was followed up for 6 months and there was no relapse.

Explanation: Enuresis is defined as involuntary and uncontrolled urination. It may be due to disharmony in the Lung, Kidney, Spleen or Bladder. Most cases are due to poor consolidation of Kidney Qi. When the Kidney Qi is Deficient, the Bladder cannot adjust the water passages.
    Chengjiang Ren 24 is the major point to regulate the water passages. Its use for this purpose is recorded as early as the Western Jin dynasty

by Huangfu Mi in the *Zhen Jiu Jia Yi Jing* (Rudiments of Acupuncture and Moxibustion): 'For reddish or yellowish urination use Chengjiang'. Later generations of doctors, however, have rarely used it for these indications. It is a meeting point of the Ren Mai with Du, Large Intestine and Stomach channels. It does regulate the water passages. The key to using it is correct insertion. The needle should be angled obliquely upwards to a depth of 0.3 cun.

Baihui Du 20 raises the Clear Yang. Guanyuan Ren 4 tonifies Kidney Qi and consolidates control of the Bladder. Zusanli ST 36 reinforces Spleen Qi. Sanyinjiao SP 6 reinforces Liver, Spleen and Kidney Yin, and at the same time consolidates the function of the Bladder to control urination.

Acupuncture and moxibustion at these points warm the Kidney, reinforce Qi, invigorate the Bladder and readjust the water passages.

Zhang Dengbu, SHANDONG TCM COLLEGE HOSPITAL
(see Shandong College Journal of Traditional Chinese Medicine, Issue 1, 1985)

97. Stress incontinence

Yu, female, age 42, accountant

Case registered: 6 September 1979

History: The patient had three children and had had three terminations of pregnancy. Her most recent termination was in the previous July, and she did housework during the time she should have been recuperating. When she returned to work after 2 weeks, the first thing she did was carry bricks. That evening she lost control of her bladder. Some water escaped if she coughed or if there was any pressure on her abdomen. This gradually got worse till she was losing water whenever she stood or walked around. She had to change her trousers several times a day. She had taken traditional Chinese drugs for 20 days without effect.

Examination: The patient's build was normal, and she seemed to have had an average diet. Vagina multiparous. Vesicovaginal wall prominence. Urinary meatus flaccid. Urine would leak out if the bladder area was touched lightly. The incontinence stopped during ureter lifting test. There were large areas of eczema on the medial aspect of the patient's thighs, with bloody strips where she had been scratching.

Diagnosis: Enuresis: Kidney Deficiency and sinking of Qi in the Middle Burner.

Treatment: Tonify the Kidney, strengthen the Qi of the Middle Burner and invigorate the function of the Bladder.

Principal Points:
1. Shenshu BL 23, Sanyinjiao SP 6, Shuidao ST 28.
2. Ciliao BL 32 or Shangliao BL 31, Weiyang BL 39, Shuidao ST 28.

Treatment was giving daily, alternating the two groups. The points were reinforced and the needles were retained for 20 to 30 minutes. A course consisted of 12 treatments. Moxibustion was given after acupuncture at Shuidao ST 28. The patient was advised to contract her anus for 3–5 minutes, 3–5 times a day, to strengthen the pelvic floor muscles. After the first treatment she was incontinent if she sat for a long time or coughed. After four treatments she was only incontinent if she squatted down and deliberately tensed her abdomen. After five treatments there was no incontinence even if she coughed forcefully. After seven treatments she had no symptoms at all. After 12 treatments she was given a rest of 3 days. When she came back she had relapsed slightly because she had caught a cold. Treatment was resumed as before, and after 24 sessions the disorder was cured. The case was followed up for 3 years and there was no relapse.

Explanation: In TCM stress incontinence is classified as enuresis. According to the *Nei Jing*, 'Stress incontinence is poor consolidation of the Bladder'. It is usually due to Kidney Deficiency and sinking of Qi in the Middle Burner.

Reinforcing Shenshu BL 23 and the eight Liao points warms and consolidates Kidney Qi. Reinforcing Sanyinjiao SP 6 tonifies Spleen Qi, regulates and invigorates the Kidney and Liver. Reinforcing Weiyang BL 39, the lower He-Sea point of the Triple Burner and Zhongji Ren 3, the Front-Mu point of the Bladder, consolidates the Lower Burner.

Wang Ghengying, PHYSIOTHERAPY DEPT, CHANGDE COUNTY PEOPLE'S HOSPITAL, HUNAN PROVINCE
(see Shanghai Journal of Acupuncture and Moxibustion, Issue 4, 1985)

98. Urinary retention

CASE 1

Wang, female, age 72, peasant

History: The patient had bacillary dysentery and was treated in hospital. Afterwards she developed urinary retention. A urinary catheter was inserted and retained for 10 days, but it had to be removed after she developed a fungal infection. She was still unable to pass water. Fibre-optic rectoscopy and various X-ray examinations revealed no abnormalities. After another 7 days the patient was still unable to pass water on her own and her lower abdomen was full. Her appetite was poor, her limbs were weak and she had lumbar pain and cold sensations in the knees.

Examination: The patient was dark skinned and emaciated. *Tongue body:* pale and scalloped. *Tongue coating:* thin and greasy. *Pulse:* deep, thin and choppy.

Diagnosis: Urinary retention: Kidney Deficiency with Bladder dysfunction.

Treatment: Reinforce the Kidney and dredge the Bladder to ease the water passages.

Principal Points: Yingu KID 10, Sanyinjiao SP 6.

The points were needled bilaterally and the needles were retained for 30 minutes. The needles were manipulated at 10 minute intervals and reinforced by alternating the angle of insertion to go with and then against the flow of the channels.

Auricular Points: Kidney, Bladder, Ureter, Adrenal, Urethra.

Wang Bu Liu Xing (vacarria seeds) were taped to the points on both ears, and the patient's family were advised to rub them gently three times a day.

Treatment was given daily. After three treatments the patient could urinate easily and the disease was cured. The case was followed up and there was no relapse.

> Gu Pinfang and Wang Jilong, SHANGHAI MUNICIPAL HOSPITAL NO. 8
> *(see Shanghai Journal of Acupuncture and Moxibustion, Issue 4, 1986)*

Editor's Note: Urinary retention is caused by impairment of the digestive and transporting functions, and obstruction of the Bladder. This can arise from different patterns: Heat stagnating in the Lung can obstruct the regulation of the water pathways; Damp Heat in the Middle Burner going down to the Bladder; Deficiency of Kidney Yang in the Lower Burner; weakness of Fire in the Vital Gate failing to transform water and Qi leading to Bladder dysfunction. The most common pattern is impairment of the Bladder and Kidney.

In this case urination was completely obstructed. The patient was old, and weak after a serious illness. Her Kidney Qi was therefore depleted, leading to Bladder dysfunction and urinary retention.

Reinforcing Yingu KID 10, the He-Sea point, tonifies the Kidney. Reinforcing Sanyinjiao SP 6, the meeting of the three leg Yin channels, nourishes the Spleen, Liver and Kidney and removes Damp. The auricular points also tonify the Kidney and induce urination.

CASE 2

Zhou, male, age 26, actor

Case registered: August 1982

History: In April 1975 the patient went on a long distance bus journey. The bus did not stop for a long time and he was unable to relieve himself. Ever since he had difficulty urinating. He could only pass water a drop at a time, and each visit to the toilet would last 3–5 hours. He felt ill, and could not sleep at night. He was prescribed medication, and tried acupuncture and moxibustion in various hospitals, but although his symptoms improved, urination would still take 1–2 hours and this prevented him from working normally.

Examination: The patient looked tired and lacklustre. *Tongue body:* pale. *Tongue coating:* thin and moist. *Pulse:* deep and thin.

Diagnosis: Urinary retention: Deficiency of Kidney and Bladder.

Treatment: Reinforce Kidney Qi and dredge the water passages.
Standard techniques were attempted at first, but without effect. Then Zhibian BL 54 was needled, and sensation was propagated to the genitals. The patient was immediately able to pass water easily. After one course of treatment the disorder was greatly improved. Another course of consolidating treatment was given: the disease was cured and the patient returned to work.

> Zhang Jianqiu, LONG MARCH HOSPITAL, ARMY MEDICAL UNIVERSITY NO. 2
> *(see Shanghai Journal of Acupuncture and Moxibustion, Issue 3, 1984).*

Editor's Note: This patient's disease was caused by circumstances which forced him to deliberately retain his urine. From the symptoms and pulse it is clear that the Kidney was Deficient and the Bladder was weak. The cure was achieved by needling Zhibian BL 54 till sensation reached the affected area. The *Zhen Jiu Jia Yi Jing* (Fundamentals of Acupuncture and Moxibustion) says Zhibian BL 54 is good for 'pain and heaviness in the genitals and difficulty in urination'. This point is therefore good not only for Bi syndrome, but for genital diseases and difficult urination. The key to success is to propagate Qi sensation to the affected area.

99. Chyluria (filariasis)

CASE 1

Xiao, male, age 33, worker

Case registered: 3 October 1968

History: 4 years previously the patient began to pass cloudy, milky urine. He was given treatment to reinforce the Kidney, but his urine became more turbid and milky, even slightly pink. Tests showed red blood cells. Sometimes he urinated clots. His appetite was good, but he began to get thin and weak. Filariasis was suspected but he tested negative. Treatment with hetrazan, antibiotics, haemostats and Chinese herbs produced temporary effects only. His condition would improve, only to relapse, especially if he ate fish, meat or greasy food. When he came to this hospital he complained that some hospitals had turned him away, and he now demanded acupuncture and moxibustion.

Examination: The patient did not look well nourished. His complexion was dark and yellow, and his skin was coarse and swollen. His urine was pink and turbid with clots, but urination was not frequent, urgent or painful. His inguinal lymph nodes were slightly swollen. Mild varicocele. *Tongue body:* pale. *Tongue coating:* white. *Pulse:* deep and hollow.

Diagnosis: Chyluria: Damp Heat in the Lower Burner.

Treatment: Clarify the Clear and dissolve the Turbid, clear Damp Heat and stop bleeding.

Principal Points: Geshu BL 17, Ganshu Bl 18, Pishu BL 20, Sanjiaoshu BL 22, Shenshu BL 23, Xiaochangshu Bl 27, Pangguangshu Bl 28, Sanyinjiao SP 6, Qihai Ren 6, Taixi KID 3.
　　These points were divided into two groups and rotated with each treatment. After 10 treatments there was a noticeable improvement. Fatty and bloody urine relates to the Kidney, so the treatment aims were adjusted to regulate the Kidney and stop bleeding.

Revised Points: Yinbai SP 1, Xuehai SP 10, Guanyuan Ren 4, Guilai ST 29.
　　After three treatments the bleeding stopped and the patient's urine became clear. Five more treatments were given and the disorder was cured.

CASE 2

Xu, male, age 45, purchasing agent

Case registered: 13 April 1975

History: The patient had had intractable chyluria since 1960. He was treated in a Zhejiang hospital for filariasis with prolonged high doses of hetrazan. Treatment was only partially effective, and he had many relapses. He was given two pelvic rinses and treatment with Chinese herbs, but the problem remained. Recently, the symptoms had got worse and he was dispirited and exhausted. He was about to have another pelvic rinse when he heard that this hospital had good results treating this disease.

Examination: The patient's build was normal, but he was malnourished. He was thin, lacklustre and was clearly in pain. No swollen lymph nodes. No oedema in the legs. His skin was not coarse. No scrotal varicocele. Urination was not painful, frequent or urgent. Urine very turbid, milky but no clots. *Tongue body:* pale. *Tongue coating:* white and greasy. *Pulse:* deep and slow.

Diagnosis: Chyluria: Damp Heat in the Lower Burner, Deficiency of Spleen and Kidney.

Treatment: Clear Damp Heat and reinforce Kidney and Spleen.

Principal Points:
1. Zhongji Ren 1, Guilai ST 29, Xuehai SP 10, Yinbai Sp 1, Sanyinjiao SP 6.
2. Shenshu BL 23, Sanjiaoshu BL 22, Qihai Ren 6, Yinlingquan SP 9.

   Treatment started on 13 April. The two groups of points were alternated and treatment given daily. After five treatments there was a clear improvement. An interval of a week was allowed after 15 treatments. When the patient returned he reported that his symptoms had practically gone. Another 15 treatments were given and the case was cured. The case was followed up for 3 years and there was no relapse.

Explanation: These two cases were difficult and intractable. The first case was chyluria with blood, which was cured with 10 treatments. In the second case the chyluria formed clots in the bladder which obstructed urination and had to be forced. After only eight treatments the obstruction was relieved and the urine became normal. This hospital has treated several of these cases, which have usually been cured after one or two courses of treatments. This is proof of the efficacy of acupuncture for the treatment of this disease.

Yang Reichun, ACUPUNCTURE AND MOXIBUSTION SECTION, SHANTOU PREFECTURAL PEOPLE'S HOSPITAL, GUANGDONG PROVINCE
(see the New Chinese Medicine, Issue 8, 1984)

100. Nephroptosis

Wu, female, age 37, peasant

Case registered: 27 September 1969

History: 7 years ago the patient had lumbar pains after jumping across a ditch whilst carrying a heavy burden. This developed into abdominal pain and poor appetite, and she started to lose weight. Ultrasound scans at a Yangzhou hospital showed her left kidney had prolapsed, and she decided to have acupuncture and moxibustion.

Examination: The patient was conscious, but looked severely ill. She could not stand or sit properly. Her abdomen was soft and sunken, and tender on palpation. The aortic pulse was clearly visible. Her entire left kidney was palpable when she was sitting. There were red blood cells in her urine (++++).

Diagnosis: Prolapsed kidney: Sinking of Qi in the Middle Burner.

Treatment: Tonify Qi of the Middle Burner, raise kidney, stop pain.

Principal Points: Shuifen Ren 9, Jiechui (Extra)[1], Sanyinjiao SP 6, Zusanli ST 36.
   The next day the patient's lumbar and abdominal pain improved. Her appetite was better but she still slept badly.

Auricular Points: Shenmen.
   After 10 treatments most of the patient's symptoms had gone. Tests found no red blood cells in the urine, ultrasound scans did not show kidney waves (sic) and the kidney was no longer palpable. 16 consolidating treatments were given, and the patient was discharged as cured. Her weight had increased from 44.5 kg to 51 kg. When she was re-examined at a Yangzhou hospital in February 1970 the position of the kidney was normal.

Explanation: Most cases of kidney prolapse seen in this hospital are on the right, and usually the patients are women. This may have something to do with childbirth. In comparative studies with two groups of patients we have found that proper rest is an essential element of the cure. Extensive propagation of needle sensation and strong stimulation are also important.
   Shuifen Ren 9 connects the Yin channels. Jiachui (Extra) is located on the abdomen. It is an empirical point for nephroptosis. Initially it was

---

[1]Jiechui (Extra) is located 3 cun medial to the anterior superior iliac spine.

selected to relieve the pain that most patients suffer, but it was later discovered that it is also effective in raising the kidney.

Yao Weiliang, YANGZHOU MUNICIPAL TCM HOSPITAL, JIANGSU PROVINCE
(see Jiangsu Journal of Traditional Chinese Medicine, Issue 1, 1981)

101. Chronic nephritis

Zhu, male, age 45, technician

Case registered: 8 January 1981

History: The patient became ill in April 1978 with fever, sore throat, slight oedema in the legs. Urinary protein (+++), urinary red blood cells (+++). This was diagnosed as acute nephritis and chronic nephrotic nephritis. He was treated with Western and traditional Chinese drugs for a year and a half. Urinary protein over a 24-hour period dropped from 6.25 g to 2.92 g, but other indices did not improve. He was then referred for acupuncture and moxibustion. His current symptoms were aching in the waist, heaviness, numbness and slight oedema in the legs.

Examination: Urinary protein (+++ to ++++) with granular casts. Red blood cells (++). Urinary protein over a 24-hour period was 2.92 g. *BP:* 17.9/12.8 kPa (134/96 mmHg). *Tongue body:* pale, slightly swollen and scalloped. *Tongue coating:* thin and white. *Pulse:* thin.

Diagnosis: Oedema: Deficiency of Kidney Yang, retention of Water.

Treatment: Tonify Kidney, Spleen and Liver. Treat Ren and Du Mai to regulate Yin and Yang.

Principal Points:
1. Ganshu BL 18, Pishu BL 20, Shenshu BL 23, Zhishi BL 52, Feiyang BL 58, Fuliu KID 7.
2. Shufu KID 27, Danzhong Ren 17, Bulang KID 22, Jiuwei Ren 15, Qihai Ren 6, Sanyinjiao SP 6, Taixi KID 3.

Ganshu BL 18, Pishu BL 20, Shenshu BL 23, Zhishi BL 52, Shufu KID 27, Danzhong Ren 17, Bulang KID 22 and Jiuwei Ren 15 were reinforced with superficial needling method. The other points were needled with reinforcing and reducing evenly method. The needles were retained for 30 minutes. The two groups of points were alternated, and treatment was given twice a week.

After a year the syndrome improved: the patient's blood pressure returned to normal, urinary protein was (++ to +++), urinary red blood cells 0–5. After another 6 months, urinary protein over a 24-hour period dropped 0.54 g and stayed between trace levels and (+). The kidney function became normal. Consolidating treatment was given once a week thereafter.

Explanation: In TCM the Kidney is considered to store Essence, taking nourishment from the other organs and storing it. Protein is one of the basic substances of life and forms the Kidney Essence. Chronic nephritis is usually a Deficiency condition. It can arise from Yin Deficiency or Yang Deficiency, but Yang Deficiency is more common. In this hospital Yang Ci (centro-square needling) technique and Ci Wei (superficial needling) technique from the *Nei Jing* and the *Nan Jing* are used.[1]

Points on the Kidney, Liver and Spleen channels and the related Back-Shu points were reinforced with superficial needling. This is because the Kidney is the Prenatal origin of Qi, and the Spleen is the Postnatal origin. The Liver and the Kidney share the same source. Danzhong Ren 17 and Qihai Ren 6 tonify Qi. When the body resistance is strengthened it removes pathogens and consolidates the Kidney, resulting in a drop in urinary protein.

From January 1980 to September 1981 this hospital saw 15 cases of chronic nephritis. These were either Yin or Yang Deficiency patterns. The same points prescription was given, with the following modifications:

Chills: moxibustion at Dazhui Du 14, Mingmen Du 4, Guanyuan Ren 4

Yin Deficiency: Jingmen GB 25, Geshu BL 17

Facial oedema: Renzhong Du 26, Yinlingquan SP 9, Sanjiaoshu BL 22, Pangguangshu BL 28

Hypertension: Taichong LIV 3, Zusanli ST 36

Insomnia: Fengchi GB 20, Yongquan KID 1

External Pathogen: Dazhui Du 14, Shenzhu Du 12, Lieque LU 7

Sore throat: Hegu L.I. 4, Tianrong SI 17

Chest pain: Shufu KID 17, Bulang KID 22

Poor kidney function: Jiaji (Extras) at T5–T7.

Results: clear effects in five cases, some effects in three cases and no effects in seven cases. In some cases immunoglobulin was measured, and low levels were seen to normalize after treatment.

We have reports on the treatment of acute nephritis with acupuncture and moxibustion, but there is little information on the treatment of chronic cases. In Western medicine there are no specific effective treatments for chronic nephritis, but it is possible that the combination of Western medicine and TCM would give relatively good results. Of the above-mentioned cases, 10 had a chronicity of 5 or more years.

---

[1]Yang Ci – centro-square needling: one needle is inserted superficially at the centre of the affected area and another four are inserted in a square around it. Indicated for widespread, superficial Cold Bi syndrome.

In our 2½ years of observation, we have concluded that acupuncture and moxibustion to 'reinforce the body resistance to resolve pathogens' can partially relieve the symptoms in chronic cases, reducing urinary protein and readjusting the immune system. It is most effective in Yang Deficiency patterns.

Case treated by Xi Yongjiang et al, case study by Pu Yunxing and Xi Depei, SHANGHAI TCM COLLEGE YUEYANG HOSPITAL
(see Correspondence, Journal of Acupuncture and Moxibustion, Issue 1, 1987)

102. Impotence

CASE 1

Zhou, male, age 32, married

Case registered: 19 February 1964

History: The patient had been impotent for 5 years. The problem started in June 1959 when his wife collapsed during intercourse. In September of that year he went to hospital many times to have his sperm tested, but found it very difficult to produce a sample. Eventually he did, but with great difficulty. Tests showed: sperm count 32 000 000/ml, motility 30%. Some sperm were malformed.

From 1960 the patient was prescribed herbal decoctions and powders as well as hormones, but none of these helped. He was also given 30 acupuncture treatments, also to no avail. In January 1964 he was given intramuscular injections of testosterone propionate: 25 mg once every 2 days. After 8 days he felt dull pain in his right abdomen and in his testicles. The treatment was discontinued and his symptoms remained unchanged. He then came to the acupuncture and moxibustion section of this hospital.

Examination: The patient looked thin and tired. *Pulse:* wiry in the middle position and weak in the proximal position.

Diagnosis: Impotence: Disharmony of Liver and Kidney, sluggish Kidney Yang.

Treatment: Clear the Liver, tonify and invigorate the Kidney Yang.

Principal Points: Qihai Ren 6, Guanyuan Ren 4, Shenshu BL 23, Mingmen Du 4, Sanyinjiao SP 6, Guilai ST 29, Ciliao BL 32, Zhongji Ren 3.

Secondary Points: Xinshu BL 15, Ganshu BL 18, Danshu BL 19, Zusanli ST 36, Taichong LIV 3, Taixi KID 3.

3–4 points were needled at a time. Needling to produce sensations of heat method was used at Qihai Ren 6, Guanyuan Ren 4, Zhongji Ren 3, Guilai ST 29, till sensation was propagated to the penis. Moxibustion was given after needling.

After four treatments the patient began to have erections in the morning and at night, or if his bladder was full. When his wife came to visit him on 25 February the couple were advised to have intercourse, to quantify any improvement. This was relatively successful: he was able to manage a partial erection, and had a premature ejaculation. He was very much encouraged by this.

During his acupuncture treatments Qi sensation was strongest at Guanyuan Ren 4, Qihai Ren 6 and Guilai ST 29. He was advised to give himself moxibustion for 10 to 15 minutes every night at one of these points. By 10 March he was much improved. When he felt aroused in the mornings or evenings he could maintain an erection for over 5 minutes. On 20 March his wife came to see him and they had sexual intercourse, which was mutually satisfactory. His sperm was tested again that day: sperm count 8 400 000/ml, sperm motility 80%. No malformation of sperm cells. *Pulse:* normal, and only slightly weak on the Kidney position. To consolidate the treatment he was told to give himself regular moxibustion at Guanyuan Ren 4, Qihai Ren 6, Mingmen Du 4 and Shenshu BL 23. The disorder was cured with 24 sessions of moxibustion.

Guan Zunhui, KUNMING MUNICIPAL TCM HOSPITAL YUNNAN PROVINCE
(see Journal of Traditional Chinese Medicine, Issue 9, 1964)

Editor's Note: Impotence and premature ejaculation can be caused by Deficiency of Kidney Qi which depletes the Kidney Yang, or impairment of Kidney Qi by fear or fright which obstructs the Kidney Yang. In this case the patient had been frightened when his wife had collapsed during intercourse, and the fear had obstructed the Kidney Yang and caused disharmony in the Liver and Kidney. Taichong LIV 3, Ganshu BL 18 and Danshu BL 19 regulate the Qi of the Liver and Gall Bladder. Shenshu BL 23, Mingmen Du 4, Guanyuan Ren 4, Qihai Ren 6 and Taixi KID 3 invigorate Kidney Yang. Moxibustion strengthens the Kidney Yang and tonifies the whole body.

CASE 2

Xu, male, age 29, sailor

Case registered: 2 April 1983

History: The patient had been married for 3 years. At first he had no problems during sex, but once when at sea he caught a fever during some cold weather. Ever since he had felt faint and weak, with dull pains in the lumbar region, knees and lower abdomen. In the last year he suffered from premature ejaculation and occasional impotence.

Examination: The patient's complexion was ashen. *Tongue body:* pale. *Tongue coating:* thin and white. *Pulse:* soft and thin.

Diagnosis: Impotence: Kidney Yang Deficiency.

Treatment: Nourish and reinforce Kidney Yang.

Principal Points: Guanyuan Ren 4, Shenshu BL 23, Ciliao BL 32, Taixi KID 3.
    The points were reinforced with lifting and thrusting method, and at Guanyuan Ren 4 sensation was propagated to the penis. The needles were retained for 15 minutes.

Secondary Points: Shenque Ren 8, Qihai Ren 6, Mingmen Du 4, Sanyinjiao SP 6.
    Reinforcing moxibustion was given. After two treatments the patient had an erection. After five treatments he could manage a partial erection if he tried to arouse himself. At this point he was asked to refrain from sex for a while. After 12 treatments he was able to have normal erections. The case was followed up 6 months later, and the patient's sex life was normal.

Explanation: Impotence is usually due to Deficiency of the Liver and Kidney. The patient was exposed to cold, and his symptoms were caused by consumption of Kidney Qi after disease.
    Ciliao BL 32 was selected because of the Exterior–Interior relationship of the Bladder to the Kidney, and was used to activate the Qi of the Bladder channel. Shenque Ren 8, Qihai Ren 6, Guanyuan Ren 4, Taixi KID 3, Mingmen Du 4, and Shenshu BL 23 invigorate the Kidney Yang and direct energy to the genitals. Sanyinjiao SP 6 works with Shenshu BL 23 and the other points to regulate the Liver and Kidney. When the Kidney Qi became strong, the disease was cured.

Zhang Weimin, NANTONG MEDICAL COLLEGE HOSPITAL
(see *Journal of Traditional Chinese Medicine, Issue 8, 1985*)

103. Impotence with testicular pain

Zhang, male, age 38, cadre

Case registered: 18 December 1981

History: Over the last 2 months the patient suffered from bouts of pain in the testicles, which felt icy cold, especially on the right. He was unable to get an erection. He also had cold pains in the lower abdomen and legs, especially early in the morning and at night. He caught colds frequently.

Examination: The patient looked tired and lacklustre. *Tongue body:* dark red. *Tongue coating:* white. *Pulse:* deep and slow.

Diagnosis: Periumbilical colic due to invasion of Pathogenic Cold.

First Treatment: Lieque LU 7, Zhaohai KID 6, Guanyuan Ren 4, Zhongji Ren 3, Mingmen Du 4.

These points were selected according to the Ling Gui Ba Fa, 'Eight Point Selection' or 'Eight Wise Turtle Methods'. The time was Stem 8, Branch 6, the date was Stem 7, Branch 7, the month was Stem 7, Branch 1, and the year was Stem 8, Branch 10.

Lieque LU 7 and Zhaohai KID 6 were opened with reinforcing method. Warm needle was used at Guanyuan Ren 4 and Zhongji Ren 3, using a G2H warm needling unit. Moxibustion was given at Mingmen Du 4. The pain improved after this treatment.

Second Treatment: Lieque LU 7, Zhaohai KID 6, Guanyuan Ren 4, Qichong ST 30.

The time was Stem 10, Branch 6, the date was Stem 8, Branch 8. Lieque LU 7 and Zhaohai KID 6 were opened with reinforcing method. Warm needle was used at Qichong ST 30, and moxibustion was given at Guanyuan Ren 4.

After four of these treatments the patient had no more pain in the testicles. After 12 treatments he felt warm in his lower abdomen and testicles. The case was followed up for 6 months: there was no relapse, and the patient's impotence also improved.

Explanation: The *Su Wen* says, 'Disease in the Ren Mai (Conception Vessel) causes the Seven Hernias' (Gu Kong Lun, Bones chapter). The *Qi Jing Ba Mai Kao* (Study of the Eight Extraordinary Vessels) says, 'Disease in the Yin Qiao Mai (Yin Heel Vessel) causes pain in the lower abdomen, contraction and pain in the genitals affecting the waist and hips. This is called scrotal hernia'. Lieque LU 7 leads to Ren Mai, and Zhaohai KID 6 leads to Yin Qiao Mai. These points are two of the Eight Confluent points. The *Mai Jing* (Pulse Classic) Vol. II says, 'When there is disease in Ren Mai (Conception Vessel) which is worse for movement, there is periumbilical pain in the lower abdomen which affects the pubic bone and causes testicular pain. Use the point 3 cun below the navel'. Warm needling at Guanyuan Ren 4, Zhongji Ren 3 and Qichong ST 30 expels

Pathogenic Cold from the channels, invigorates Qi and supports Yang. When the Cold was expelled the pain went.

Guan Zunhui, KUNMING MUNICIPAL TCM HOSPITAL, YUNNAN PROVINCE
(see Journal of Traditional Chinese Medicine, Issue 3, 1987)

104. Contraction of the penis

CASE 1

Lan, male, age 42, technician

History: The patient had a previous history of masturbation. After getting married he experienced impotence and premature ejaculation. Recently he had sensations of cold and constriction in the lower abdomen. A few days later his penis contracted. He had chills and was averse to cold. His limbs were cold, but he had no fever.

Examination: The patient was nervous and looked pale. His penis was contracted. *Tongue coating:* thin and white. *Pulse:* deep, rapid and thin.

Diagnosis: Flaccid constriction of the penis: Stagnation of Cold in the vessels and tendons, Deficiency of Kidney Yang.

Treatment: Tonify Kidney Yang, warm the channels to disperse Cold, relax the tendons and activate the collaterals.

Principal Points: Guanyuan Ren 4, Shenshu BL 23, Sanyinjiao SP 6, Taichong LIV 3, Neiguan P 6.

The points were reinforced, and the needles were retained for 20 minutes, with manipulation every 10 minutes. Moxibustion was given after needling at Guanyuan Ren 4 and Shenshu BL 23. After the first treatment the patient felt an improvement in the contraction, chills and aversion to cold. After 3 days all his symptoms were gone. The disease was completely cured after 20 days of treatment. The patient was advised to apply moxibustion regularly to Guanyuan Ren 4 and Shenshu BL 23 to reinforce the Kidney and his general health. The case was followed up for 6 years and there was no relapse.

Explanation: Flaccid constriction of the penis is usually due to congenital deficiency, or excessive sex damaging the Kidney Qi. The symptoms are usually feelings of cold, cold limbs, pale complexion, impotence, premature ejaculation, and a deep, thin pulse. The Yang is weak and exhausted, and cannot warm the body, so Pathogenic Cold stagnates in the tendons and vessels. Cold contracts things, which leads to arthralgia and constriction of the tendons and muscles.

The *Ling Shu* says, 'The tendons of the Liver channel . . . join in the genitals and are related to the collateral . . . when exposed to Cold the genitals contract' (Jing Jin, Channels and Tendons chapter). The *Su Wen* says, 'All Cold and constrictions are in charge of the Kidney' (Zhi Zhen Yao Da Lun, The Truest and Most Important chapter). The Liver channel goes through the genitals, to which all the large tendons lead. The Kidney opens at the two Yin orifices. When the Liver and Kidney are heavy and cold there will be flaccid constriction of the penis.

The classics stress the interrelation between the Liver and Kidney. Kidney disease can cause Liver disease. In this case weakness of the Kidney Yang caused dysfunctional Liver Blood, which then did not nourish the tendons and caused the symptoms. The root of the disease was in the Kidney, and the symptoms were in the Liver.

Treatment used the principle of 'treating disease by addressing the root', reinforcing the Kidney Yang, warming the channels, dispersing Cold, relaxing the tendons and activating the collaterals.

Kidney Qi flows to Shenshu BL 23, the Back-Shu point. so it can be used to reinforce Kidney Yang. Guanyuan Ren 4 is where the congenital Yin and Yang are housed. Located on the lower abdomen it is an important point to reinforce the Kidney Yang. Sensation can be propagated from here to the genitals, causing redness or heat in the local area and relieving the contraction. Sanyinjiao SP 6 is the meeting point of the three leg Yin channels and treats diseases in all three channels. When used together with Taichong LIV 3, the Yuan-Source point, it removes cold from the Liver, relaxes the tendons and activates the collaterals. Neiguan P 6, the Luo-Connecting point, nourishes the Heart and calms the Mind.

Shi Jiaping, ACUPUNCTURE AND MOXIBUSTION SECTION, JIANXI TCM COLLEGE
(see Journal of Traditional Chinese Medicine,Issue 5, 1987)

CASE 2

Yu, male, age 38, cadre

Case registered: 2 December 1967

History: The patient's wife reported that the problem started at about 10.00 p.m. the previous night. The initial symptoms were general weakness, aching in the waist and knees, cold limbs and chills followed by contraction of the penis.

Examination: The patient looked weary and lacklustre. His voice was low and weak. His penis and scrotum were contracted and his lower abdomen was very tender. There were no other abnormal findings. *Tongue body:* pale. *Tongue coating:* thin and white. *Pulse:* deep, thin and weak.

Diagnosis: Flaccid constriction of the penis: Invasion of Pathogenic Cold into the Liver channel.

Treatment: Warm the channels to disperse Cold and relax the tendons.

Principal Points: Jimai LIV 12, Qihai Ren 6, Guanyuan Ren 4, Zusanli ST 36, Shenshu BL 23, Sanyinjiao SP 6.
   At Jimai LIV 12, Qihai Ren 6 and Guanyuan Ren 4, 1–3 cun needles were used. These were angled towards the penis and inserted 0.5–1 cun deep, and sensation was propagated to the penis. At Zusanli ST 36 the needle was inserted 1.5 cun deep. The needles at the above points were retained for 15 minutes. At Shenshu BL 23 the needles were inserted quickly, to a depth of 0.5–1 cun, and withdrawn immediately without rotation. At Sanyinjiao SP 6 the needle was inserted obliquely upwards to a depth of 0.5–1 cun deep, and retained for 15 minutes. Moxibustion was given at Shenshu BL 23 and Sanyinjiao SP 6 for 15 minutes, using seven moxa cones. The treatment was given three times, with a rest of 15 minutes in between treatments. The patient's penis gradually grew back to size and the disorder was cured.

Explanation: Flaccid constriction affects the genitals in both men and women. In this case Pathogenic Cold invaded the Liver channel, stagnating Qi and Blood which caused contracture of the tendons and muscles. Jimai LIV 12 disperses Pathogenic Cold in the Liver channel to stop contracture. Qihai Ren 6 and Guanyuan Ren 4 warm the Yang, and reinforce and regulate Qi and Blood. Zusanli ST 36 and Sanyinjiao SP 6 strengthen the Spleen and Stomach. Shenshu BL 23 strengthens the organs, especially the Kidney. The combination of moxibustion with acupuncture reinforced the effect of both therapies to warm the Kidney Yang.

Peng Yuge, NANCHENG COUNTY PEOPLE'S HOSPITAL, JIANXI PROVINCE
(see Shenxi Traditional Chinese Medicine, Issue 7, 1984)

CASE 3

Fu, male, age 32, cadre

Case registered: 2 March 1982

History: 6 months previously the patient's penis had contracted after a fit of anger. He took herbs for 2 days and the problem disappeared. Recently he had been angry again and the problem recurred. This time it did not respond to herbs and he called this hospital for an emergency home visit.

Examination: The patient was flushed and sweating on his forehead and face, but his hands and feet were cold. He was anxious and looked as if he was in considerable pain. His penis was contracted to 2 cm and he felt cold. *Tongue body:* dark red and contracted. He was unable to protrude it. *Tongue coating:* thin and white. *Pulse:* deep, wiry and rapid.

Diagnosis: Flaccid constriction of the penis: Liver Qi Stagnation, disturbance of Functional Qi, Deficiency and Cold in the Lower Burner.

Treatment: Relieve Stagnation of Liver Qi, regulate Functional Qi by reinforcing and reducing at the same time.

Principal Points: Baihui Du 20, Yintang (Extra), Zhongchong P 9, Ximen P 4, Dadun LIV 1, Guanyuan Ren 4, Qihai Ren 6.

Dadun LIV 1 was bled, and the other points were first reinforced, then strongly reduced with lifting and thrusting. The patient's symptoms improved after 10 minutes. His colour became normal, he sweated less, his hands and feet became warm and contracture disappeared. The patient was then brought to the hospital for more treatment to address the root. He had a mild relapse after an hour, but this was controlled with a repeat prescription. After 2 weeks in hospital he was completely cured. The case was followed up for a year and there was no relapse.

Explanation: Flaccid constriction is a functional disturbance of the Liver channel. The *Ling Shu* says, 'When the Qi of the Liver channel is dead, the tendons are dead. The Liver channel is where the tendons join. The tendons converge in the genitals and connect with the tongue through the collaterals. When the channel is not nourished the tendons contract, causing the tongue and the genitals to contract and the lips to become dark'. In this case anger had disturbed the flow of Liver Qi. Symptoms were Heat in the upper part of the body and Cold in the lower part, and contracture of the tongue and penis.

Liu Leigeng, ACUPUNCTURE AND MOXIBUSTION SECTION, DAXIAN PREFECTURAL TCM HOSPITAL SICHUAN PROVINCE
(see Shenxi Traditional Chinese Medicine, Issue 7, 1984)

CASE 4

Mo, male, age 74

Case registered: 28 September 1974

History: The previous night the patient watched a film, then suddenly felt discomfort and lower abdominal fullness. By 3.00 p.m. the next day, he had contracture of the penis with difficulty in urination. After 5 hours the fullness in the lower abdomen was very severe, and his penis had completely retracted into his body. He also had pain in the waist, difficulty talking and was only able to lie on his side. Modern drugs had no effect.

Examination: Blood pressure, temperature, pulse and respiration normal. The patient was lying on his left side with his knees bent. He was conscious, but looked pale, nervous and lacklustre, and was clearly in great pain. Heart sounds were normal. Respiration sounds were slightly thin on both sides. His abdomen was flat, and the abdominal wall was slightly tense. His penis was completely withdrawn, only skin was visible.

Diagnosis: Flaccid constriction of the penis: Kidney Yang Deficiency.

Treatment: Reinforce the Kidney Yang and relieve contracture.

Principal Points: Guanyuan Ren 4, Changqiang Du 1.
The points were stimulated strongly, and the needles retained for 8 minutes. 5 minutes after Guanyuan Ren 4 was needled the patient was feeling better. By the time the needles were withdrawn he had regained his facial colour and was healthy, cheerful and able to speak. The next day he still felt fine.

Xie Mingde, GUANGXI BOTANY INSTITUTE CLINIC
(see Guangxi Traditional Chinese Medicine, Issue 6, 1982)

Editor's Note: In this case the patient was an old man in his seventies, whose Kidney Qi was weak. When he was tired and exposed to cold, Pathogenic Cold invaded the Liver channel. The Liver is in charge of the tendons which go around the genitals, which gave rise to these symptoms.
Guanyuan Ren 4 is the meeting of Ren Mai with the three leg Yin channels, and is an important point to reinforce the Kidney Yang. Changqiang Du 1 is the Luo-Connecting point, and a meeting point of Du Mai with the Kidney and Gall Bladder. It therefore nourishes and reinforces the Lower Burner. Together these points strongly tonify the Kidney Yang, expelling Cold and relieving contracture.

105. Priapism

D, male, age 25, soldier, foreigner

Case registered: 23 November 1979

History: The patient was admitted to hospital on 12 November 1970 after he had had an erection for a whole week. He was prescribed diazepam, and given intramuscular injections of wintermin, as well as blocking anaesthesia in the lumbosacral vertebrae, but there was no improvement. He was then referred for acupuncture and moxibustion. By now he had had an erection for over 20 days, even when he was asleep. The erection was painful and he was distressed and restless. He was not married, but was sexually experienced.

Examination: The patient was large and strong. His penis was erect and 16 cm long (6.3"), causing difficulty putting on clothes and with other activities. There was no emission. Urine was yellowish. *Tongue body:* slightly red at the tip. *Tongue coating:* thin, white and dry. *Pulse:* wiry and slightly rapid.

Diagnosis: Pathogenic Heat in the Liver, Gall Bladder and Heart, Deficiency of Kidney Yin.

Treatment: Nourish Kidney Yin, clear Heat in Liver and Gall Bladder.

Principal Points:
1. Taichong LIV 3 through to Yongquan KID 1, Taixi KID 3, Ciliao BL 32.
2. Sanyinjiao SP 6, Zhaohai KID 6, Shenmen HT 7, Huiyin Ren 1.

Treatment was given every day, rotating the two groups of points. All the points were needled bilaterally and reduced strongly, then connected to an electro-acupuncture unit. After six treatments there was a noticeable improvement in the erection and pain. The patient's penis reduced in size to 8 cm (3.1") and was no longer rigidly erect. After 12 treatments it was normal. He was detained for observation for 2 weeks, but there was no relapse and he was discharged as cured.

Explanation: This disease has been recorded in many generations of medical literature. The *Ling Shu* says, 'In diseases of the Liver channel, Pathogenic Heat causes persistent erections' (Channels and Tendons chapter). Herbal prescriptions for this disease have been recorded, but in clinic acupuncture has rarely been used.

Diseases of the penis are rooted in the Ren, Du and Liver channels. Many different channels pass through the genitals: the Liver main channel, divergent channel, tendino-muscular channels and collaterals all pass through here. Liver Wood is the house of Ministerial Fire. In a strong youth Heat is Exuberant. Exuberant Heart Fire triggers Ministerial Fire, which burns upwards causing priapism. In other cases Excess Heat harms the Yin, so the tendons are not adequately nourished and kept moist. This can also lead to priapism.

The Liver and Gall Bladder are an Interior–Exterior pair. The Gall Bladder also leads to the Heart, so the patient was restless and anxious.

The pain in the patient's penis, yellowish urine, dry tongue with red tip, and wiry and rapid pulse are all signs of Exuberant Heat in the Heart and Liver Channel.

Taixi KID 3, Zhaohai KID 6, Taichong LIV 3 through to Yongquan KID 1 were used to clear Pathogenic Fire and Heat. Shenmen HT 7 clears Heart Fire and calms the Mind. Ciliao BL 32 clears Pathogenic Heat in the Bladder and activates the channels and collaterals. Huiyin Ren 1 activates Ren and Du Mai and regulates the Functional Qi. All these points nourish Yin to clear Fire, according to the principle of 'strengthening Yin to suppress Yang'. When Yin Water is sufficient, the Fire is controlled, the Liver Wood is soothed and the disease is cured.

Yang Jiebin, CHENGDU TCM HOSPITAL
(see Correspondence Journal of Acupuncture and Moxibustion, Issue 2. 1987)

106. Hypersensitivity of the glans penis

Male, age 58

Case registered: 12 March 1987

History: For the last year the patient had had two points on the glans of his penis which were extremely sensitive and painful. Initially he felt shocking pain when he touched them, but later even the touch of his clothes became painful. The condition was diagnosed as 'balanic hyper-algia' and he was prescribed medication, and eventually referred for acupuncture and moxibustion. He had no relevant previous history. His reproductive functions were normal.

Examination: The patient was overall in good condition. Examination of his genitals found nothing abnormal, except two bean-sized hypersensitive areas. One was by the urinary meatus, and the other was lateral to the coronary sulcus of the balanus.

Treatment: Dredge the channels and collaterals and regulate the Functional Qi. Stop medication.

Principal Points: Guanyuan Ren 4, Sanyinjiao SP 6.
  Both points were reduced with twirling, lifting and thrusting method to move Qi. At Guanyuan Ren 4 sensation was propagated to the glans. The needles were manipulated to maintain sensation for 10 minutes. The tenderness improved after the treatment. Treatment was given once a day for 10 days, and the disease was cured. The case was followed up after 3 months and there was no relapse.

Explanation: This is a very rare disease. Tests ruled out the possibility of organic disease.

Guanyuan Ren 4 and Sanyinjiao SP 6 are closely related to the Liver channel, which travels through the genitals. Guanyuan Ren 4 is where the three leg Yin channels meet Ren Mai, the governor of all diseases in the Yin channels. Sanyinjiao SP 6 is the group Luo -Connecting point of the three leg Yin channels, and is an important point for urogenital diseases. Together these two points activate the channels and collaterals and regulate the Functional Qi. When the Qi moves freely the pain is relieved.

Xu Shibiao, NANNING TCM MUNICIPAL HOSPITAL, GUANGXI
(see Guangxi Traditional Chinese Medicine, Issue 6, 1987)

107. Spermatorrhoea, persistent

Yuan, male, age 51, cadre

History: The patient had had spermatorrhoea three or four times a month since he was a young man. Medication had not helped. Recently the problem had got worse because he had had a relapse of hepatitis. He felt dizzy, his head felt dull and heavy and he had lower backache. His appetite was poor and he was losing weight.

Examination: The patient looked thin and tired. *Tongue body:* red tip and edges. *Tongue coating:* thin, yellow and greasy.

Diagnosis: Spermatorrhoea: Accumulation of Damp Heat with underlying Kidney Yin Deficiency.

Treatment: Nourish the Qi of the Middle Burner, nourish Kidney Yin, clear Damp Heat.

Principal Points: Shenshu BL 23 (bilateral), Zhishi BL 52 (bilateral), Guanyuan Ren 4, Qihai Ren 6, Sanyinjiao SP 6 (bilateral).

Secondary Points: Zhongji Ren 3, Ciliao BL 32 (bilateral), Zusanli ST 36 (bilateral).

The points were reinforced with twirling method, the needles were reinforced for 15 minutes, then moxibustion was given. Treatment was given daily. After a week the patient had no spermatorrhoea, and his lumbar pain and appetite improved. Laboratory tests showed that his transaminase levels had dropped from 400 to 190. Over the following 2 weeks points from the two prescriptions were alternated and treatment was given every other day. 20 treatments over a period of 4 weeks were given in total, and the patient had no further loss of sperm. Re-examination showed that his liver function was now normal. The case was followed up for a year and there was no relapse.

Explanation: In this case the disease had lasted for 30 years. It was aggravated by the bout of hepatitis, which indicated that it was due to Deficiency of Yin which was unable to control the sperm. There were also signs of accumulation of Damp Heat.

Qihai Ren 6, Guanyuan Ren 4 and Zhongji Ren 3 nourish the Kidney Qi. Sanyinjiao SP 6 and Shenshu BL 23 nourish the Kidney Yin. Qihai Ren 6 and Zusanli ST 36 tonify the Qi of the Middle Burner and clear Damp Heat. Zhishi BL 52 is also known as Jinggong, 'the house of sperm' and is an important point to treat spermatorrhoea, especially when used together with Ciliao BL 32.

Zhang Weimin, NANTONG MEDICAL COLLEGE HOSPITAL

108. Spermatorrhoea, acute

Zhang, male, adult, trainee

Case registered: December 1984

History: For 6 months after entering college the patient experienced dizziness and poor appetite. He slept badly and his memory became poor. These symptoms got worse as the midterm examinations drew near, and he became anxious about doing badly. At the start of the actual exam he was nervous and shaky, then suddenly felt weak in the waist and knees. At this point the spermatorrhoea began, and lasted for about 10 minutes. He felt dizzy and weak, and was unable to continue the exam. Every 5 or 6 minutes he would lose more semen. The invigilator called the doctor, who was unable to help. I arrived there an hour later, after all the other examinees had left.

Examination: The patient was sitting at his desk, unable to move. The front of his trousers was wet with semen. *Tongue body:* red at the tip. *Tongue coating:* thin. *Pulse:* deep and thin.

Diagnosis: Spermatorrhoea: Mental fatigue harming the Spleen and Kidney Yin. Fright harming the Kidney, which fails to retain the sperm.

Treatment: Calm the Mind, nourish Spleen and Kidney Yin, tonify Kidney Qi.

Principal Points: Shenmen HT 7, Sanyinjiao SP 6, Taixi KID 3.

The points were reinforced and the needles were retained for 15 minutes. By then the patient was feeling much more calm, and the spermatorrhoea had almost completely stopped. The needles were withdrawn, the patient was advised to come for treatment the next day, then sent to his room to rest.

In the hospital the next day the patient reported that he had slept better the previous night, but he had had some more milder spermatorrhoea, accompanied by weakness in the waist and knees and aversion to cold in the limbs. He was given more treatment based on the previous day's prescription.

Principal Points: Shenmen HT 7, Sanyinjiao SP 6, Taixi KID 3, Shenshu BL 23, Guanyuan Ren 4, Mingmen Du 4.

Guanyuan Ren 4 and Mingmen Du 4 were not needled, but treated with moxibustion. The other points were reinforced. After seven treatments all his symptoms went, and his memory improved.

Explanation: The *Su Wen* says, 'Fright damages the Kidney' (Yin Yang Ying Xiang Da Lun, Concept of Yin and Yang chapter). In this case fatigue damaged the Heart and Spleen, and fear damaged the Kidney. Shenmen HT 7, the Yuan-Source point, nourishes Heart Yin and calms the Mind. Sanyinjiao SP 6 is the meeting point of the three leg Yin channels, and regulates and nourishes the Spleen and Kidney. Taixi KID 3, the Yuan-Source point, reinforces the Kidney and controls nocturnal emission. The Back-Shu points are where the essence of the Zang-Fu organs gathers, so Shenshu BL 23 was selected to nourish the Kidney. Moxibustion at Guanyuan Ren 4 and Mingmen Du 4 reinforces Kidney Qi.

Li Zhenlin, PEOPLE'S LIBERATION ARMY POLITICAL COLLEGE CLINIC, NANJING
(see Shanghai Journal of Acupuncture and Moxibustion, Issue 4, 1986)

109. Non-ejaculation

Chen, male, age 25, peasant

History: The patient and his wife had not conceived after 3 years of marriage. The couple had regular sex, both were healthy and strong and their tests were normal.The patient was able to maintain an erection for long periods, but was unable to ejaculate during intercourse. Sometimes he would have nocturnal emissions. He had seen many different doctors who had prescribed him traditional Chinese drugs to tonify the Kidney and calm the Mind, and he had also prescribed some for himself, but none had helped.

Examination: No prostatic hyperplasi. No abnormal findings in the genitals. *Tongue body:* red. *Tongue coating:* think and yellow. *Pulse:* wiry and slippery.

Diagnosis: Persistent erection: Exuberant Liver Fire, impairment of Kidney Qi.

Treatment: Purge Liver Fire and nourish the Kidney.

Principal Points: Zhongji Ren 3, Xingjian LIV 2, Sanyinjiao SP 6, Shenshu BL 23.

The points were needled bilaterally and reduced. The needles were retained for 10 to 20 minutes, and manipulated twice to strengthen the stimulation. Treatment was given daily. After 4 days the patient went away on business for 10 days, and by the time he got back he was already able to ejaculate. His wife became pregnant 2 months later and in due course gave birth to a baby boy.

Explanation: The key symptoms in this case were normal sexual appetite, persistent erections and inability to ejaculate. This disorder can be differentiated into several patterns:
1. Exuberant Liver Fire or Ministerial Fire impairs the Kidney Yin.
2. Deficiency of Spleen and Kidney.
3. Stagnation of Qi, which disturbs the passage of sperm and inhibits ejaculation.

In this case Exuberant Liver Fire impaired Kidney Yin. The Zhang Shi Yi Tong (Zhang's Medicine) says, 'Persistent erection is by nature persistent Ministerial Fire in the Liver'. Treatment should purge Liver Fire and nourish Kidney Yin.

Xingjian LIV 2 purges Liver Fire. Zhongji Ren 3 and Sanyinjiao SP 6 regulate the house of sperm (testes). Zhongji Ren 3 is the Front-Mu point of the Bladder, and thus purges Liver Fire through the Bladder. Shenshu BL 23 and Sanyinjiao SP 6 nourish Kidney Yin. Together they purge Liver Fire, nourish Kidney water, activate the collaterals and open the orifices.

110. Male sterility (azoospermia)

Male, age 39, school teacher

History: The patient had been married for 14 years. Throughout this time he was neurotic and sexually impotent. His semen was tested and was found to contain no sperm (azoospermia). He also suffered from dizziness, palpitations, insomnia, lumbar pains, depression, pain and heavy sensations in the testicles. His appetite was poor, and his memory was getting gradually worse.

Examination: The patient looked pale and lacklustre. *Tongue body:* pale. *Pulse:* deep, thin and weak.

Diagnosis: Male sterility: Kidney Yang Deficiency.

Treatment: Strengthen Kidney Yang, refresh and calm the Mind.

Principal Points:
1. Shenmen HT 7, Taixi KID 3, Shenshu BL 23, Yinjiao Ren 7, Jinggong (Extra), Shiguan KID 18, Ganshu BL 18, Taichong LIV 3, Ligou LIV 5.
2. Zusanli ST 36, Sanyinjiao SP 6, Xuehai SP 10, Qihai Ren 6, Guanyuan Ren 4, Zhongji Ren 3, Mingmen Du 4.

The points were needled with slow-fast reinforcing and reducing method. The needles were inserted deep and retained for 30–50 minutes, but the main emphasis of the treatment was moxibustion rather than needle manipulation. The two groups of points were rotated, and treatment was given once every other day. One course consisted of 10 treatments. After three courses of treatment the patient's symptoms went and he was cured. Tests showed the presence of sperm in his semen. His wife conceived after 3 months, and later gave birth to a baby boy.

Explanation: The Heart houses the Mind (Shen) and the Kidney houses the Will (Zhi). Disharmony between the Heart and Kidney causes distress, insomnia and excessive dreaming. Shenmen HT 7 and Taixi KID 3, the Yuan-Source points, were selected to rebalance the relationship between Heart and Kidney.

The Liver and Kidney are the sources of energy for the genitals. The Liver houses the Blood and the Kidney houses the sperm. Water generates Wood, Kidney generates Liver. Shenshu BL 23 and Jinggong (Extra) affect the Water. Taichong LIV 3, Ligou LIV 5 and Ganshu BL 18 affect the Wood. In this way Yin and Yang were harmonized to generate sperm.

The Spleen and Stomach are the Postnatal sources of Qi. They belong to Yin Earth. They are the primary organs of digestion and the source of Qi and Blood. Zusanli ST 36, the He-Sea point, and Sanyinjiao SP 6, the meeting point of the three leg Yin channels, reinforce the Spleen and Stomach, tonify Qi and Blood and are used for all consumptive and deficiency diseases.

Xuehai SP 10 is also called Baichongke (Nest of One Hundred Worms), and has a direct effect on sperm.

The Du Mai, the Sea of Yang, travels along the back and governs all the Yang channels. The Ren Mai, the Sea of Yin, travels along the front and governs all the Yin channels. Both channels have a common point of origin, which is a meeting point of Yin and Yang, Heaven and Earth.

Thus selecting Qihai Ren 6, Guanyuan Ren 4 and Zhongji Ren 3 on the Yin and Mingmen Du 4 on the Yang balances Yin and Yang, reinforcing both Yang Qi and Yin Essence.

Shiguan KID 18 is a meeting point between the Kidney and Chong channels, and is an important point for lack of sperm. The *Bai Zheng Fu* (Songs of the One Hundred Diseases) says 'When there is no child treat Yinjiao Ren 7 and Shiguan KID 18'.

Xiao Shaoqing, NANJING TCM COLLEGE
(see Tianjin Traditional Chinese Medicine, Issue 5, 1986)

111. Mumps orchitis and parotitis

Zeng, male, age 47, worker

Case registered: 23 November 1971

History: The patient had high fever with parotitis and was hospitalized. His parotid glands were painful and swollen. On examination his left testicle was also discovered to be swollen and tender to touch.

Examination: Temperature: 41°C. *Pulse rate:* 104/min. *Blood:* WBC $8.4 \times 10^9/l$ ($8.4 \times 10^3/mm^3$), neutrophil 88%, lymphocyte 12%.

Diagnosis: Hernia: Accumulation of Heat in the Lower Burner, Stagnation of Qi in the Liver, Kidney, Ren and Du channels.

Treatment: Clear Heat in the Lower Burner, regulate Qi in the Liver, Kidney, Ren and Du channels.

Principal Points: Yangchi TB 4.

Supplementary Treatment: Intravenous drip: 500 ml of 5% glucose saline and 5% glucose. 2 grams of vitamin C.

Three pea-sized cones were burned on the left Yangchi TB 4. No antibiotics were prescribed. The next day the patient's temperature was 37°C, his testicle was reduced in size and he had less pain. The same treatment was repeated, and on the third day moxibustion was given alone. The day after this the parotitis was much improved, and the orchitis was completely gone. seven moxibustion treatments were given in total, and the patient was cured. The case was followed up for 16 years and there was no relapse.

Yang Dinglin, SHANGRAO MUNICIPAL TCM HOSPITAL, JIANXI PROVINCE

Editor's Note: In TCM acute orchitis is classified as hernia. Usually it is due to accumulation of Heat in the Lower Burner, Stagnation of Qi in the Liver, Kidney, Ren and Du channels.

In this case the doctor achieved good results by using moxibustion on the left Yangchi TB 4. The Japanese doctor Sawada Takashi has also got good results with moxibustion at this point when treating uterine flexion. This is the Yuan-Source point of the Triple Burner, so moxibustion here clears accumulated Heat in all three Burners, and regulates the Functional Qi in the Triple Burner.

ENDOCRINE DISORDERS

112. Diabetes mellitus

Li, female, age 62, cadre

Case registered: 1 April 1987

History: Since 15 September 1986 the patient had unquenchable thirst, hunger and general weakness. She was diagnosed with diabetes in a provincial hospital. Blood sugar on an empty stomach 8.1 mmol/l (148 mg%), urinary glucose (++++). She was prescribed oral Glyburide (glibenclamide) and her condition improved after a month. Urinary glucose was reduced to (++). She was given medication to reduce her hunger and thirst from February 1987, but these persisted and she still felt weak. At this point she came for acupuncture and moxibustion.

Examination: The patient was generally in good shape. No conjunctival xanthochromia. There were traces of urinary glucose. *Tongue coating:* thin and white. *Pulse:* leisurely.

Diagnosis: Diabetes (Xiao Ke) : Kidney Deficiency Fire.

Treatment: Tonify Kidney Yin and promote production of Body Fluids.

Principal Points: Yongquan KID 1, Taixi KID 3.
   The patient's medication was stopped. The points were stimulated bilaterally with a magnetic hammer, tapping gently 50 times at each point. Treatment was given daily. After 5 days her thirst and weakness improved. After 7 days her sleep improved and her strength was almost fully restored. After 13 days, tests showed no urinary glucose, and blood sugar on an empty stomach was reduced to 5.6 mmol/l (102 mg%). After 21 days all her symptoms had gone and she was able to do light physical work.

Xu Benren, ACUPUNCTURE AND MOXIBUSTION SECTION, SHENYANG AIR FORCE HOSPITAL

Editor's Note: Diabetes or 'Xiao Ke' can be caused by excessive fat and sugar in the diet, excessive alcohol intake, excessive sex, or physical and emotional factors. Heat accumulates and impairs the Yin, consuming the Lung, Stomach and Kidney, which results in excessive intake of water and food, with diuresis and emaciation. The root of the disease is in the Kidney. When Water (Kidney) and Fire (Heart) are in balance, Body Fluids circulate to the Lung and Stomach and down to the Bladder, where they turn to Qi. The person's appetite and thirst will be normal.

Deficiency of Water causes excess Fire resulting in a Fire–Water imbalance and the above symptoms. Diabetes can exist in the Upper, Middle or Lower Burners, but whichever pattern it is, it is most important to treat the Kidney.

In this case the doctor selected two Kidney points, Yongquan KID 1 and Taixi KID 3, to nourish the Kidney Yin and tonify the production of Body Fluids. Patients much prefer tapping with a magnetic hammer to needling, as there is no pain.

113. Diabetes insipidus

Cai, female, age 64, member of staff

Case registered: 1972

History: The patient had had frequent headaches since 1960. These headaches were usually temporal. They got worse after 1970, and were accompanied by sickness. Her eyesight started to deteriorate, and she began to have frequent and copious urination, up to 20 times a day. She was prescribed triamterine, Pituitrin (powdered pituitary, posterior lobe), liquid extract of liquorice, and a long-acting anti-diabetic agent (sic – possibly anti-diuretic hormone), which had to be stopped because it caused her to collapse.

Examination: BP: 17.3/10.7 kPa (130/80 mmHg). *Pulse rate:* 72/min. Field of vision in both eyes had concentric contraction. Vision 0.4 in both eyes. Papilloedema present. Blood sugar 4.9 mmol/l (88 mg%). Urinary specific gravity 1.0005. No urinary sugar. 17-hydroxycorticosterone 11 mg/24 hours, 17 ketosteroid 3.8 mg/24 hours. Basal metabolic rate –14%. Lateral X-ray of the head showed the sella turcica was round in shape, and the dorsum showed slight absorption. *Tongue body:* pale. *Tongue coating:* thin. *Pulse:* deep and thin.

Diagnosis: Diabetes: Deficiency of Kidney Yin and Kidney Yang.

Treatment: Nourish Kidney Yin, warm and consolidate Kidney Yang.

Principal Points: Baihui Du 20, Guanyuan Ren 4, Zusanli ST 36, Sanyinjiao SP 6, Taixi KID 3.

These points were needled for a considerable time, but without effect. By November 1973 the patient was very weak and was urinating more than 30 times a night. *BP:* 14.7/9.33 kPa (110/70 mmHg). Her field of vision in both eyes was severely diminished and head X-rays showed the sella turcica was expanding like a ball.

Revised Treatment: After long discussion and study it was decided to needle Jingming BL 1 deeply.

After needling Jingming BL 1 the patient's frequency of urination was reduced to four times per night. This disease had not responded to any treatment over a 10-year period, but this one point had marked effects.

Explanation: This case of diabetes fits the description of Lower Burner pattern diabetes in the *Jin Gui Yao Lue* (Prescriptions from the Golden Chamber): In diabetes the symptoms are copious urination; drinking large quantities and urinating large quantities.

It can be differentiated into two types: Kidney Yin Deficiency, and Kidney Yin and Yang Deficiency. In this case the treatment was to nourish Kidney Yin, warm and consolidate Kidney Yang but the patient did not respond. Jingming BL 1 was then selected according to Western medical theories, and was very effective. It is the starting point of the Bladder channel, and the meeting of the Bladder, Small Intestine, and Yin and Yang Chiao channels. Deep needling at this point regulates the function of the pituitary gland.

Ma Reiyin, ACUPUNCTURE AND MOXIBUSTION SECTION, SHANGHAI TCM COLLEGE HOSPITAL, SHUGUANG
(see Shanghai Journal of Acupuncture and Moxibustion, Issue 3, 1983)

114. Sheehan's syndrome

Liu, female, age 29, nurse

Case registered: 15 January 1986

History: The patient had an induced labour in May 1984, and collapsed after massive haemorrhaging. Later she became anaemic with loss of hair on her head and all over her body. She became emaciated, with aversion to cold and sensations of cold, palpitations, poor appetite, fatigue and oedema in the legs. She was given diethylstilboestrol and other hormones, but she got steadily worse.

Examination: Temperature: 35°C. *BP:* 10.7/6.67 kPa (80/50 mmHg). Weight

35 kg. *Pulse rate:* 45/min. *Blood:* RBC $2.5 \times 10^{12}/1$ $(2.5 \times 10^6/mm^3)$, haemoglobin 80 g/1 (8 g%). Blood sugar (fasting) 3.3 mmol/1 (60 mg%). Serum protein-bound iodine 2.5 mg%. Urinary 17-hydroxycorticosterone 3 mg/24 h. Urinary 17-ketosteroid 4mg/24 h. Basal metabolic rate –20%. Radioiodine absorption 13% (24 hours). Cytological examination with vaginal smear showed reduced keratin cells, mostly blue cells, low cell glycogen, high levels of white cells and bacteria, reflecting low hormone level.

The patient was thin, pale and lacklustre. Her limbs were cold and her skin was dry, with very few hairs. She had pitting oedema on her legs. *Tongue body:* pale. *Tongue coating:* thin. *Pulse:* deep, thin and slow.

Diagnosis: Loss of hair: Exhaustion of Qi and Blood, Deficiency of Spleen and Kidney.

Treatment: Tonify Yang, reinforce Spleen and Kidney.

Principal Points:
1. Guanyuan Ren 4, Zhongwan Ren 12, Zusanli ST 36, Sanyinjiao SP 6.
2. Geshu BL 17, Pishu BL 20, Weishu BL 21, Shenshu BL 23, Taixi KID 3.

Treatment was given daily, alternating the two groups of points. A course consisted of 10 treatments, with a 3 day rest between courses. Sanyinjiao SP 6 and Taixi KID 3 were needled only, but the other points were treated with warm needle, burning cun long segments of moxa stick or moxa cones on the handles. The needles were retained for 30 minutes.

After three courses of treatment the patient's spirits improved, her appetite was better and her limbs were warmer to the touch. Her body temperature and blood pressure became normal. After four courses her hair started to grow, and after five courses she gained 4 kg in weight, and no longer felt any discomfort.

Red blood cells were now $3.5 \times 10^{12}/1$ $(3.5 \times 10^6/mm^3)$, haemoglobin 100 g/1 (10 g%). She had a period on 6 April: the flow was medium and lasted 4 days. Another course of consolidating treatment was given. She was discharged from hospital on 25 April. Her last examination showed: urinary 17-hydroxycorticosterone 6 mg/24 h. Urinary 17-ketosteroid 8 mg/24 h. Basal metabolic rate –2%. Radioiodine absorption 18% (24 hours).

Explanation: Sheehan's syndrome is caused by ischaemia of the anterior pituitary following postpartum haemorrhage. The manifestations are hypofunction of the thyroid, sex glands and adrenal cortex. The disease is consumptive and chronic. In Western medicine the treatment is hormone replacement therapy, which gives poor results.

In TCM the disease is seen to be due to Deficiency of Spleen and Kidney. Qi and Blood become exhausted after massive loss of blood. Chong and Ren Mai are malnourished, and the five Zang are Deficient, so there are no menses.

The Kidney is the Prenatal source of Qi, and the Spleen is the Postnatal source. Guanyuan Ren 4 and Shenshu BL 23 were used to rescue the Fire at Mingmen (the Gate of Life), Zhongwan Ren 12 and Pishu BL 20 tonify the Spleen, Sanyinjiao SP 6 and Taixi KID 3 nourish the Spleen, Kidney and Liver. Geshu BL 17 regulates the Blood and vessels to restore Yang Qi. The sources for the creation of Qi and Blood were thus restored, and Ren and Chong Mai were reharmonized.

In Western medical terms it is possible that acupuncture and moxibustion could be used to improve the blood supply to the anterior pituitary and thus restore its function, but we have treated only a few cases so far and further observation is needed.

Zheng Shaoxiang, ACUPUNCTURE AND MOXIBUSTION SECTION, SHENXI TCM COLLEGE HOSPITAL
(see The New Chinese Medicine, Issue 4, 1987)

115. Subacute thyroiditis

Zhu, female, age 56, worker

Case registered: 22 June 1982

History: 6 months ago the patient had fever, which was worse in the afternoon, then a painful mass developed in her neck. After 3 months she was diagnosed in this hospital with thyroiditis, and prescribed hormones and other medication. The pain got worse recently, and she also had palpitations and felt restless. Her appetite was poor, she was losing weight and she felt faint.

Examination: Temperature: 38.5°C. *Pulse rate:* 120/min. *BP:* 13.3/8.0 kPa (100/60 mmHg). Facial oedema. The patient seemed in very low spirits. The mass was on the right anterior neck, and was 1.5 cm × 2.5 cm, and medium hard to the touch. It moved when she swallowed.

Haemoglobin 110 g/l (11 g%). *WBC:* 13.5×10^9/litre (13.5×10^3/mm³). Neutrophils 86%, lymphocytes 14%. 89 mm in 1 hour. Serum thyroxine 34 milli-mg/ml (sic). Auto-antibody all normal. Isotope 131 absorption rate reduced.

Diagnosis: Qi goitre: Deficiency Fire transforming to Toxic Fire.

Treatment: Purge Heat, remove goitre, reinforce and regulate Spleen and Stomach.

Principal Points: Renying ST 9, Hegu L.I. 4, Zusanli ST 36.

Renying ST 9 was reduced, and the other points were reinforced. Treatment was given every other day and a course consisted of 10 treatments.

After the first course the patient's symptoms improved. *Temperature:* 36.5°C. *Pulse rate:* 88/min. *BP:* 14.7/10.7 kPa (110/80 mmHg). *WBC:* 8.5 × 10 9/1 (8500/mm³). ESR 20 mm in 1 hour. Isotope 131 absorption rate normal. The mass now measured 0.5 cm × 0.5 cm. It was soft and no longer tender. All her other symptoms went. The case was followed up the following October. The patient reported that she had had no fevers since the treatment, and the mass had disappeared after 1 month. Her appetite was good and she was working full-time.

Explanation: The patient was weak and Deficient in Yin fluids. There was Exuberant Deficiency Fire. When the Fire stagnated it transformed into Toxic Fire causing fever and headache. The Toxic Fire rose and caused Stagnation at Renying ST 9, with swelling and pain at the neck. The channel Qi of the Large Intestine and Stomach was obstructed, disturbing the Functional Qi. The patient was thin and weak as a result, with poor appetite and loose stool. Hormone therapy is usually effective for this disease, but in this case it did not help because the patient was so weak. Her Yin and Blood were exhausted, and her body resistance was unable to expel the pathogen.

Hegu L.I. 4 and Zusanli ST 36 clear Qi in the Yang Ming channels, reinforce the Spleen and increase the body's resistance. Renying ST 9 clears Heat, purges toxins and removes goitre. This treatment was successful because it treated both the root and the symptoms.

Chen Jixiang, ACUPUNCTURE AND MOXIBUSTION SECTION, XI'AN MEDICAL COLLEGE HOSPITAL NO. 1
(see Shenxi Traditional Chinese Medicine, Issue 7, 1984)

116. Hyperthyroidism

CASE 1

Gu, female, age 42

Case registered: 10 September 1981

History: The patient had suffered from an overactive thyroid for more than 2 years. She was prescribed thyroid suppressant drugs but they caused a marked drop in her white blood cell count, as well as skin rashes. She currently had a dry mouth, with a desire for cold drinks, sensations of heat in her stomach. She ate a lot but was losing weight, and was irritable and restless.

Examination: The patient was thin. *BP:* 17.3/8.0 kPa (130/60 mmHg). III° thyroid enlargement. The swelling was diffuse and fairly firm on palpation. Vascular murmur positive. Hands shaky. Weight 42 kg. Serum T3 4.0 milli-micro-grams/ml (sic). Serum T4 260 milli-micro-grams/ml (sic). Basal metabolic rate +66%. *Tongue body:* red. *Tongue coating:* scanty. *Pulse:* thin and rapid, rate 120/min.

Diagnosis: Kidney Yin Deficiency, Heart Fire.

Treatment: Nourish Kidney Yin, purge Heart Fire, remove swelling.

Principal Points: Jianshi P 5, Shenmen HT 7, Taixi KID 3, Fuliu KID 7, Shuitu ST 10, Pingying (Extra)[1].

Jianshi P 5 and Shenmen HT 7 were reduced to protect the Yin by purging the Heart Fire. Taixi KID 3 and Fuliu KID 7 were reinforced to pull down Deficiency Fire. Shuitu ST 10 and Pingying (Extra) were added to dredge the Phlegm and Stagnation. The points were needled bilaterally, and treatment was given once every other day.

At Shuitu ST 10 the needles were inserted at 45° into the centre of the gland. At Pingying (Extra) the needles were inserted perpendicularly to a depth of 0.8–1 cun. When Qi sensation was obtained both needles were manipulated at the same time using 'slowly in and slowly out' method to induce Qi, till sensation reached the swollen gland and the throat.

After 3 weeks the patient's hands were more steady, and her intolerance of heat, excessive sweating, restlessness and bad temper were considerably better. After a further 3 weeks the thyroid enlargement was I°, and the gland was much softer.

The patient still felt hungry and ate large quantities. Her mouth was dry and her tongue was red. Shenmen HT 7 was dropped from the prescription and Neiguan P 6 and Sanyinjiao SP 6 were added. Neiguan P 6 was reduced and Sanyinjiao SP 6 was reinforced. After a further 3 weeks most of the patient's symptoms had gone: serum T4 96 milli-micro-gram/ml (sic), serum T3 2 milli-micro-gram/ml (sic). Basal metabolic rate +10. *Pulse rate:* 71/min. *BP:*14.9/10.7 kPa (112/80 mmHg). Thyroid enlargement I°. No bruit audible. Her hands no longer shook, and her weight had increased to 50 kg. She was discharged as cured and went back to work. The case was followed up for 6 months and there was no relapse.

Case treated by Jin Shubai, article by He Jinshen, SHANGHAI INSTITUTE OF ACUPUNCTURE, MOXIBUSTION AND CHANNELS
(*see Journal of Traditional Chinese Medicine, Issue 9, 1984*)

[1]Pingying (Extra) is located 0.7 cun lateral to the point midway between C4 and C5 vertebrae.

Editor's Note: In TCM hyperthyroidism can be classified as Qi goitre or diabetes. It is related to emotional factors, Kidney Yin Deficiency, fatigue or congenital weakness. The Liver is in charge of purging and discharging. It likes movement and dislikes Stagnation. When it is affected by emotional factors the Functional Qi stagnates. Stagnation of Liver Qi can transform into Fire, which in turn can impair the Yin. When the Yin is impaired Deficiency Fire agitates inside, impairing the Heart in the Upper Heater and the Kidney in the Lower Heater. If this condition lasts for a long time the Yin of the Heart, Liver and Kidney are consumed, and they act on each other, depleting each other further.

The disease is caused by Deficiency but its symptoms are Excess. The cause is Deficiency Fire and the symptoms are Exuberant Fire. Heat in the Heart transforms to the Stomach, accelerating metabolism and causing hunger. At the same time Heat in the Stomach and Liver condenses the Essence in the Yang Ming channel into Phlegm. Phlegm and Qi rise to the neck to form goitre, the swollen thyroid. When the Phlegm gets to the Liver channel and lodges in the eyes it causes bulging eyes.

Doctor Jin emphasized regulating the functions of the organs and balancing Qi and Blood, Yin and Yang. The key to this disease was Deficiency Liver Fire, which he treated according to the principle of 'Reinforcing the Mother when the Son is deficient, and reducing the Son when the Mother is in excess'. Jianshi P 5 and Shenmen HT 7 purge the Heat in the Heart, relieve the Heat in the Liver and nourish the Stomach. When the Heat in the Heart is purged, the Fire (Heart) does not burn the Metal (Lung), so the Metal can control the Wood (Liver).

Taixi KID 3 and Fuliu KID 7 nourish Kidney Yin. When the Water is full it nourishes the Liver. When the Mother organ is nourished and the Son organ is purged, the organs are regulated and Yin and Yang are harmonized. Shuitu ST 10 clears the channel Qi of the Stomach and removes Stasis of Phlegm in the neck.

CASE 2

Pang, female, age 22

Case registered: 2 June 1978

History: A month previously the patient started to have palpitations and noticed swelling on both sides of her neck. Examination showed III° enlargement, mixed pattern, with warm nodule on the right lobe. Right side murmur. Pulse regular, 140 b.p.m. Shaking hands. The condition was diagnosed as hyperthyroidism and she was given Tapazole (methimazole) for a week. Her palpitations improved temporarily, but her thyroid continued to enlarge. Her eyes started to protrude more noticeably. At this point she came for acupuncture and moxibustion.

Examination: The patient's neck was swollen and thickened, especially on the right. Her eyes were protruding and her hands were shaking. *Tongue body:* red at the edges. *Tongue coating:* thin and white. *Pulse:* wiry and rapid.

Diagnosis: Qi goitre: Stagnation of Qi and Blood.
    Treatment: Dredge the channels and collaterals, invigorate Qi and Blood, remove Stasis.

Principal Points: Two Ashi points (bilateral), approximately 0.5 cun above and below Renying ST 9. 3–4 local points in the swelling.

Secondary Points: Hegu L.I. 4, Neiguan P 6, Zusanli ST 36.
    Treatment was given once a day, and the needles were retained for 20–30 minutes. After 5 days the patient felt more comfortable in the neck and her palpitations were better. Treatment was then given every other day. A course consisted of 10 sessions, and a week was allowed between courses. Three courses of treatment were given between early June and the middle of August, and her neck became almost normal in size. All her other symptoms improved. The hyperthyoidism was controlled and she was able to go back to work. To date there has been no relapse.

Explanation: In TCM hyperthyroidism is classifed as Qi goitre. It is important to reassure the patient. Ashi points may be selected according to the size of the swelling. Multiple needling at the site of the disease dredges the channels and collaterals, invigorates Qi and Blood and removes Stasis. Hegu L.I. 4 and Zusanli ST 36 dredge the channel Qi of Yang Ming to disperse Stagnation of Qi and Blood. Neiguan, the Luo-Connecting point, regulates the Triple Burner and the Heart Qi, and can slow down the heart rate. The four Ashi points remove swelling in the neck, regulate the heart rate and improve the symptoms.

Shao Jingming, HENAN TCM COLLEGE

MISCELLANEOUS

117. Uncontrollable laughter

CASE 1

History: 3 days before the consultation the patient had suddenly burst into uncontrollable laughter. This happened several times during the day and at night, and each outburst lasted between 15–30 minutes. Afterwards she would feel exhausted. She was given tranquillizers, but their only effect was to make her sleep.

Examination: The patient burst into laughter as soon as she arrived. She giggled and chuckled uncontrollably with venous engorgement in the neck and urinary incontinence. *Tongue body:* red. *Tongue coating:* scant. *Pulse:* thin and rapid.

Diagnosis: Deficient Yin failing to control Yang, Fire–Water imbalance between Heart and Kidney.

Treatment: Nourish Kidney Yin and calm the mind.

Principal Points: Daling P 7, Renzhong Du 26, Lieque LU 7, Yongquan KID 1, Taixi KID 3.

Daling P 7 and Renzhong Du 26 were reduced, Lieque LU 7 and Yongquan KID 1 were needled with reinforcing and reducing evenly method and Taixi KID 3 was reinforced. The needles were retained for 45 minutes and manipulated every 15 minutes. After 5 minutes the patient's laughter began to subside, and she was able to stop after the third manipulation. Treatment was suspended for observation for 5 hours, and she did not have another outburst during this time. She slept fairly well that night, with no outbursts and was given one more consolidating treatment the next day.

Explanation: The Shao Yin division governs the Heart and Kidney, i.e. Fire and Water. If the Heart and Kidney Yin are Deficient the Yin will not control the Deficiency Heat, and 'the Spirit disperses and cannot be housed' (*Ling Shu*, Ben Shen chapter, Spirit). The uncontrollable laughter indicates uncontrolled Yang. Lieque LU 7, Renzhong Du 26 and Daling P 7 are all important points for this disorder. Lieque LU 7, a Confluent point of the Extra Vessels and one of the four general points, expels Heat from the Lung and clears the throat and chest. Renzhong Du 26 coordinates the Kidney channel with Du Mai and expels Yang pathogens to calm the mind. Daling P 7 nourishes the mind and Spirit and soothes distress in the chest. Yongquan KID 1 and Taixi KID 3 nourish the Water and tonify the Yin of the body. This prescription 'strengthens the Water to control Exuberant Yang'. The problem resolved when Fire and Water were harmonized.

CASE 2

Chen, female, age 38

Case registered: 12 April 1981

History: The patient had suffered a high fever a week before. It was now receding but her appetite was poor and she needed spicy foods to interest her palate. She laughed uncontrollably, felt hot and restless, and was unable to sleep. She felt distress in the chest, fullness in her upper abdomen, nausea, and heaviness in the head. She was thirsty and red-eyed.

Examination: The patient was red-faced and laughing uncontrollably. *Tongue body:* red. *Tongue coating:* yellow. *Pulse:* wiry and full, especially on the left.

Diagnosis: Obstruction of the chest by Phlegm and Heat from Stagnation of Qi turning to Fire.

Treatment: Cool Heat, regulate Rebellious Qi and relieve distress in the chest.

Principal Points: Zusanli ST 36, Hegu L.I. 4, Quchi L.I. 11, Neiguan P 6.

As these points were needled the patient burst into laughter and comical gestures. Her face became more red and it was hard to tell if she was crying or laughing. The points were needled with reinforcing and reducing evenly method, but she became worse and the disturbance attracted a crowd of onlookers.

At this stage it was obvious that the original diagnosis was incorrect. The left distal pulse corresponds to Fire. The *Su Wen* says (Yin Yang Ying Xiang Da Lun chapter, Concept of Yin and Yang) this position 'is related to the Heart in the organs, red in the colours ... laughter in the sounds ... happiness in the state of mind'. As the laughter had got worse when the Heart oriented points were needled, it was obvious that there was Heat and Phlegm in the Heart, and that this was an Excess condition.

Revised Treatment: Clear the Heart, cool Fire, eliminate Phlegm.

Revised Points: Shenmen HT 7, Fenglong ST 40, Dazhui Du 14, Jiuwei Ren 15, Laogong P 8.

The needles from the previous formula were removed and the new points were all reduced. Jiuwei Ren 15 was needled obliquely downwards.

The patient's laughter began to subside after 10 minutes. The needles were manipulated a second time after 15 minutes, after which she stopped laughing. The needles were retained for an hour. The patient was left under observation for 3 hours, with no incident. The next day she felt an improvement in her nausea but was still very distressed. The treatment was repeated, and the disorder was cured.

Explanation: This disorder was caused by Stagnation of Perverse Heat turning into Yang Fire. The Heart is the Fire organ, and therefore cannot tolerate Heat. When Heat becomes excessive, it turns into Wind and rises up with Phlegm.

The first prescription was designed to clear Heat, regulate Rebellious Qi and soothe the chest, and was by no means an inappropriate treatment. It is extremely rare for the energy to react in this way. The second prescription was designed to clear the Heart, resolve Phlegm and calm the mind. Laogong P 8 is good for uncontrollable laughter. Dazhui Du 14 is the meeting point of the three leg Yang channels, and Jiuwei Ren 15 is the Luo-Connecting point of Ren Mai. These two points in combination correct imbalances of Yin and Yang.

Jiang Liji and Jiang Yunxiang, DAISHAN HOSPITAL, DINGYUAN COUNTY, ANHUI PROVINCE
(see Journal of Traditional Chinese Medicine, Issue 10, 1982)

118. Uncontrollable yawning

Sha, female, age 32

Case registered: 5 October 1976

History: The patient was depressed. She had quarrelled with her family 3 days previously. The day after the argument she started to yawn uncontrollably. Her doctor had diagnosed the condition as 'neurosis', and she was given an intramuscular injection of luminal (phenobarbitone). She was also given acupuncture at Hegu L.I. 4, Neiguan P 6 and Shaoshang LU 11, but neither of these treatments was effective.

Examination: The patient's hair was unkempt. Her eyes were shut and her head tilted backwards. She was yawning uncontrollably, and tears were streaming down her face. *Pulse:* wiry, but not rapid.

Diagnosis: Stagnation of Yang, disturbed Spirit (Shen).

Treatment: Activate Yang and invigorate the Spirit.

Principal Points: Renzhong Du 26.

A 25 mm needle was used, and manipulated with rapid twirling for about 30 minutes. From time to time during the treatment the yawning would stop. By the time the needle was withdrawn the patient was asleep and the yawning had stopped. The case was monitored for 7 years and there was no relapse.

Explanation: The *Jin Gui Yao Lue* (Pulse, Signs and Treatment of Women's

Diseases) says, 'women are inclined to be emotional because their Qi tends to be restless. Symptoms associated with the Spirit such as yawning are commonplace, and can be regulated with Gan Mai Da Zao Tang' (Liquorice, Wheat and Jujube decoction)'.

This disorder arose from physical weakness and fatigue, combined with an emotional upset which caused Stagnation of Qi and Blood, and depressed the Yang Qi and the Spirit, which ceased to function properly.

Du Mai, the Sea of Yang, is connected to all six Yang channels. Renzhong Du 26 is a major point of Du Mai and moves Stagnation of Qi and Blood. The yawning was cured when the Spirit functioned properly once again.

Guo Kun, TCM SECTION, YINGFANG COMMUNE CLINIC, RUGAO COUNTY, JIANGSU PROVINCE
(see Jiangsu Journal of Traditional Chinese Medicine, Issue 3, 1982)

119. Hiccup

CASE 1

Zhang, male, age 49, doctor

Case registered: 26 March 1982

History: 2 weeks previously this patient had taken some medication for a recurrence of rheumatoid arthritis. He felt nauseous the next day and developed hiccups, which did not respond to a variety of medicines or to acupuncture and moxibustion. He was hiccuping continuously and had a feeling of stuffiness in the chest.

Examination: Barium X-ray showed no organic disease in the upper digestive tract.

Diagnosis: Hiccup: Rebellious Stomach Qi.

Treatment: Relieve the oppression of the chest and diaphragm, and regulate the Stomach Qi.

Principal Points: Auricular points Ge (bilateral), Erzhong and Shenmen.[1]

Secondary Points: Neiguan P 6 (bilateral), Zusanli ST 36 (bilateral).

After routine sterilization the points were injected with vitamin B_1 0.05 ml for each ear point and 1 ml for each body point. After 3½ hours the hiccups were less frequent and less intense, and by the following

---

[1]Both Ge and Erzhong correspond to the diaphragm. Ge is located directly above the external auditory meatus on the antihelix crus, and Erzhong is on the midpoint of the helix crus.

morning they were gone. The case was followed up for 3 months and there was no relapse.

Explanation: In this case the hiccups were caused by medication. They were severe and persistent, but were successfully treated by using both auricular and channel points with hydro-acupuncture to provide strong and lasting stimulation.

The auricular points relieved the oppression in the chest and diaphragm. Neiguan P 6 sends down Rebellious Qi and regulates the Stomach, and Zusanli ST 36 reinforces the Spleen and the Middle Burner.

> Case treated by Cai Chongsan, case study by Shen Xiangfeng
> ZHOUKOU PREFECTURE HYGIENE SCHOOL CLINIC, HENAN PROVINCE
> *(see Henan Traditional Chinese Medicine, Issue 4, 1983)*

CASE 2

Guo, male, age 40, cadre

Case registered: 14 February 1982

History: This patient had been healthy and strong until the middle of October 1980, when he developed hiccups at intervals of 3–5 minutes. The hiccups persisted day and night, affecting both his speech and his sleep; it was aggravated by exposure to rain or cold. Barium X-ray examination at his local hospital showed no disease or abnormality of the stomach or intestines. He did not respond to treatment so he was transferred to another hospital where various other therapies were tried to no avail, including point injection of atropine. By the time he was transferred here he had had hiccups for 16 months.

Examination: Frequent hiccups with low sound.

Diagnosis: Hiccup: Spleen and Stomach Deficiency with Rebellious Stomach Qi.

Principal Points: Tiantu Ren 22, Zhongwan Ren 12, Zusanli ST 36 and Neiguan P 6. This prescription was given for 10 days, with no improvement.

On 26 February the patient was prescribed one dose of chive seeds, but this provided temporary relief only: The hiccups recurred 4 days later and further doses of chive seeds proved ineffective.

From 7 March the principle of 'assisting the Back-Shu points with the Front-Mu points' was used.

Principal Points: Zhongwan Ren 12, Weishu BL 21, Zhangmen LIV 13, Pishu BL 20, and Zusanli ST 36, with moxibustion on the areas around the points. The disease was cured after 15 days. The case was followed up for 2 months and did not relapse.

Explanation: Both Excess and Deficiency conditions may give rise to hiccups. The Excess conditions most commonly implicated are Stomach Fire or Cold in the Stomach, and the Deficiency conditions are usually Spleen and Stomach Qi Deficiency, Spleen and Stomach Yang Deficiency, or Stomach Yin Deficiency.

In this case the disorder was caused by weakness of the Spleen and Stomach with Rebellious Qi. The main aim was to reinforce the Spleen and Stomach, and treatment was successful once acupuncture and moxibustion were used at the same time.

> Liu Minyong, ACUPUNCTURE AND MOXIBUSTION SECTION, JIANXI TCM COLLEGE HOSPITAL
> *(see Jianxi Traditional Chinese Medicine, Issue 2, 1983)*

CASE 3

Zhang, male, age 56, cadre

History: The patient suddenly developed heart pain 4 days previously. Electrocardiograph indicated infarction of the posterointerior wall, and he was hospitalized for emergency treatment and monitoring. After 2 days he developed persistent hiccup. Various medications were tried, including atropine, but these did not help and he went on to develop urinary retention.

He was treated with acupuncture at Neiguan P 6, Zhongwan Ren 12, Liangmen ST 21, Zusanli ST 36 and Yinlingquan SP 9 but the hiccups persisted. It was at this point that I was brought in for a joint consultation.

Principal Points: Futu L.I. 18.

Futu L.I. 18 was needled on the right, producing an electric sensation from the neck, down the arm and into the thumb and index finger. The needle was retained for 20 minutes. The hiccups stopped immediately, but began again after 3 hours.

The treatment was repeated the next day with the same sensation propagated to the fingers. Once again the relief was immediate, this time lasting for 6 hours.

The treatment was repeated the next day, and for the remainder of the emergency the hiccups did not recur.

Explanation: Hiccup is usually episodic and inconsequential, but persistent hiccup can lead to sudden collapse of Heart Yang and death. The patient was in a critical condition and the hiccup was therefore very dangerous. The effectiveness of Futu L.I. 18 in this case can be attributed to two mechanisms: firstly it is a point on the Hand Yang Ming channel; and the disorder was in the Foot Yang Ming channel, and secondly, Futu L.I. 18 regulates Qi and resolves Phlegm, clears the throat and soothes the diaphragm. Although this treatment was symptomatic, it was essential to stabilize the patient's condition.

Jiang Youguang, GUANG'ANMEN INSTITUTE OF TCM HOSPITAL
(see Journal of Traditional Chinese Medicine, Issue 2, 1985)

CASE 4

Shi, male, age 60, peasant

History: 10 days after an operation for cancer of the pancreas this patient started to feel a sensation of fullness in the abdomen, nausea and distress in the chest. He received gastrointestinal decompression, in which 500 ml of fluid and 200 ml of gas were drawn out. Immediately afterwards he began to hiccup, and developed a fever of 37.4°C. Intramuscular injections of maxolon (metoclopramide) had no effect and after 10 days he was referred for acupuncture.

Examination: The patient was very thin. *Tongue body:* pale. *Tongue coating:* white and greasy. *Pulse:* wiry, soft and weak.

Diagnosis: Postoperative hiccup: Rebellious Stomach Qi.

Treatment: Regulate Rebellious Qi, relieve the chest and soothe the diaphragm.

Principal Points: Neiguan P 6, Zusanli ST 36 and Fenglong ST 40.
    The points were needled bilaterally, reduced, and the needles retained for 30 minutes.
    The hiccuping stopped for half a day, during which time the patient's stitches were removed, but recurred the following morning.

Secondary Points: Hegu L.I. 4 and Taichong LIV 3.
    These points were added to the prescription, and reduced bilaterally. All the points were retained for 30 minutes, but this time the principal points were manipulated twice with reinforcing and reducing equally method. The hiccup stopped and the patient was able to get out of bed and walk around.
    The case was followed up for 2 months and the hiccups did not recur.

Explanation: Hiccups often occur with cancers of the digestive system or after surgery. This is due to impairment of the functions of the Stomach and Spleen, which causes Stomach Qi to rebel upwards.

Neiguan P 6, Zusanli ST 36 and Fenglong ST 40 relieve the chest and regulate Stomach Qi. Hegu L.I. 4 and Taichong LIV 3 send down Rebellious Qi and readjust the Qi in the Yang Ming channels.

Qian Jifeng, ACUPUNCTURE AND MOXIBUSTION SECTION, SUZHOU
MUNICIPALITY PEOPLE'S HOSPITAL NO. 4

CASE 5

Wang, male, age 50, peasant

Case registered: Autumn 1975

History: The patient had had persistent hiccup for 7 months, which was interfering with his work, meals and sleep. It had been diagnosed as 'gastric neurosis', but the patient had not responded to either traditional Chinese or Western medication.

The hiccups had started when the patient was upset by a family dispute at dinner and had persisted since then, getting worse after meals. His appetite was poor, he sighed a lot and felt weak.

Examination: The patient looked thin and depressed and hiccuped with a dull sound. *Pulse:* deep and wiry.

Diagnosis: Hiccup: Stagnation of Liver Qi and Rebellious Stomach Qi.

Treatment: Relieve the Liver and regulate Rebellious Stomach Qi.

Principal Points: Geguan BL 46, Geshu BL 17.

Secondary Points: Zusanli ST 36 (reinforced), Taichong LIV 3 (reduced) and E Ni (Extra).[1]

Treatment was given daily, alternating the two prescriptions. A single course lasted 7 days, with a 3-day rest between courses.

After five courses the hiccups were far less frequent, occurring for only an hour after meals. The patient's appetite and sleep also improved. After 11 courses the disorder was completely cured. The case was monitored for 9 years and there was no relapse.

Explanation: The Spleen and Stomach belong to the Earth element. Positioned in the Middle Burner they govern the rising and falling of Qi. When the Spleen is healthy Qi rises, and when the Stomach is regulated

---

[1] E Ni (Extra) is located on the mammillary line in the seventh intercostal space. E ni literally means 'Hiccup'.

Qi descends. The Liver belongs to the Wood element. It hates depression and governs the free flowing of Qi.

This case was caused by emotional upset oppressing the Liver, which affected the Stomach and Spleen. Qi no longer moved up and down normally, but rebelled to attack the diaphragm. Jingyue Quan Shu says 'Rebellious Qi causes hiccup' *(The Complete Works of Zhang Jingyue)*.

In this case, the primary aim was to regulate Qi and relieve Stagnation in the diaphragm. Geguan BL 46, Geshu BL 17 and E Ni (Extra) are local points which do this. Neiguan P 6 opens the chest and diaphragm and sends down Rebellious Qi, Zusanli ST 36 strengthens the Spleen and Stomach and regulates the Middle Burner, Taichong LIV 3 opens up and regulates the flow of Qi in the Liver and Gall Bladder channels, and soothes depression.

Case treated by Xie Linyuan, case study by Xieleye, WENDENG COUNTY BONE SETTING HOSPITAL, SHANDONG PROVINCE
(see Journal of Traditional Chinese Medicine, Issue 1, 1984)

120. Anaphylactic shock

Quan, female, age 45, worker

Case registered: 10 July 1982

History: The patient had pain in the elbow joint for 6 months. She came here in October 1981, and the condition was diagnosed as tennis elbow. She was treated with local blocking injections of procaine and prednisolone acetate. She returned in July 1982. Her elbow was swollen, hot and painful. It was tender on palpation and movement was difficult. She reported that the previous treatment had been effective, so she was given an injection of 6 ml of 0.5% procaine and 25 ml of prednisolone into the tender area (Tianjing TB 10). She immediately felt distress in the chest, with faintness and palpitations and became nauseous with cold sweat on her limbs.

Examination: The patient looked pale. *BP:* 8.00/4.00 kPa (60/30 mmHg). Semicoma. *Pulse rate:* 100/min., slightly thready and rapid.

Diagnosis: Jue syndrome.

Treatment: Resuscitate the Mind.

Principal Points: Neiguan P 6 (bilateral).

The needles were inserted immediately and twirled for 5 minutes, then retained. The patient's feeling of distress in the chest improved, and her nausea and other symptoms soon went. After 15 minutes her blood pressure was 12.0/8.00 kPa (90/60 mmHg), and her pulse was down to 90 b.p.m. After 40 minutes all her symptoms had gone and she was able to get out of bed and move around.

At this point she admitted that the last time she had been given this treatment she had experienced the same symptoms and had been resuscitated by emergency treatment. She had been advised not to use this therapy again, but because it was so effective she had concealed this part of her history to get another treatment.

4 days later she returned to report that her pain was much better and that she wanted a repeat treatment. She added that during the needling she had felt heat moving from her palm along the anterior surface of the arm. When the sensation reached her stomach she immediately felt more comfortable.

It was decided that although the treatment was dangerous, experimentation is necessary if the body of knowledge of Traditional Chinese Medicine is to expand. Preparation was made for emergency treatment, and Neiguan P 6 was needled bilaterally with strong stimulation for 5 minutes before the injection. After 5 minutes the patient once again felt distress in the chest for 2 minutes. Strong stimulation was given at the points by twirling the needles, and the distress was relieved.

Later a third and fourth injection were given in the same way, and there were no untoward reactions.

Explanation: In TCM allergic shock is classified as Jue syndrome (fainting). Neiguan P 6, the Luo-Connecting point and Confluent point of Yin Wei Mai, resuscitates the Mind and activates Blood and the collaterals. It is suggested that this point could be used as a preventative for patients with a past history of allergic shock.

Fang Fengping, ZHANGJIANG PREFECTURAL HOSPITAL, GUANGDONG PROVINCE
(see The New Chinese Medicine, Issue 6, 1984)

121. Tuberculosis of the lymph nodes

Wang, female, age 42, homemaker

Case registered: 28 July 1955

History: The patient had had several nodes beneath her right ear for 16 years. Each node was about the size of an apricot stone. There was a larger one above the left supraclavicular fossa. In the last few months she had developed fever, which was worse in the afternoons, and the nodes in her neck had enlarged. This was diagnosed as tuberculosis of the lymph nodes, and surgery was suggested. The patient was unable to afford this, and instead came for acupuncture and moxibustion. She had high fever, severe pain, poor appetite, insomnia, and scanty reddish urine.

Examination: The patient was thin and yellow-looking. There was a fist-sized lump on the left side of her neck. Below her right ear there were several walnut-sized lumps. From her knees down to her feet there were also many purple coloured nodes, which were painful and itchy. *Temperature:* 39°C. *Tongue coating:* yellow, and thick in the middle. *Pulse:* deep and slightly rapid in the proximal positions, superficial in the middle and distal positions.

Diagnosis: Deficiency of Lung Yin, Stagnation of Heat and Phlegm.

Treatment: To treat the symptoms: Remove Heat and stop pain. To treat the cause: Nourish Lung Yin, regulate Qi, dissolve Phlegm, soften and resolve hard masses.

Principal Points: Dazhui Du 14, Feishu BL 13, Gaohuangshu BL 43, Shaohai HT 3, Zhoujian (Extra), Zusanli ST 36, Yanglingquan GB 34, Sanyinjiao SP 6.

Secondary Points: Jianwaishu SI 14, Huantiao GB 30, Yinlingquan SP 9, Ganshu BL 18, Jianjing GB 21.

The two groups of points were treated on alternate days. Birdpecking and twirling method was used and the needles were retained for 10 minutes. Moxibustion was administered at the local sites of disease and at Gaohuangshu BL 43 and Zhoujian (Extra) for 10 minutes,

After the first treatment the patient's pain improved and she was able to sleep. After two treatments the fever began to subside and her appetite improved. After treatments the lumps were markedly reduced in size and the systemic symptoms improved. After 26 days all the systemic symptoms had gone: the fist-sized node was now pea sized, and the smaller nodes had disappeared completely. The patient's appetite was good and her energy was much better.

Du Dewu, ACUPUNCTURE AND MOXIBUSTION SECTION, SHANGHAI TCM COLLEGE HOSPITAL
(see Proceedings of the Symposium for Traditional Chinese Medicine and Channels, Acupuncture and Moxibustion, Shandong Province, 1960)

Editor's Note: Tuberculosis of the lymph nodes is mostly due to Kidney and Lung Yin Deficiency and Stagnation of Liver Qi. This predisposes the body to invasion of toxic pathogens, which accumulate to consume the Yin. When the Water is Deficient, Deficiency Fire develops inside. The Lung cannot descend and disperse fluids, which congeal and become

Phlegm. The disease is caused by the accumulation and Stagnation of Fire and Phlegm.

Acupuncture at Feishu BL 13, Dazhui Du 14 and Sanyinjiao SP 6, and moxibustion at Gaohuangshu BL 43 nourishes the Lung Yin and clears Heat. Jianwaishu SI 14, Huantiao GB 30, Yanglingquan GB 34, Jianjing GB 21 and Ganshu BL 18 dredge the Functional Qi of the Liver and Gall Bladder and the neck area. Zusanli ST 36 and Yinlingquan SP 9 nourish and reinforce the Spleen and Stomach. When the Functional Qi flows without obstruction and the Spleen and Stomach are active, the Phlegm will resolve. Zhoujian (Extra) and Shaohai HT 3 are important points to treat tuberculous lymph nodes. The moxibustion was added to enhance the effect of the acupuncture and make it more specific.

122. Cysticercosis (bladderworm infestation) of the muscle and subcutaneous tissue

Wang, male, age 28, peasant

Case registered: 30 January 1979

History: The patient had subcutaneous nodules all over his body. This had been diagnosed as cysticercosis 6 months previously. He was generally in good condition. He had no previous history of intestinal disease or epilepsy, and no problems with his vision.

Examination: 44 hard, mobile oval cysts could be palpated under the skin on the patient's head, neck, trunk and limbs. Each was the size of a peanut.

Treatment: The cysts were used as points. A 26 gauge 1 cun needle was either inserted into the centre of each and twisted in one direction for 10 revolutions, or inserted with a twist and twirled back and forth through a large angle before withdrawal. Treatment was given once every other day, sometimes less frequently. During the first treatment 31 cysticerci were needled. The remainder were treated during the second session, and on two other occasions. After a month they had all disappeared. The case was followed up after some time and the patient was found to be in good health.

Explanation: Cysticercosis is caused by ingestion of tapeworm eggs in contaminated food or drink. These develop into larvae and can affect any of the body's tissues. In this case acupuncture was tried, and it proved effective. It is important to hold the cysts firmly to ensure good insertion, and to twist the needle through a large angle. For those on the chest and back or over important organs, oblique insertion should be used.

Guan Xiaoxian, LONGTAN DISTRICT PEOPLE'S HOSPITAL, JILIN
(see Jilin Traditional Chinese Medicine, Issue 2, 1983)

123. Scorpion sting

Sun, female, age 40, cadre

Case registered: 22 May 1987

History: The patient was stung by a scorpion at about 6.00 a.m. whilst doing some housework. She came for emergency treatment.

Examination: The sting was on the patient's right index finger. It was swollen and painful and her whole arm was painful. She was groaning with pain.

Principal Points: Hegu L.I. 4, Waiguan TB 5, Quchi L.I. 11, Ashi point on the right hand, between the 2nd and 3rd metacarpophalangeal joints and slightly posterior (approximately at the location of Luozhen (Extra) point).

The points were needled on the affected side, and continuous lifting, thrusting and twirling was given to produce strong stimulation. After 10 minutes the pain began to subside. After 30 minutes it was much improved and tolerable. The needles were then manipulated at intervals of 10 minutes. After 50 minutes there was no pain at all, only a sensation of heaviness in the finger.

Explanation: Acupuncture is effective for scorpion sting. The principle is to select local and distal points and get strong sensation. The therapy is easy to apply, quick acting, and has no side effects. The mechanism is under study. We have two theories:

1. Acupuncture is effective because it relieves the pain. There are many cases where acupuncture has been shown to increase the pain threshold, e.g. acupuncture anaesthesia.
2. Acupuncture relieves Stagnation of Qi and Blood, improves the circulation of blood in the local area, regulates the immune response and accelerates the decomposition of the scorpion poison proteins. It therefore activates the Blood, removes poison, relieves pain and swelling.

Case treated by Sun Xuequan, case study by Yang Liyong,
MENGYIN COUNTY HOSPITAL, SHANDONG PROVINCE

124. Acute gas poisoning

Gao, female, age 27, worker

Case registered: 12 January 1981

History: On 11 January neighbours observed the patient's husband carry a coal stove with no stovepipe into their room and go to bed with the doors and windows closed. The patient had had a baby 4 days previously. At noon the next day the neighbours forced their way in to find the patient lying unconscious.

Examination: The patient was comatose and did not respond to any stimuli. Her build was average and did not appear malnourished. BP normal. Neck flaccid. Eyes rolled upwards. Pupils were the same size. Reflex to light slightly sluggish. Corneal reflex slightly sluggish. Complexion pale and yellow, lips dark red. Her mouth was tightly closed, and her arms and legs were in spasm. Her arms trembled paroxysmally and both hands were clenched. Heart and lungs were normal. Respiration rapid. *Pulse:* thin and rapid (90/min).

Treatment: Open the doors and windows to ventilate the room. Loosen the patient's clothing at the neck and clear secretions from the mouth and nose. Give acupuncture alternating with massage.

Principal Points: Renzhong Du 26, Hegu L.I. 4.
   These points were needled. Strong stimulation was applied by twirling.
   Massage was applied at Chengjiang Ren 24, Zhongchong P 9, Neiguan P 6, Waiguan TB 5, Tai Yang (Extra) and Yintang (Extra). Friction (Gua Sha Liao Fa)[1] was also given at the sides of the neck and the base of the throat, until the skin became purple and congested. The patient was thus revived without any medication.
   After 40 minutes she turned red, and the spasm and tremor lessened. Her jaw relaxed and she was able to swallow some boiled water. Massage was continued at the same points. By 5.00 p.m. the patient was resuscitated. She felt weak, with headache and pain in her cheeks. After 3 days of bedrest she was fully recovered. A month later she reported some occasional ringing in her ears, but this disappeared without medication. Her baby grew well and when the case was followed up a year later, she was in good health.

Explanation: The success of this treatment for gas poisoning is due to the efficacy of acupuncture in treating coma and shock. Animal tests have

---

[1]This technique consists of rubbing certain areas slowly with the back of a spoon or the back of the middle joint of the middle finger. The skin is rubbed in one direction only until it goes red.

shown that needling can promote the disassociation of carboxyhaemo-globin from gas poisoning. Renzhong Du 26, Hegu L.I. 4 and Zusanli ST 36 have been used on hares to shorten their resuscitation time from anaemia. Renzhong Du 26 is also an important point of Du Mai. It readjusts the Yin and Yang of the whole organism and harmonizes the functions of the different parts of the body.

Li Jinxiang, HENAN PROVINCIAL NO. 2 TEXTILE FACTORY CLINIC ,
(see Journal of Traditional Chinese Medicine, Issue 11, 1982)

125. Sequelae of gas poisoning

CASE 1

Zhao, male, age 56, worker

Case registered: February 1978

History: The patient was poisoned by gas fumes during the night on 27 December 1977. He was found unconscious the next day and resuscitated with emergency treatment in hospital. By the end of January however, he seemed listless, taciturn, slow in his movements and gait, and was making mistakes in his work. His appetite was poor, and he lost control of his bowels and bladder. When he went out he could not find his way back home. He had previously been weak, but had no history of mental disease.

Examination: BP: 16.0/10.0 kPa (120/75 mmHg). Heart and lungs normal. Weakness of the limbs. Excessive tendon reflex, but no pathological reflex. *Tongue body:* pale. *Tongue coating:* thin and white. *Pulse:* deep, thin and weak.

Diagnosis: Deficiency of Kidney Qi.

Treatment: Refresh the mind, activate the Blood and collaterals, tighten Kidney Qi.

Principal Points: Two groups of points were used:
1. Fengchi GB 20 (bilateral), Dazhui Du 14, Quchi L.I. 11 (bilateral), Zusanli ST 36 (bilateral).
2. Shenmen HT 7 (bilateral), Guanyuan Ren 4, Sanyinjiao SP 6 (bilateral).
    Fengchi GB 20 and Dazhui Du 14 were reduced with strong stimulation, but the needles were not retained. At Quchi L.I. 11 and Zusanli ST 36, the needles were retained for 15–20 minutes. After two treatments the patient was talking in a louder voice and was in better spirits. After four treatments his strength, spirit, appetite and movement were all restored.

He was still incontinent, however, so the second group of points was needled. After two of these treatments he was cured. The case was followed up for 2 years and there was no relapse.

Explanation: The first prescription was to refresh the mind and activate the Blood and collaterals. The second group was to calm the mind and tighten the Kidney Qi.

CASE 2

Dong, male, age 72, peasant

Case registered: March 1978

History: The patient had a previous history of hypertension, but had generally been healthy and frequently did farm work. He was poisoned by fumes during the night of 23 January 1978, and was found in a coma. He was revived in hospital and the next day seemed completely normal. On 5 April he began to act strangely: sleeping little but talking frequently when he did. He showed no inclination to eat or drink, began to make mistakes at work and walk erratically. His speech became illogical, sometimes emotional or offensive, and he felt faint.

Examination: BP: 22.7/13.3 kPa (170/100 mmHg). Heart and lungs normal. Abdomen normal. Hypermyotonia. Physiological reflex present. Bilateral ankle clonus. Unsteady gait. *Tongue body:* red. *Tongue coating:* yellow. *Pulse:* wiry and strong.

Diagnosis: Hyperactive Liver Yang.

Treatment: Refresh the mind, regulate Qi and Blood, dredge the channels and collaterals, soothe the Liver and suppress hyperactivity of Yang.

Principal Points: Two groups of points were used:
1. Fengchi GB 20 (bilateral), Dazhui Du 14, Shenmen HT 7 (bilateral), Sanyinjiao SP 6.
2. Hegu L.I. 4, Taichong LIV 3.
    Fengchi GB 20 and Dazhui Du 14 were reduced with strong stimulation, but the needles withdrawn quickly. At Shenmen HT 7 and Sanyinjiao SP 6 they were retained for 20 minutes.
    After four treatments with the first group of points the patient's spirits and sleep improved. He was able to walk normally, but was still unnaturally garrulous. The second group was now needled, and after three treatments all his symptoms had gone. The case was followed up for 3 years and there was no relapse.

Explanation: The above cases are both sequelae of brain damage after carbon monoxide poisoning. Both cases are different, however, in that the first was Yin and static, and the second was Yang and active. The first patient had previously been weak, and his sequelae were incontinence of stool and urine arising from weakness of Kidney Qi, which was unable to hold or consolidate. The second patient had a previous history of Exuberance of Liver Yang, so his sequelae were restlessness, insomnia and offensive language, all symptoms of mania. Treatment in both cases followed the principle of 'Reducing what is Exuberant and reinforcing what is Deficient'.

The first patient had been weak so besides using Shenmen HT 7, the Yuan-Source point to refresh the mind, Quchi L.I. 11 and Zusanli ST 36 were selected. As He-Sea points, they activate Qi and Blood and strengthen the Spleen and Stomach. Guanyuan Ren 4, the Front-Mu point of the Small Intestine, and Sanyinjiao SP 6, the meeting point of the three leg Yin, were used to tighten the Kidney Qi.

The second patient had a previous history of hypertension, which was aggravated by the poisoning, so Sanyinjiao SP 6 and Shenmen HT 7 were used to refresh the mind. Taichong LIV 3 and Hegu L.I. 4 were used to suppress the hyperactivity of Liver Yang. These two points used together are known as 'Si Guan' or 'Four Gates'. Both are Yuan-Source points: one nourishes Yin, the other suppresses Yang. Together they soothe Liver Yang, harmonize Liver Qi and Blood and activate the channels and collaterals.

Lu Xingzhai, ANYANG PREFECTURAL HYGIENE SCHOOL, HENAN PROVINCE
(see Henan Traditional Chinese Medicine, Issue 3, 1982).

126. Coma from electric shock

Lahebi, male, age 16, peasant, foreigner

Case registered: March 1982

History: The patient was hit by lightning when he was caught in a rainstorm.

Examination: The patient was semicomatose. *BP:*18.7/14.7 kPa (140/110 mmHg). His head was burned. A 6 cm square patch of hair around Fengchi GB 20 had been scorched away, the adjacent skin was dark red and there was obvious haematoma. His limbs tremored paroxysmally. Physiological reflex present. *Tongue body:* bluish purple. *Pulse:* 86 per minute, deep and choppy.

Diagnosis: Injury of the head with Blood Stagnation. Loss of consciousness, sense organs shut.

Treatment: Resuscitate the Mind, invigorate the Blood and collaterals to remove Stagnation.

Principal Points: Neiguan P 6, Renzhong Du 26, Sanyinjiao SP 6, Shixuan (Extras).

At Renzhong Du 26 the needle was inserted obliquely upwards to a depth of 0.5 cun. The Shixuan (Extras) were bled. Neiguan P 6 and Sanyinjiao were needled with strong stimulation. Electro-acupuncture was given at Neiguan P 6, with continuous wave electric stimulation at a frequency of 100–120 per minute, and at an appropriate intensity. After 5 minutes the patient groaned. The intensity was increased for another 5 minutes. At this point the patient cried out, complaining of heaviness and pain behind his ear. The current was switched off immediately, and he recovered after another 5 minutes.

Zheng Yugang, WUCHANG COUNTY TCM HOSPITAL, HUBEI

Editor's Note: In this case of coma from electric injury, the doctors gave symptomatic treatment to resuscitate the Mind and open the sense organs. Renzhong Du 26 and the Shixuan (Extras) are important points for resuscitation. Together with Neiguan P 6 and Sanyinjiao SP 6 they invigorate the Blood, channels and collaterals, remove Blood Stagnation and resuscitate the Mind. Electric stimulation was used to reinforce the effect of the needles.

127. Hernia, inguinal

Chen, male, age 28, worker

Case registered: 20 August 1981

History: The patient was admitted with high fever and chills, which were reduced after emergency treatment. In the night, however, a lump the size of a rat appeared in his groin on the left. It was painful, and the pain radiated into his abdomen and testicles, which were wet and cold. This happened about four times during the night, and the pain was very severe. While the lump was there the patient was unable to urinate or defaecate. He was referred for acupuncture and moxibustion the next day.

Examination: The lump reappeared just before the patient was examined. It was soft when pressed, and there was dull pain when more pressure was exerted. When percussed it sounded like a drum. Liver and spleen were not enlarged. *Tongue body:* pale. *Tongue coating:* white and moist. *Pulse:* deep, wiry and leisurely.

Diagnosis: Chong Hernia: Pathogenic Cold in Chong Mai.

Treatment: Warm the Middle Burner and expel Pathogenic Cold, redirect Rebellious Qi in Chong Mai downwards.

Principal Points: Qugu Ren 2, Yinjiao Ren 7, Taichong LIV 3 (left), Qichong ST 30 (left).
   Lifting, thrusting and twirling manipulation was used, and the points were rubbed after the needles were withdrawn. Moxibustion was given. During moxibustion at Qugu Ren 2 and Yinjiao Ren 7 the patient felt tingling and numbness. These sensations penetrated deeper into the points and along the midline of the abdomen to the stomach. At this point the pain was relieved. There were similar sensations at Taichong LIV 3 and Qichong ST 30. At the end of the treatment the patient felt warmth all over his abdomen. Treatment was given once every 2 days. After the first session the lump only appeared once a day. After four treatments the condition was cured.

Explanation: The *Su Wen* says, 'The disease is characterized by pain rising up and invading the heart, and the patient has difficulty passing stool and urine. This is called Chong Hernia' (Gu Kong Lun, Bones chapter). Wang Bing mentions that, 'The course of the disease indicates that it is in the Ren Mai (Conception Channel). It is called Chong Hernia because it rises upwards (Chong)', i.e. this disease rises upwards and causes pain. Gao Shizong observes that, 'Diseases in Ren Mai manifest in men as the seven kinds of hernia, and in women as stasis of menstrual flow. If a man cannot pass stool or urine it is Chong hernia. This means that not only is there internal disease, but also obstruction of stool and urine. The energy accumulates inside and rises upwards'. Zhang Jiebin mentions that this disease is called Chong Hernia, 'because it affects both Ren and Chong Mai'. From the above we can conclude the following:
1. The disease is in Ren and Chong Mai.
2. It is caused by Exuberance of Yin Cold, which leads to imbalance and malnourishment of Ren and Chong Mai.
3. The symptoms are Rebellious Qi rising from the lower abdomen causing pain, and inability to pass stool or urine.
4. Treatment should aim to relieve and regulate the Chong Qi.
   Chong Hernia is the main disease of Chong Mai. The *Nan Jing* says, 'Hernia is Qi in nature. All hernias are stagnation of Qi causing disease' (Hui Zhu Jian Zheng, Medical Problems chapter). The treatment principle should be primarily to warm the vessels and dispel the Pathogenic Cold to redirect Rebellious Qi downwards. Points on Ren Mai, the Liver and Stomach channels should be used with reinforcing and reducing evenly

method to dredge and regulate the Stasis of Qi and relieve the pain. Moxibustion after needling disperses the accumulated Cold.

The Liver channel 'goes around the genitals and lower abdomen ... Ren and Chong Mai originate in the lower abdomen, and pass up along the abdomen when they reach the superficial level'.

Qugu Ren 3 is a meeting point of Ren Mai with the Liver channel. Yinjiao Ren 7 is a meeting point of Chong Mai, Ren Mai and the Liver.

Many generations of doctors have stressed the importance of Taichong LIV 3 and Qichong ST 30 in the treatment of hernia, e.g. the *Tong Ren* (Bronze Figure) records the use of Qichong 'for Rebellious Qi in the abdomen rising to assault the Heart', and the *Tu Yi* (The Diagrams) observes that, 'It is good for Rebellious Qi, sensations of gas rushing in the abdomen, and hernias'.

The *Qian Jin Yi Fang* (Supplement to the Important Prescriptions Worth a Thousand Gold Pieces) mentions that Taichong LIV 3 is 'good for all cases of Cold in the upper body' and recommends treatment with 'as many moxa cones as it takes to stop the pain'.

Used in combination, these points regulate Rebellious Qi in the channels and collaterals, clearing Stagnation and relaxing the tendons, so that the Cold is dispersed and the pain is relieved.

Li Licheng, JINAN MUNICIPAL CENTRAL HOSPITAL, SHANDONG PROVINCE
(see Journal of Traditional Chinese Medicine, Issue 4, 1984)

128. Hernia, femoral

Li, female, age 46, peasant

History: The patient had paroxysmal abdominal pain for 7 hours. She had a spherical mass in the right inguinal region. It was painful and did not disappear when pressed. She had vomited twice, and was unable to pass stool.

Examination: Temperature normal. *Pulse rate:* 86/min. *BP:* 14.9/11.2 kPa (112/84 mmHg). Heart and lungs normal. The patient was moaning, and clearly in great pain. Her abdomen was slightly distended, but soft. There was no tenderness, and no rebound tenderness. There was visible peristalsis and excessive bowel sound.

Diagnosis: Pathogenic Cold in the Liver channel.

Treatment: Dredge Liver Qi, warm the channel and disperse Cold.

Principal Points: Dadun LIV 1.

Initially manual repositioning was attempted, but this was ineffective.

Next Dadun LIV 1 was needled on the affected side with reinforcing and reducing evenly method. The needle was retained, and moxibustion was applied until the impacted mass was reduced. The mass was massaged during the treatment to help disperse it. After 15 minutes there was no more pain and the mass was reduced.

Explanation: In TCM incarcerated hernia can be due to Cold, Damp or Heat. The disease affects the Liver channel. The *Ling Shu* says, 'The Liver channel has a branch called Ligou LIV 5, 5 cun superior to the medial malleolus which leads to the Shao Yang channel. This branch goes along the shins to the testes and joins at the penis. Adversely rising Qi causes swollen testicles and hernia. Excess symptoms are persistent erections and deficiency symptoms are severe itching' (*Miraculous Pivot*, Channels chapter). Many generations of doctors have therefore treated hernia with Liver points which dredge the channel.

Dadun LIV1, the Jing-Well point, dredges Liver Qi and redirects it downwards to relieve pain. Moxibustion warms the channel and disperses Pathogenic Cold. Acupuncture and moxibustion are simple and economical therapies for incarcerated hernia, but are not indicated for chronic cases with intestinal necrosis and peritonitis.

Ying Hao, ACUPUNCTURE AND MOXIBUSTION SECTION, JIANNING COUNTY HOSPITAL, FUJIAN PROVINCE
(see *Chinese Acupuncture and Moxibustion, Issue 4, 1982*)

Part Two
GYNAECOLOGY

129. Breast lump

Zhang, female, age 34, cadre

Case registered: August 1975

History: The patient had a mass in her left breast 3 years previously. The mass and the whole left breast were removed in the surgical department of this hospital. Pathological examination afterwards showed mammary hyperplasia. She now had a mass in her right breast, and was anxious that it might be malignant. The surgical department were unable to make a definite diagnosis, but suggested removal of the whole breast for later pathological examination. The patient was opposed to this and it was decided that she undergo a course of medication with hormones and traditional Chinese drugs instead. The mass continued to grow, however. She lost her appetite, and developed sensations of fullness and pain on the right.

Examination: There was a 6 × 4 cm mass above the areola of her right breast. It was medium hard in texture, fairly smooth and tender on palpation. The skin was normal in colour. *Tongue body:* dark. *Tongue coating:* yellow and greasy. *Pulse:* wiry.

Diagnosis: Breast nodule: Stagnation of Liver Qi.

Treatment: Dredge and regulate Liver Qi, activate circulation of Blood, resolve Stasis.

Principal Points: Taichong LIV 3, Danzhong Ren 17, Yingchuang ST 16, Zusanli ST 36.
   The points were needled on the affected side, and reduced. Electro-acupuncture was given with a G6805 unit, and the needles were retained for 30 minutes. Treatment was given daily. Sensation from Zusanli ST 36 was propagated to the breast. The mass started to reduce in size, and after 28 treatments completely disappeared. The case was followed up for 11 years and there was no relapse.

Explanation: In TCM the nipples are controlled by the Liver channel, and the breasts belong to the Stomach channel. Thus breast disease is usually ascribed to Stomach and Liver dysfunction. In this case the patient presented with pain in the left side, poor appetite, and a mass in the breast. Together with her tongue and pulse these pointed to Stagnation of Liver Qi affecting the Qi and Blood of the Spleen. The treatment principle was therefore to dredge the Liver Qi, invigorate the Blood to resolve Stasis and swelling. The points selected were mostly on the Liver and Stomach channels.

Dai Yuqin, NINGXIA MEDICAL COLLEGE HOSPITAL,
(see Ningxia: Scientific Papers in Traditional Chinese Medicine, Vol 1)

130. Tremor of the genitals at night

Li, female, age 19, peasant

Case registered: 10 August 1967

History: The patient developed a severe tremor in her genitals at night. It woke her up from intense dreaming between 1.00 and 2.00 a.m. Her appetite, bowels and urination were all normal.

Examination: Gynaecological examinations were normal. The patient was healthy looking and well fed, but her demeanour was quite anxious. *Tongue body:* pale. *Tongue coating:* thin and white. *Pulse:* deep, wiry and choppy.

Diagnosis: Stagnation of Liver Qi causing agitation of Liver Wind.

Treatment: Nourish the Liver and Kidney to calm Liver Wind.

Principal Points: Ganshu BL 18, Taichong LIV 3, Taixi KID 3, Sanyinjiao SP 6.
    At Ganshu BL 18 the needle was inserted 0.7 cun deep with reinforcing and reducing evenly method, then three pea-sized moxa cones were applied. At Taichong LIV 3 and Taixi KID 3 the needles were inserted 1 cun deep. Taichong LIV 3 was reduced and Taixi KID 3 was reinforced. Sanyinjiao SP 6 was needled with reinforcing and reducing evenly method to a depth of 1.5 cun. Treatment was given once every other day. After the first treatment there was a marked improvement and the continuous tremor was reduced to a slight intermittent tremor. She was able to sleep at night, but still dreamed a lot. After two treatments the tremor disappeared and she was able to sleep peacefully. She was given five treatments in total and was completely cured. The case was followed up for 6 months and there was no relapse.

Explanation: 'All Wind syndromes, tremor and faintness belong to the Liver channel', which governs the tendons and goes around the genitals.

The symptoms manifested at Shou time (Branch 2), so treatment was directed at the Liver channel.

Ganshu BL 18 and Taixi KID 3 nourish the Liver and Kidney. Sanyinjiao SP 6 regulates the Liver, Kidney and Spleen channels. Taichong LIV 3 soothes Liver Wind.

Feng Wenhua, ACUPUNCTURE AND MOXIBUSTION SECTION, LUOYANG COUNTY HOSPITAL, CHENGGUAN, SHENXI PROVINCE
(*see Shanghai Journal of Acupuncture and Moxibustion, Issue 3, 1984*)

131. Genital itching

Fu, female, age 54

History: The patient had genital itching for more than 10 years. It was mild at first, but when it got worse she went to her local hospital for treatment. She was given medication, and fumigated the area regularly with steam from herbal decoctions. Although the itching came and went it was never cured. When it was severe she was unable to sleep, and became restless and irritable. There was no local swelling or leucorrhoea, but she had dry stools and yellow urine.

Examination: Tongue body: dry. *Tongue coating:* thin and greasy. *Pulse:* wiry and rapid.

Diagnosis: Stagnation of Liver Qi transforming to Heat, Damp Heat flowing downwards.

Treatment: Clear Heat, soothe the Liver and resolve Damp.

Principal Points: Zhongji Ren 3, Sanyinjiao SP 6, Ququan LIV 8, Taichong LIV 3.

Eight treatments were given over a 20-day period and the needles were retained for 30 minutes. The itching was completely cured. The case was followed up a month later and there was no relapse.

Explanation: Zhongji Ren 3 clears Heat and resolves Damp. Ququan LIV 8 clears Damp Heat and regulates the Lower Burner. These two points are important points for genital itching. Taichong LIV 3 regulates the Liver Qi. Sanyinjiao SP 6 treats diseases in the digestive and urogenital systems.

This is a good formula for itching inside or outside the vagina, and has rarely been known to fail. Together these four points clear Damp Heat, dredge the Lower Burner, regulate Liver Qi and relieve genital itching.

Shao Jingming, HENAN TCM COLLEGE
(see *China's Countryside Medicine. Issue 6, 1981*)

132. Bleeding gums during menstrual cycle

Wang, female, age 35, married, worker

Case registered: 9 July 1985

History: For the last 13 months the patient had not menstruated. Instead she bled from her front lower gums and spat out red saliva. She was also faint and restless, with sensations of fullness and pain in her chest and sides. She was constipated, and her mouth was dry, foul and bitter tasting.

Examination: Tongue body: normal. *Tongue coating:* thin and slightly yellow. *Pulse:* wiry.

Diagnosis: Accumulated Heat in the Liver causing the Blood to rush upwards.

Treatment: Clear Liver Heat and induce Blood to flow downwards.

Principal Points: Quchi L.I. 11, Hegu L.I. 4 through to Houxi SI 3, Yanglingquan GB 34, Taichong LIV 3 through to Yongquan KID 1, Jiexi ST 41.

All the points were reduced. The next day the patient's period began, and the bleeding from her gums stopped. The flow was medium in quantity and dark red with clots. She was in good spirits. Hegu L.I. 4 and Taichong LIV 3 were mildly reduced. The case was followed up for a year, and her menstruation was normal in quantity and colour.

Explanation: The Liver houses the Blood, controls the dispersal of Blood and regulates the quantity of Blood flow. Energy flows smoothly through Chong and Ren Mai when they are filled periodically. When the Liver fails to disperse, Heat accumulates which drives Blood upwards. In this case this was what caused the bleeding gums.

The Large Intestine channel has a branch which goes from the supraclavicular fossa up to the neck, through the cheeks, down into the teeth. The Yang Ming channels are rich in Qi and Blood. Selecting points on the arm and leg Yang Ming channels is therefore very effective to clear accumulated Heat.

Yanglingquan GB 34 is the He-Sea point of the Gallbladder channel and Taichong LIV 3 is the Yuan-Source point of the Liver channel. The two channels are a Yin–Yang pair, so these points are used together to regulate Liver Qi and relieve Stagnation, send down Blood in the channels and stop the gums bleeding.

Gu Zhaojun, ACUPUNCTURE AND MOXIBUSTION SECTION, NANJING TCM
COLLEGE
(see Jianxi Traditional Chinese Medicine, Issue 3, 1987)

133. Metrostaxis

Li, female, age 31, member of staff

History: The patient's health had generally been good. After her menarche at 17, her menstrual flow was slightly excessive and lasted 7 to 8 days. 2 weeks ago she started another period. This was very heavy and did not stop, and she had some moderate dark yellow discharge. She felt weak and faint and her appetite was poor.

Examination: Her complexion was yellow and dry. She was restless, and dreamed a lot at night. Bowels and bladder normal. *Tongue body:* pale. *Tongue coating:* scanty. *Pulse:* thin and rapid.

Diagnosis: Liver Qi Stagnation, Spleen Qi Deficiency.

Treatment: Clear Heat, reinforce the Spleen to stop bleeding.

Principal Points: Hegu L.I. 4, Yinlingquan SP 9, Sanyinjiao SP 6.
Treatment was given once a day. There was no improvement after the first treatment, but she felt a little stronger. After the second treatment there was a marked reduction in the amount of bleeding, and the discharge lightened in colour. After the third treatment the bleeding stopped and all her other symptoms disappeared.

Explanation: In this case the Spleen and the Liver failed to control and house the Blood. Her fatigue and pale yellow complexion were symptoms of Deficient Spleen Qi, and her poor sleep were due to Stagnation of Liver Qi.
Sanyinjiao SP 6 regulates and reinforces Spleen Qi and nourishes Liver Yin to stop bleeding. Yinlingquan SP 9 reinforces the Spleen and regulates the Middle Burner. Hegu L.I. 4 clears Heat and regulates Qi.

Zhang Shanchen, SHANDONG TCM COLLEGE HOSPITAL

134. Chronic pelvic inflammatory disease and infertility

Guo, female, age 32

Case registered: 7 October 1983

History: Since 1974 the patient began to have delayed periods, with sensations of hypochondriac pain and fullness, and dull lower abdominal pain, especially during her periods. Her abdomen was not tender and felt better for warmth. She had profuse leucorrhoea: the discharge was watery and did not smell. She had not become pregnant during 7 years of marriage. The condition was diagnosed as chronic pelvic inflammatory disease with primary infertility. She had a previous history of early morning diarrhoea.

Examination: The patient looked pale. She weighed 40 kg. Her voice was thin and weak. *Tongue body:* pale. *Tongue coating:* thin. *Pulse:* deep, thin and weak.

Diagnosis: Leucorrhoea: Cold and Damp in the Lower Burner, Deficiency of Kidney and Spleen Qi.

Treatment: Reinforce Spleen and Kidney, nourish and invigorate Chong and Ren Mai.

Principal Points: Guanyuan Ren 4, Zusanli ST 36.

Treatment was given once a day, with a 1-day break on Sundays between courses. Moxibustion was applied at the points for 20 minutes at a time.

After 1 month the patient's symptoms were much improved. After another 2 months her periods were regular, she had no more pain in her abdomen and waist and she had put on 11 kg in weight. The leucorrhoea was normal. Uterine examination was normal, and 2 months later she became pregnant. She later gave birth to a baby boy.

Explanation: In TCM chronic pelvic inflammatory disease is usually held to be due to maladjustment of Chong Mai and lack of astringency in Ren Mai, which allows the penetration of Pathogenic Cold and Damp into the Lower Burner. Spleen Deficiency and Damp in the Spleen lead to Deficiency of Kidney Qi.

Moxibustion at Guanyuan Ren 4 nourishes the Kidney, consolidates the Origin of Life, and regulates and restores Yang. This point houses sperm in men and Blood in women.

Zusanli ST 36, the He-Sea point, regulates and reinforces the Spleen and Stomach, nourishes Qi and Blood, and reinforces deficiency and debility.

Moxibustion at these two points reinforces the Spleen and Stomach, regulates and invigorates Chong and Ren Mai to cure the disease gradually.

Xu Zheng, SHIJIAZHUANG MUNICIPAL GLASS FACTORY CLINIC, HEBEI PROVINCE

135. Infertility

CASE 1

Shi, female, age 34, worker

Case registered: 29 November 1977

History: The patient had been married for 10 years but had never been pregnant. Her husband was healthy and they had a normal sex life. Examination in a local hospital in March 1977 showed the uterus was normal in size and not displaced, and the cervix and vagina were smooth. Uterine curettage showed that the endometrium was in secretory phase. Fluid infusion revealed blockage of both fallopian tubes. When she came here she had fullness of the breasts before her period and tenderness of the nipples, with severe sensations of heaviness in her lower abdomen. Her menstrual blood was dark and scanty. She also had pain in the lower back and knees. She felt tired and her appetite was poor.

Examination: The patient was emaciated. *Tongue body:* normal. *Tongue coating:* thin. *Pulse:* thin and wiry.

Diagnosis: Infertility: Deficiency and impairment of Chong and Ren Mai, Stagnation of Liver Qi.

Treatment: Regulate Liver Qi, regulate and dredge Ren and Chong Mai.

Principal Points: Guanyuan Ren 4, Qihai Ren 6, Shuidao ST 28, Guilai ST 29, Zusanli ST 36, Neiguan P 6, Taichong LIV 3, Sanyinjiao SP 6, Gongsun SP 4.

   The points were rotated, and electric stimulation was added. Treatment was given once every other day.

   After the second treatment she developed heaviness and pain in her right shoulder. She had no previous history of shoulder pain. After 17 treatments all her symptoms had improved except the shoulder pain. She was re-examined at her local hospital. Carbon dioxide was passed into both fallopian tubes. When the pressure was increased to 200 mmHg, bubbling sounds could be heard on both sides of her abdomen. At the same time she experienced oppression in the chest and pain in her shoulder, which indicated that her fallopian tubes were unblocked. Acupuncture was continued. 7 months after her initial consultation she reported that she had not had a period for a month. Her appetite was poor and she felt sick and tired. Her pulse was wiry and slippery. A urine test showed her to be pregnant.

Explanation: In TCM infertility is believed to be related to Kidney Qi, Blood, Chong Mai and Ren Mai. Guanyuan Ren 4 and Qihai Ren 6 regulate and strengthen both Ren and Chong Mai. Neiguan P 6 and Taichong LIV 3 regulate Liver Qi. Sanyinjiao SP 6 strengthens the Liver, Spleen and Kidney, and nourishes Chong and Ren Mai. Zusanli ST 36, Guilai ST 29 and Shuidao ST 28 regulate Stomach Qi and regulate the channels and vessels. Gongsun SP 4 dredges and regulates the Sea of Blood, because of its connection with Chong Mai.

> Case treated by Zhu Rugong, case study by Ju Xianshui and Lu Yanyao, SHANGHAI TCM COLLEGE HOSPITAL
> *(see Shanghai Journal of Traditional Chinese Medicine, Issue 7, 1981)*

CASE 2

Sun, female, age 32, saleswoman

Case registered: 8 November 1980

History: The patient had been married for 3 years. Her husband was healthy and their sex life was normal, but she had not managed to get pregnant. An examination in March 1980 found that her left fallopian tube was blocked. She took 60 doses of Chinese herbs, which relieved the abdominal pain she had been suffering, but she was still unable to get pregnant. Before her periods she suffered fullness and burning pain in the breasts, tenderness of the nipples, and fullness and pain of the lower abdomen. Her menstrual blood was dark, scanty and contained clots. She also suffered from fatigue, and pain in the lower back and knees.

Examination: The patient looked emaciated, and was dark around the eyes. *Tongue body:* normal. *Tongue coating:* thin and white. *Pulse:* wiry and thin.

Diagnosis: Infertility: Deficiency and impairment of Chong and Ren Mai, Stagnation of Liver Qi.

Treatment: Soothe Liver Qi, regulate and reinforce Ren and Chong Mai.

Principal Points: Guanyuan Ren 4, Qihai Ren 6, Taichong LIV 3, Gongsun SP 4, Shangjuxu ST 37, Xiajuxu ST 39.
    Taichong LIV 3, Gongsun SP 4, Shangjuxu ST 37 and Xiajuxu ST 39 were needled on the left. Lifting, thrusting and twirling technique was used to elicit Qi sensation, then the needles were retained for 15 minutes, and manipulated again once. Her period came after the 10th treatment, and her symptoms were markedly better. X-rays showed the left fallopian tube was unblocked. The patient came for 10 more consolidating

sessions, then treatment was suspended to observe the effects. After 2 weeks she returned to say that she had missed a period. Her appetite was poor, she felt tired and nauseous. Her tongue was red with a thin yellow coat, and her pulse was wiry and slippery. She craved sour and salty food. A urine test showed her to be pregnant, and she was advised to go home and rest.

Explanation: The Su Wen says 'A woman starts her period at the age of fourteen, when Ren Mai is unblocked and the pulse at Taichong LIV 3 is full. She is then capable of having a child . . . At the age of forty-nine Ren Mai is empty, and the pulse at Taichong LIV 3 is forceless. Menstruation is exhausted and she cannot have a child' (Familiar Conversations, Innate Vitality chapter). These observations show that fertility is closely related to Ren and Chong Mai. Deficiency or impairment of these two vessels can lead to different gynaecological diseases. Qi Deficiency in Chong Mai can lead to leucorrhoea or vaginal bleeding in pregnancy. Maladjustment of the two vessels can lead to infertility, disease in the two vessels can lead to agalactia, protracted discharge of lochia or severe haemorrhage. This is because Chong Mai is the Sea of Blood, and connects the Shao Yin channels. It connects the 12 channels and links the Zang-Fu to the womb. Thus the Blood of all the organs and channels belongs to Chong Mai. Chong and Ren Mai are thus always important to keep in mind when treating gynaecological disease. The key to their treatment is regulation of menstruation, and the key to regulation of menstruation is readjustment of these two vessels. In this case regulating Liver Qi was also a priority.

Guanyuan Ren 4 and Gongsun SP 4 regulate and nourish the two vessels. Guanyuan Ren 4 is a meeting point of the three leg Yin channels and Ren Mai, and Gongsun SP 4 is one of the Eight Confluent points and opens into Chong Mai. Taichong LIV 3 regulates Liver Qi and Blood. Qihai Ren 6, Shangjuxu ST 37 and Xiajuxu ST 39 nourish Qi and Blood, regulate and reinforce the intestines, Spleen and Stomach to reinforce the source of Postnatal Qi. When Qi and Blood were regulated and circulating well, and Chong and Ren Mai were full the patient was able to get pregnant.

CASE 3

Wu, female, age 27, married

Case registered: 4 May 1982

History: The patient had been married for a year and had not managed to get pregnant. She was born when her mother was 40 years old, and grew up weak and thin. Her menses started when she was 17. They were usually late and the flow was dark and scanty, lasting 2 or 3 days. She also had lower abdominal pain during menstruation. Generally her vagina was dry. An examination showed that her genitals were underdeveloped: she had no pubic hair, her womb was underdeveloped with no appendages. Her condition was diagnosed as 'uterine hypoplasia' and she was told she could not become pregnant. She then tried placental tissue fluid and traditional Chinese drugs, but without success, and eventually decided to try acupuncture and moxibustion.

Examination: The patient was emaciated and weak. She had no appetite and felt weak. *Tongue body:* pale and slightly swollen. *Pulse:* deep, thin and weak.

Diagnosis: Deficiency and impairment of Chong and Ren Mai.

Treatment: Regulate Chong and Ren Mai.

Principal Points: Shenshu BL 23, Ganshu BL 18, Pishu BL 20, Zusanli ST 36, Ciliao BL 32, Guanyuan Ren 4.

Point Injection Therapy: 0.5 ml of Dang Gui solution was injected into the points. Only two points were used in one treatment, then moxibustion was given at Guanyuan Ren 4.

After five treatments her vagina was less dry, and her spirits and appetite improved. After 20 treatments she missed a period. Treatment was suspended for observation. A test confirmed that she was pregnant, and after 9 months she gave birth to a baby girl.

Explanation: Female infertility is defined as failure to conceive after 1 year of married life when the husband has normal sperm. It can be caused by Deficiency Cold, Phlegm Damp or accumulation of Heat. Whatever the cause, the key to the disease is regulation of Chong and Ren Mai. To readjust both vessels it is important to nourish the Spleen and Stomach to reinforce the source of Postnatal Qi, and to tonify the Liver and Kidney.

We usually use Pishu BL 20, Zusanli ST 36 and Zhongwan Ren 12 to reinforce the Middle Burner. Shenshu BL 23, Ganshu BL 18 and Guanyuan Ren 4 nourish the Liver and Kidney. Ciliao BL 32 regulates the womb. All these points together readjust Chong and Ren. Point injection therapy with Dang Gui enhances these effects.

The treatment of this case was characterized by the approach of treating the Zang-Fu, with special emphasis on the Spleen and Stomach. This approach originates from the *Nei Jing*, and was further developed in the writings of Hua Tuo and Qian Yi. The theory was fully developed in the Jin dynasty when Zhang Yuansu designed the model of treatment based on Excess and Deficiency, and Root and Branch manifestations of specific Zang and Fu. This approach has been followed by generations of doctors.

Case treated by Zhang Heyuan, case study by Liu Mingyi,
GUIYANG TCM COLLEGE

136. Severe morning sickness

Sheng, female, age 25, cadre

Case registered: 30 April 1984

History: The patient had not menstruated for 50 days. She also felt faint and tired, was sick and had no appetite. Over the past 2 weeks she frequently vomited coffee-like liquids, and was unable to eat or drink. Tests showed no pathology, but she was found to be pregnant. Treatment with fluid infusion and anti-emetics was unsuccessful, and she was referred for acupuncture and moxibustion.

Examination: The patient was emaciated and sleepy. Her eyes were deeply sunken. *Tongue body:* pale. *Tongue coating:* white. *Pulse:* slow, slippery and weak.

Diagnosis: Pernicious vomiting: Deficiency of Stomach Qi.

Treatment: Reinforce the Stomach, regulate the Qi of the Middle Burner and redirect Rebellious Qi downwards.

Principal Points: Jinjin (Extra), Yuye (Extra), Shangwan Ren 13, Zhongwan Ren 12, Tiantu Ren 22.
   At Shangwan Ren 13, Zhongwan Ren 12 and Tiantu Ren 22 the needles were twirled to reinforce and then withdrawn. Next, 0.5 ml of a solution of vitamins B_1 and B_6 was injected. Jinjin and Yuye were bled. Treatment was given once a day.
   After the first treatment the patient's vomiting was much less. After five treatments she was completely cured, with no relapse at the time of writing.

Explanation: Vomiting during pregnancy is called pernicious vomiting in TCM. The symptoms are loss of appetite, choosiness at mealtimes, nausea, vomiting, or even constant vomiting and inability to eat. It is caused by Deficiency of Stomach Qi, Stasis of Phlegm, or Stagnation of Liver Qi causing Rebellious Qi to rise. In this case the vomiting arose from Deficiency of Stomach Qi. Chong Mai belongs to Yang Ming. When menstrual blood is not discharged during pregnancy Chong Mai becomes Exuberant and its Qi rises to attack the Stomach. This in turn is unable to send down Qi, and instead the Stomach Qi rises with the Rebellious Chong Qi, causing nausea and vomiting.

Jinjin (Extra) and Yuye (Extra) are effective for vomiting. Zhongwan Ren 12 is the Gathering point of the Fu and the Front-Mu point of the Stomach, and Shangwan Ren 13 is the meeting point of the Stomach and Ren Mai. Together these two points regulate and strengthen the Stomach and Spleen to redirect Rebellious Qi downwards. Tiantu Ren 22 regulates Qi in the chest and diaphragm, so that the Qi in the Upper Burner moves freely and the Stomach Qi can descend freely.

Point injection of vitamins B_1 and B_6 enhances the effects of the points. The medication also helps maintain the normal functioning of the digestive system and is nutritious: it is thus very useful in the treatment of morning sickness.

Kong Lingju and Qiu Xiurong, JILIN FARM PRODUCT SCHOOL

137. Eclampsia

CASE 1

Hu, female, age 24, peasant

Case registered: 6 September 1964

History: The patient was pregnant. Shortly before the baby was due she became very nervous and felt faint, with oppression in the chest. Later she became semiconscious, with muscle tremors, numbness of the hands and feet and tremor of the corners of the mouth. Her eyes were fixed straight ahead. This happened 2–3 times a day. She gave birth to a baby girl, but the symptoms returned during labour. In the 2 days following delivery she was often semiconscious. She had paroxysmal tremor, opisthotonos, and faecal and urinary incontinence. Her condition was diagnosed as eclampsia, but symptomatic allopathic treatment had no effect.

Examination: The room smelled. The patient was lying in bed and did not answer when spoken to. She was short and fat, with a dark complexion and dark red lips. Her eyes were tightly shut and her jaw and fists were clenched. Her limbs were trembling and her back was very tense. She had oedema of the ankles. There were sounds of sputum in her throat and her mouth was running with saliva. Her lower abdomen was full, hard and very hot. Her mouth needed to be forced open to examine her tongue. *Tongue coating:* thick, yellow, slightly dry and rough. *Pulse:* deep and choppy.

Diagnosis: Pathogenic Wind, Blood Stasis, Turbid Yang obstructing the orifices.

Treatment: Resuscitate the Mind, activate the vessels, relieve pain and stop spasm.

Principal Points: Renzhong Du 26, Yongquan KID 1 (bilateral).
   Strong stimulation was used. After a short time the patient turned her head and showed that she was in pain. The needles were then withdrawn.

Secondary Points: Zusanli ST 36, Hegu L.I. 4, Sanyinjiao SP 6, Quchi L.I. 11, Xuehai SP 10 (all bilateral), and Zhongwan Ren 12.
   Medium strong stimulation was used, and the needles were retained for 20 minutes, with occasional manipulation during that time to maintain the level of stimulation. The patient groaned during the treatment and wet the bed. Her spasm began to improve and the tremor did not recur. By the time the needles were withdrawn she was already able to look around and moan quietly. Her consciousness was now restored, but she looked dull and her lower abdomen was still full and hard.
   Early the next morning she was given one dose of modified Sheng Hua Tang (Generation and Transformation Decoction). She discharged dark red blood clots several times after this, and then felt much more comfortable in her lower abdomen and was able to help herself to porridge. All her symptoms were gone and she was discharged from hospital to go home and rest. The case was followed up for several years, and both mother and child remained healthy.

Explanation: This is a serious disease where any delay in treatment puts both mother and child at risk. The earliest record of the disease is found in the *Chao Shi Bing Yuan* (General Treatise on the Causes and Symptoms of Disease): 'The disease manifests as periodic loss of consciousness. It is spasm caused by Wind invading the Tai Yang channels'. Treatment for this disease is described in the *Yi Xue Xin Wu* (The Understanding of Medicine): 'Before delivery it is necessary to reinforce Qi and Blood and soothe Wind. After delivery it is important to tonify Qi and Blood strongly'.
   Generally speaking, eclampsia before and during birth is due to Deficient Yin which cannot control the Yang, so Liver Yang rises up, or Exuberant Heat leads to stirring up of Wind, which rises up with the Qi of the fetus. Postnatal eclampsia is usually due to weakness of the vessels and

Deficiency of Blood: the Spirit is not housed, or the weakness leaves the person susceptible to Pathogenic Wind.

I would suggest that the above are only generalizations and may not be appropriate for specific cases. Of course there is no doubt that after giving birth a woman displays many symptoms of Deficiency, to such a degree that the classics say, 'After labour a woman is a basin of ice', and 'all diseases after childbirth should be treated with the emphasis on reinforcing Qi and Blood', but can cases of retention of lochia, Putrid Blood invading the Heart, or Wind stirring within leading to disturbance of the Spirit really be considered Deficiency diseases? In these cases the doctor must waste no time moving Stagnation by dredging the orifices and purging pathogens to calm the Mind. The last thing he or she should do is add fuel to the fire by reinforcing. The difference between Excess and Deficiency here is no less than the difference between Heaven and Hell, and the doctor must use the symptoms and signs to differentiate the two.

In this case the patient had symptoms of eclampsia before and after the birth, and there was retention of the lochia and Blood Stasis after the birth. This obstructed the Functional Qi and disturbed the function of sending the Clear Yang up and the Turbid Yang down. Pathogenic Qi invaded and rose up, causing spasm and semiconsciousness. This could be seen from the patient's dark lips, choppy pulse, clenched fists and the hardness of her lower abdomen.

Zhang Zhongjing needled Qimen LIV 14 on women with 'Heat invading the Chamber of Blood causing hallucinations'. This supports the ideas I have proposed above. Zhang Zhongjing was treating cases affected during menstruation. This case was postpartum. The aetiology is, however, the same, as the chamber of Blood is empty following loss of Blood, which leaves the patient susceptible to Pathogenic Qi. The difference in this case is that the symptoms before and after labour were urgent, and needed to be treated symptomatically.

For these reasons tonics were not administered, and acupuncture was used to resuscitate the patient, activate the channels, relieve pain and stop spasm. Renzhong Du 26 and Yongquan KID 1 are important emergency points to resuscitate and revitalize. Zusanli ST 36, the Lower He-Sea point of the Stomach channel, is an important point to readjust the functions of the Spleen and Stomach. Hegu L.I. 4, the Yuan-Source point, activates and regulates Qi and Blood and restores the actions of raising the Clear and descending the Turbid. Zhongwan Ren 12 is one of the Thirteen Ghost points: it redirects Rebellious Qi downwards and eases the Triple Burner. Sanyinjiao SP 6, Xuehai SP 10 and Quchi L.I. 11 treat syncope from disturbance of Yin and Yang, soothe Exuberant Liver Qi and move Stasis in the collaterals. When the Wind is stilled, the Liver is soothed so the spasm is relieved. Sheng Hua Tang removes old Blood and helps to generate new.

Wang Yin and Wang Qihui, ACUPUNCTURE AND MOXIBUSTION SECTION, NINGDU COUNTY PEOPLE'S HOSPITAL, JIANXI PROVINCE

CASE 2

Hu, female, age 22, peasant

Case registered: 14 February 1984

History: The patient had been pregnant for 20 weeks but she had had no morning sickness or fetal movement. This was her first pregnancy. Her last period had been turbid. By the end of the 12th lunar month of 1983 she had worsening oedema of the legs and body, faintness, headache and sickness. She was eventually admitted to hospital in a coma, with eclampsia and suspected fetal death. She was prescribed medication to calm the Mind, relieve spasm, reduce blood pressure and induce urination. The next day she gave birth to a stillborn baby boy. After 5 days her blood pressure was normal and the oedema subsided, but she was only semiconscious and seemed lacklustre: unable to speak or get out of bed. She had urinary and faecal incontinence.

Examination: Coma. Oedema (+++). *Temperature:* 36.6°C. *Pulse rate:* 88/ min. *Respiration:* 22/min. *BP:* 20.0/14.7 kPa (150/110 mmHg). Neck soft. Heart negative. Mucus could be heard in her lungs. *Blood test:* RBC $4.92 \times 10^{12}/l$ ($4.92 \times 10^6/mm^3$), *WBC:* $12 \times 10^9/l$ ($12 \times 10^3/mm^3$), neutrophils 85%, lymphocytes 15%, haemoglobin 140 g/l (14 g%). Urinary protein (+++).

Diagnosis: Deficiency of Kidney and Liver Yin, Heart Fire, Liver Yang rising causing Wind.

Treatment: Nourish Yin and suppress Yang, soothe Wind and calm the Liver.

Principal Points: Baihui Du 20, Fengfu Du 16, Yamen Du 15, Tiantu Ren 22, Lianquan Ren 23, Tongli HT 5, Zhaohai KID 6, Yongquan KID 1, Neiguan P 6, Sanyinjiao SP 6, Taixi KID 3, Taichong LIV 3, Yanglingquan GB 34, Zusanli ST 36, Quchi L.I. 11.

The points were rotated and needled in compatible groups. After two treatments the patient was in better spirits. She was able to open her mouth more and her tongue was more flexible. After three treatments her urination became normal. After six treatments she was able to speak a little. After 30 treatments her speech was clear. She could get out of bed and walk unaided, so she was discharged as cured.

Explanation: Du Mai governs the Yang of the whole body, so Baihui Du 20 regulates Yin and Yang and calms the Mind. Fengfu Du 16 is located just beneath the Sea of Marrow (i.e. the brain), and is where Du Mai and the Bladder channel meet. Yamen Du 15 is where Du Mai and Yang Wei Mai meet. It activates the channels and opens the orifices. Tiantu Ren 22 and Lianquan Ren 23 are where Ren Mai and Yin Wei Mai meet. They help restore the function of the tongue. These five points are important points to calm the Mind and treat aphasia.

Tongli HT 5 clears Heart Fire and opens the sense organs. Zhaohai KID 6 and Yongquan KID 1 send Yin up to nourish the sense organs. They also control excess Yang, nourish the Yin, purge Fire and are good for constipation.

Neiguan P 6, the Luo-Connecting point and one of the Eight Confluent points, nourishes the Mind and refreshes the spirits. Sanyinjiao SP 6 benefits the Stomach and urination. Taixi KID 3 and Taichong LIV 3 together nourish Liver Yin. Taixi KID 3 and Yanglingquan GB 34 together nourish the Liver, and reinforce the tendons and the marrow. These five points nourish the Kidney and Liver, and are therefore important in the treatment of Wei syndrome.

Zusanli ST 36 and Quchi L.I. 11 were selected according to the classical principle of 'treating Wei syndrome by selecting points solely on the Yang Ming channels'.

Li Shuxuan, ACUPUNCTURE AND MOXIBUSTION SECTION, GAN DAQING, OBSTETRICS AND GYNAECOLOGY DEPARTMENT, QINGYANG PREFECTURAL PEOPLE'S HOSPITAL, GANSU PROVINCE
(see Hebei Traditional Chinese Medicine, Issue 3, 1986)

138. Retention of dead fetus

Shen, female, age 25, peasant

Case registered: 5 February 1981

History: The patient had been married for a year and pregnant for over 9 months. Previously her periods were normal and regular. 3 days previously she had a sudden painless discharge of water and the umbilical cord came out. At first she was too shy to go to hospital, but the next day the cord became yellow and the fundus of the uterus became enlarged. She had severe pain and nausea. On the third day the pain improved, but she felt faint and tired, and vomited frequently.

Examination: The patient's complexion was pale. Her breathing was deep and rapid, and she was restless. There was uterine contraction, but no fetal heart sound. *Pulse:* rapid and thin.

Diagnosis: Missed labour.

Treatment: 15 units of oxytocin were given intramuscularly. 150 ml of sodium bicarbonate solution were given as fluid infusion to correct acidosis. This treatment had no effect and preparations were made for caesarean section. Both the patient and her family were very anxious about this, so acupuncture was suggested instead.

Principal Points: Hegu L.I. 4, Sanyinjiao SP 6, Zusanli ST 36.

All the points were needled bilaterally. The patient had strong Qi sensation and started sweating. Medium strong stimulation was given, and the needles were retained for 20 minutes. 30 minutes after they were removed the patient gave birth to a stillborn baby. The fetus weighed 4.5 kg and was already rotten and smelly. The patient recovered fully.

> Wu Xiebing, DONGPING TOWNSHIP HOSPITAL, ANHUA COUNTY, HUNAN PROVINCE
> *(see The New Chinese Medicine, Issue 10, 1984)*

Editor's Note: Missed labour is not often seen clinically. Acupuncture was successfully tried after the medication failed. The points were well chosen. Hegu L.I. 4, the Yuan-Source point, is the place where Qi and Blood converge. It can be used to treat both Cold and Heat symptoms. Sanyinjiao SP 6 is the meeting point of the Liver, Spleen and Kidney channels. It nourishes the three leg Yin channels and activates the Blood. Reducing it impairs the Liver, Spleen and Kidney to induce abortion. Hegu L.I. 4 raises and disperses. Reinforcing Hegu L.I. 4 and reducing Sanyinjiao SP 6 activates Blood and promotes abortion. Zusanli ST 36 regulates Qi and Blood and reinforces the body's resistance, so it is not damaged by the abortion.

139. Severe haemorrhage
during termination of pregnancy

Su, female, age 36, teacher

Case registered: 3 November 1965

History: The patient underwent an abortion after a 4-month pregnancy. During the operation it was discovered that the cervix was too narrow for the fetus to pass through, so a laparouterotomy was performed. The patient was in poor health and very frightened. She could not bear the operation, and as the fetus was taken out she had a sudden massive haemorrhage. The operating table was covered in blood. The operation was halted at once and emergency measures were taken to stop the bleeding. Sterilized gauze was inserted into her vagina. Haemostatic drugs were injected and low molecular weight dextran was added to her intravenous drip. The bleeding did not stop, however. Fresh blood gushed out through the gauze, and her condition deteriorated rapidly. Her blood pressure could not be measured. She was in shock and covered in cold sweat. It was 11.00 p.m. and there was no blood available for transfusion. At this point the duty doctor contacted the acupuncture department.

Examination: The patient was comatose and pale with ashen lips. Her body felt wet and cold. *Tongue body:* pale. *Tongue coating:* dry and grey. *Pulse:* deep, slow and barely palpable.

Diagnosis: Yang collapse.

Treatment: Rescue depleted Yang and revive patient.

Principal Points: Baihui Du 20, Renzhong Du 26, Hegu L.I. 4 (bilateral), Neiguan P 6 (bilateral), Xuehai SP 10 (bilateral).
    All the points were reinforced with gentle twirling technique, then the needles were connected to an electro-anaesthesia unit. When the needles were inserted there was no resistance at all, but after 5 minutes' manipulation they felt more gripped. The patient's lips and eyelids showed signs of movement, and the bleeding lessened. The needles were retained without manipulation for a further 20 minutes. The patient regained her facial colour, and regained consciousness. Her pulse was restored and the sweating stopped. *BP:* 11.5/7.33 kPa (86/55 mmHg). When the gauze was removed from her vagina the bleeding had stopped completely. The operation was completed under general anaesthetic. She was discharged after 2 weeks' treatment with medication, blood and fluid transfusion.

Wang Yin and Wang Qihuai, TCM DEPARTMENT, NINGDU COUNTY PEOPLE'S HOSPITAL, JIANXI PROVINCE
(see *Jianxi Traditional Chinese Medicine, Issue 4, 1984*)

Editor's Note: This case history demonstrates the effectiveness of acupuncture for haemorrhagic shock. Baihui Du 20, Renzhong Du 26 and Hegu L.I. 4 rescue depleted Yang and revive the patient. Neiguan P 6 and Xuehai SP 10 nourish the Blood and refresh the Mind. Reinforcing technique restores the Yang and resuscitates the spirits.

140. Postpartum urinary incontinence

Shen, female, age 24, peasant

Case registered: 20 January 1980

History: The patient had discharged small amounts of lochia for over 2 months. She also had pain in her lower abdomen. She was prescribed Chi Shao, Wu Ling Zhi, Tao Ren, Dang Gui Wei, Dan Shen and Chuan Xiong. The lochia stopped and her pain improved, but she developed urinary incontinence, especially when walking, coughing or laughing. She felt cold and tired, with aching and sensations of heaviness.

Examination: Tongue body: pale. *Tongue coating:* thin and moist. *Pulse:* weak.

Diagnosis: Kidney Yang Deficiency.

Treatment: Warm Kidney Yang and astringe the Lower Burner.

Principal Points: Feishu BL 13, Mingmen Du 4, Zhongliao BL 33, Qihai Ren 6, Zhiyin BL 67.
   Warm needle technique was used at Feishu BL 13, Mingmen Du 4 and Zhongliao BL 33, with two cones on each needle. Direct moxibustion was given at Qihai Ren 6 and Zhiyin BL 67, using three pea-sized cones at each point.
   After three treatments the patient was aware of pressure in her bladder, but still lost control if she coughed. This was still so severe that her trousers were soaked. After five treatments she had regained control, and felt well when passing water. She was able to do light work, with just a little dampness if she coughed. Her lumbar pain also improved. She came for a further seven treatments, and the problem was completely cured.

Explanation: In this case the Yang was depleted after protracted discharge of the lochia. When the Qi is Deficient and sinks down the Bladder is unable to control the passage of urine.
   Mingmen Du 4, Qihai Ren 6 and Zhiyin BL 67 warm Kidney Yang. Zhiyin BL 67 is the Mother point of the Bladder channel and was selected to tonify the Bladder according to the principle of 'reinforcing the Mother when an organ is Deficient'. Moxibustion here was used to turn water into Qi. Zhongliao BL 33 astringes the Lower Burner. Feishu BL 13 regulates Lung Qi and disperses water from above. Thus the treatment addressed both the cause and the symptoms. When the Vital Qi is restored, the cold in the body Yin is relieved and the function of the Bladder is restored.

Cai Guohong, ZHANGPU TOWNSHIP CLINIC, KUNSHAN COUNTY, JIANGSU
PROVINCE
(see Jiangsu Journal of Traditional Chinese Medicine. Issue 3, 1985)

Part Three
PAEDIATRICS

141. Nasal obstruction

Wei, male, age 18 days

History: The baby was admitted to hospital with pneumonia, which was cured with antibiotics. The day he was scheduled to be discharged he caught a cold and developed nasal obstruction and sneezing. He cried when feeding because his nose was blocked. He was given medication for his cold but did not respond, so he was given diluted naphazoline nose drops. The effect was only temporary, and his nose would become blocked minutes later.

Examination: There were no abnormal findings except some nasal discharge.

Diagnosis: Deficiency of Defensive Qi.

Treatment: Reinforce Defensive Qi.

Principal Points: Baihui Du 20.
  Mild moxibustion was given at the point with a moxa stick. The doctor monitored the temperature at the point with his index and third finger. Treatment was given three times a day, for 10 minutes at a time. After the first treatment the obstruction was relieved, and the baby was able to sleep quietly and feed without any problem. Treatment was continued for another 2 days, and he was discharged as cured. The problem recurred if he caught a cold, but responded quickly when his parents repeated the treatment.

Explanation: The Yin and Yang of the newborn are very fragile. The interstices of the skin are not strong enough to defend the body from external attack. External pathogens invade easily, stagnating the flow of the exterior Yang Defensive Qi. In turn this obstructs the flow of air of the Lung at the nose.
  Du Mai is the governor of all the Yang, and is known as the Sea of Yang. Baihui Du 20 is located on the top of the head. In TCM it is thought that moxibustion is good for strengthening the defensive functions of the body, so moxibustion at Baihui Du 20 is therefore effective for nasal obstruction of the newborn.

Long Jinlang, tiandeng COUNTY PEOPLE'S HOSPITAL, GUANGXI
(see Journal of Traditional Chinese Medicine, Issue 8, 1987)

142. Abdominal pain

Jiang, male, age 12, schoolboy

Case registered: 7 August 1984

History: The patient had paroxysmal abdominal pain for 2 years. He would have several attacks a day, each one lasting from several minutes to as much as 2 hours. The pain was very severe. Each attack would stop spontaneously. He tried many different treatments but without success, and came here during his holidays, when the pain got particularly bad.

Examination: He had severe colicky pain. When it was at its worst his face turned pale and his lips became dark. His hands were cold and his abdomen was tense and warm. His symptoms were slightly better for warmth.

Diagnosis: Abdominal pain: Invasion of Pathogenic Cold in the Interior, disease in the tendons of the Yang Ming channel.

Treatment: Expel Yin Cold from Triple Burner.

Principal Points: Zusanli ST 36, Sanyinjiao SP 6, Taibai SP 3, Taichong LIV 3, Ashi points.
   This treatment was given several times without effect.

Scarring Moxibustion: Shimen Ren 5.
   The pain was worst at Shimen Ren 5. Scarring moxibustion was given once only, and the pain was cured.

Explanation: The patient had paroxysmal abdominal pain characterized by abdominal tension without tenderness. The *Ling Shu* says, 'The tendons of the Stomach channel join at the genitals and are distributed at the abdomen . . . when they are ill there is tension of the abdominal muscles' (Channel Tendons chapter). It also says, 'The Stomach channel has a branch which starts from the Stomach and goes down along the inside of the abdomen'. The ancients said that, 'The points on the skin are related to where the channels go'.
   In this case Yin Cold pathogens had invaded the Stomach channel tendons. The key to successful treatment to such a disease is 'selecting the painful areas as the point' and 'puncturing with a red-hot needle'. Applying moxibustion at Shimen Ren 5 followed these principles. Moreover, Shimen Ren 5 is the Front-Mu point of the Triple Burner, so moxibustion there warms and activates the Triple Burner itself, clearing the Upper and Lower Burners of obstruction and expelling Pathogenic Cold. The *Qian Jin Fang* (Golden Prescriptions) records the use of Shimen

Ren 5 for colicky pain in the lower abdomen. In this case, a disease of 2 years' duration was rapidly cured.

Xie Zipiang, JIESHOU HOSPITAL, GAOYOU COUNTY, JIANGSU PROVINCE
(see Jiangsu Journal of Traditional Chinese Medicine, Issue 12, 1985)

143. Volvulus of the stomach

Male, age 11

Case registered: 7 February 1983

History: 20 days previously the patient had a severe bout of vomiting 2 hours after gorging himself at dinner. Following this he developed pain and discomfort in his upper abdomen and became unable to keep his food down. The fullness and pain were relieved by vomiting. His condition was diagnosed in a hospital as acute gastritis, and he was given fluid infusion, gentamicin, and vitamin B_6, but his condition did not improve. He had no previous history of stomach problems.

Examination: He was conscious. He looked slightly dehydrated and quite ill. Heart and lungs normal. Barium meal X-ray: chest, diaphragm and oesophagus negative. A small amount of fluid was retained in the stomach. The stomach was shaped like a coiled shrimp. There were two fluid levels. The greater curvature of the stomach turned upwards to form the upper margin. Together with the pyloric canal and the duodenal bulb they formed an arch pointing down to the right. The lesser curvature formed the lower margin. The oesophageal and gastric mucosa crossed over. *Blood test:* WBC $8.9 \times 10^9/1$ ($8.9 \times 10^3/mm^3$), neutrophils 72%, lymphocytes 28%, serum potassium 2.4 mmol/l (9.6 mg%), serum sodium and chlorides normal.

Diagnosis: Vomiting.

Treatment: The patient was given daily infusion of potassium and oral metoclopramide. These had no effect and he began to get thinner.

Auricular Points: Stomach.
   The point was needled. While the needle was retained the boy was put on his back with his knees on his chest and his chest was shaken gently several times from left to right. He felt better after this and his symptoms disappeared. A barium meal X-ray 5 days later showed his digestive tract was normal. The case was followed up for a month after his discharge and there was no relapse.

Explanation: The basic cause of volvulus is abnormal flaccidity of the supporting ligament of the stomach. The examination had revealed that volvulus was on the central axis of the stomach. The ear point regulates gastric peristalsis, while the shaking from left to right was because most volvulus on the central axis is a twisting of the stomach body on the axis between the cardia and the pylorus.

> Zhang Zhizhu and Wen Qiuhua, LIAOCHENG PREFECTURAL PEOPLE'S HOSPITAL, SHANDONG PROVINCE
> (see Shandong Journal of Traditional Chinese Medicine, Issue 6, 1984)

144. Acute infantile convulsion

Feng, male, age 4 months

Case registered: 28 June 1958

History: The baby started to have convulsions a few days after birth. This happened several times a day. The problem was diagnosed as convulsions from calcium deficiency, and he was given calglucon intravenously. The convulsions did not abate, however, and the frequency increased to every 1 or 2 hours, sometimes every few minutes. The baby's appetite was poor and he was constipated.

Examination: He went into convulsions at the start of the consultation. He had spasms and contraction in the limbs, clenched fists, opisthotonos and lockjaw. He looked pale and was semiconscious, with his eyes turned up. The superficial venule of his index finger was dark red.

Diagnosis: Stagnation of Heat causing Liver Wind, Phlegm obstructing the orifices.

Treatment: Disperse Heat, resolve Phlegm, calm the Mind and soothe Wind to open the orifices.

Principal Points: Renzhong Du 26, Yintang (Extra), Baihui Du 20, Fengfu Du 16, Dazhui Du 14, Ganshu BL 18, Neiguan P 6, Hegu L.I. 4, Zhongwan Ren 12, Zusanli ST 36.

Secondary Points: Quchi L.I. 11, Shousanli L.I. 10, Shenmen HT 7, Yanglingquan GB 34, Yongquan KID 1, Yamen Du 15.

Strong birdpecking technique was used, and the needles were not retained. Treatment was given daily.

After the first treatment his symptoms improved greatly: the incidence of convulsions was reduced by half. After three more treatments the disorder was cured. The case was followed up for many years, and there was no relapse.

Du Dewu, ACUPUNCTURE AND MOXIBUSTION SECTION, SHANDONG TCM
COLLEGE HOSPITAL

Editor's Note: From the examination it is apparent that this case was due
to irregular feeding causing Stagnation of food in the Stomach and
Intestines. Heat and Phlegm resulted, causing obstruction of the Functional
Qi. When the baby was frightened or exposed to External Pathogens,
the Phlegm obstructed the Mind and the stagnated Heat agitated Liver
Wind, causing the convulsions.

Renzhong Du 26 and Yintang (Extra) open the orifices and calm the
Mind. Baihui Du 20 and Fengfu Du 16 soothe Wind and calm the Mind.
Dazhui Du 14, Hegu L.I. 4, Zhongwan Ren 12 and Zusanli ST 36 resolve
Heat, Phlegm and Stagnation of food in the Stomach and Intestines.
Ganshu BL 18 and Neiguan P 6 relieve the Liver and regulate the
functions of the Stomach to nourish the Blood and relieve the Middle
Burner. Yamen Du 15, Shenmen HT 7 and Yongquan KID 1 calm the
Mind by nourishing the Heart and Kidney. Yanglingquan GB 34, the Hui-
Converging point of tendons, Quchi L.I. 11 and Shousanli L.I. 10 relieve
the tendons and vessels to regulate Qi and Blood. Rapid results were
achieved in this case by using all these points and strong birdpecking
technique.

145. Chronic infantile convulsion

Zhen, female, age 7 months

Case registered: 20 May 1980

History: This baby was her mother's first child, and the birth had been on
time and without incident. The mother was not able to produce much
milk, however, and the baby was fed irregularly. When she was 3 months
old she developed abdominal distension, poor appetite and frequent
bowel movements, 5–7 times a day. There was undigested food in the
stool. She began to lose weight and when she was 4 months old she
began to have convulsions. She would have 15–20 attacks in the early
morning. Each episode would last 2–3 minutes, and occasionally as long
as 30 minutes. During an attack she had spasm in the limbs, mild
tremors in her body, and her eyes would roll up. Her lips were dark and
her breathing became difficult. Examinations at the County and Prefectural
hospitals found no signs of organic disease. She was given Western
medication but her condition did not improve.

Examination: The baby was conscious. She looked pale, thin and underdeveloped. The whites of her eyes were slightly blue. Her abdomen was

distended. The superficial venule of her index finger was blueish. She was unable to sit or stand.

Diagnosis: Chronic infantile convulsion due to Deficiency of Spleen.

Treatment: Nourish the Spleen and Stomach to reinforce the sources of Qi and Blood.

Principal Points: Zhongwan Ren 12, Zhangmen LIV 13 (bilateral), Tianshu ST 25 (bilateral), Danzhong Ren 17, Sifeng (Extras, bilateral), Zusanli ST 36 (bilateral).

The Sifeng points were bled with a three-edged needle. Mild stimulation was given at the other points, and the needles were withdrawn after twirling, lifting and thrusting 11–13 times. Treatment was given daily, and the parents were advised to feed her more regularly and make sure she was kept warm.

June 2nd: Her appetite and abdominal distension improved. She now passed stool 3–4 times a day. Treatment was now given every other day.

June 20th: Her appetite was much better and the abdominal distension was improved. She looked more healthy and less pale. The spasms were less frequent, of shorter duration and much less severe.

Principal Points: Zhongwan Ren 12, Zhangmen LIV 13 (bilateral), Tianshu ST 25 (bilateral), Zusanli ST 36 (bilateral).

July 14th: The baby had received a total of 29 treatments. The spasm had stopped and she was quite healthy. Treatment was stopped.

Explanation: This disease is also known as slow infantile convulsion. The symptoms conform to Wind syndrome, and the cause is Deficiency of Spleen and Stomach. It is characterized by slow onset. Although it is called Jing Feng (Alarm and Wind), it is not really related to Alarm and Wind.

The points were selected according to the principle of treating the symptoms during the attacks and the cause during remission. Zhongwan Ren 12, the Hui-Converging point of the Fu and Front-Mu point of the Stomach, strengthens the Middle Burner. Zhangmen LIV 13, the Hui-Converging point of the Zang and the Front-Mu point of the Spleen, reinforces the Spleen Earth. Tianshu ST 25 readjusts the Middle Burner, refreshes the Spleen and stops diarrhoea. Danzhong Ren 17, the Hui-Converging point of Qi, controls the Upper Burner. It invigorates the circulation of functional Qi and spreads essential substances to the whole body. The Sifeng points are effective for chronic infantile malnutrition. Zusanli ST 36, the He-Sea point, is an important point to strengthen the whole body. It reinforces the Postnatal source of Qi by tonifying and regulating the Stomach and Spleen. When the Stomach and Spleen had become healthy and there was sufficient Qi and Blood, the Wind syndrome from Spleen Deficiency was relieved.

Li Qinming, ACUPUNCTURE AND MOXIBUSTION SECTION, LIAOCHENG PREFECTURAL TCM HOSPITAL

146. Fever with spasm and coma

Wu, male, age 1

Case registered: Summer 1970

History: The baby was admitted to a local hospital with high fever. The fever got steadily worse, and after a week he lost consciousness in the morning and his limbs went into spasm. The condition was diagnosed as viral encephalitis, and the parents were urged to take him swiftly to a provincial hospital for emergency treatment. They brought him here for acupuncture at dusk the same day.

Examination: The boy was in a semicoma. The alae nasae were moving. He had spasm in his hands and feet, and his lips and fingers were very pale. The superficial venule of the index finger went through all three passes (Wind Pass, Qi Pass and Life Pass).

Diagnosis: Acute convulsion: External Summer Heat and accumulation of Phlegm Heat.

Treatment: Clear Heat, disperse Phlegm, soothe Wind and open the clear orifices.

Principal Points: Renzhong Du 26, Shixuan (Extras), Zusanli ST 36 (bilateral), Neiguan P 6 (bilateral), Sanyinjiao SP 6 (bilateral).
About 30 minutes after the treatment the spasm stopped. By midnight the fever began to subside and the baby was able to sleep peacefully. When he was brought here the next day he looked very different: he was feeding in his mother's arms and looked up every now and then to listen to what was being said. Zusanli ST 36 was needled again to consolidate the result. The case was followed up and there were no relapses or sequelae. Medication is too slow for such serious cases, whereas acupuncture is clearly very effective.

Hu Yuanmin, JIANXI MEDICAL COLLEGE HOSPITAL NO. 2
(see Jianxi Traditional Chinese Medicine, Issue 4, 1984)

Editor's Note: This disease arose from Summer Heat pathogens on the outside and accumulation of Phlegm Heat on the inside. The Spirit was obstructed by Phlegm and Liver Wind was agitated by Exuberant Heat, resulting in symptoms of Wind such as spasm and coma.

Renzhong Du 26 and the Shixuan points clear Heat, soothe Wind, refresh the Spirit and open the clear orifices. Zusanli ST 36, Neiguan P 6 and Sanyinjiao SP 6 purge Heart Fire and resolve Turbid Phlegm. When the Heat is cleared and the Phlegm resolved, the Spirit is restored and the convulsions stop.

147. Measles, cerebritis and coma

Zhao, female, age 3

Case registered: 16 March 1981

History: The patient was admitted to hospital in a coma with measles and cerebritis. She got steadily worse: her neck was hard on palpation, her breathing was shallow and rapid, and her abdominal reflex was dulled. She was given nasogastric feeding and her parents were informed that she was critically ill. She was given Western and traditional Chinese drugs, but did not respond. At this point her parents asked for acupuncture and moxibustion.

Examination: The patient's pupillary reflex was dulled. Vision and hearing were impaired. Her limbs were stiff. Weak plantar reflex.

Treatment: Refresh the Mind and open the clear orifices.

Principal Points: Yintang (Extra), Nijiao (Extra), Naoqing (Extra), Shaoshang LU 11, Yongquan KID 1.

At Yintang, Nijiao and Naoqing needle sensation was propagated after insertion. Shaoshang LU 11 and Yongquan KID 1 were reduced. Treatment was given once a day.

After the first treatment the patient was able to swallow. After the second treatment the nasogastric tube was removed and she was given liquid food.

Secondary Points: Yinbai SP 1, Jiexi ST 41.

These two points were added to the original prescription.

Auricular Point: Brain.

A vacarria seed was taped in place.

After nine treatments the child's spirits had improved and her breathing was normal. Treatment was given once every other day.

Additional Points: Hegu L.I. 4, Quchi L.I. 11, Biguan ST 31, Zusanli ST 36.

A month after starting acupuncture she was discharged as cured.

Explanation: The *Su Wen* says: 'When external pathogens invade the Heart, Kidney, Lung, Spleen and Stomach channels, all five channels are impaired, causing agitation in the vessels of the whole body and loss of consciousness ... the illness is also called dead syncope' (Miu Ci Lun, Contralateral Needling chapter).

The use of Yinbai SP 1, Shaoshang LU 11 and Yongquan KID 1 is described in the *Su Wen.* Yongquan, the Jing-Well point treats collapse, syncope, hypertension and infantile convulsion. Xi Hong Fu says, 'Needling Yongquan KID 1 will save the patient's life' (Songs of Xi Hong Fu). The *Zhen Jiu Da Cheng* (Great Compendium of Acupuncture and Moxibustion) says that the point is effective for corpselike syncope (Shi Jue). Shaoshang LU 11, the Jing-Well point, treats coma from Wind stroke. Together these two points join Prenatal Qi and Postnatal Qi. The extra points refresh the Mind and open the clear orifices.

Jiao Zengwen, HANDAN PREFECTURAL HOSPITAL, HEBEI PROVINCE
(see Hebei Traditional Chinese Medicine, Issue 1, 1985)

148. Athetosis

CASE 1

Liu, female, age 13, student

Case registered: 19 March 1983

History: The patient's mother reported that the child had begun to bend, stretch or twist her limbs or whole body involuntarily. She had difficulty speaking or swallowing, which was worse if she was excited. All her symptoms stopped when she was asleep.

Examination: Her torso was slumped. She looked lacklustre, but continually made faces and stuck out her tongue, and was emotional and restless. *Temperature:* 36°C. Diminished muscle power. Diminished muscle tone. No knee reflex. Her joints were stiff. Her skin was hypersensitive. *Blood test:* WBC 11×10^9/l (11×10^3/mm³), neutrophils 72%, ESR 10 mm in 1 h.

Diagnosis: Tremor and dizziness: Liver Wind agitating within.

Treatment: Soothe Liver Wind, expel Damp, relieve spasm.

Principal Points: Taichong LIV 3, Fengchi Du 20, Yanglingquan GB 34, Hegu L.I. 4, Zusanli ST 36, Baihui Du 20, Dazhui Du 14.
    5–7 points were selected at a time. Moxibustion was added with a moxa stick at each point. Treatment was given once a day, and a course consisted of seven treatments. The patient's symptoms improved consid-

erably after three sessions. The point prescription was changed at this point, according to her presentation. After 10 days she was completely cured. The case was followed up for a year and there was no relapse.

Explanation: The *Ling Shu* says, 'When there is disease in the five Zang, treat the twelve Yuan-Source points . . . the Liver originates from Taichong LIV 3' (Jiu Zhen Shi Er Yuan, Nine Needlings and Twelve Source Points chapter).

Taichong LIV 3 soothes Liver Wind. Fengchi GB 20 relieves Wind and is good for all Wind syndromes. It is also a meeting with the Gallbladder and Yang Qiao Mai, and nourishes Yin and suppresses Yang. Yanglingquan GB 34, the Hui-converging point of tendons and He-Sea point, relieves the Liver and relaxes the tendons. Dazhui Du 14 is where all the Yang meet. It expels Pathogenic Wind and strengthens the body's resistance. Zusanli ST 36 and Neiguan P 6 regulate Qi and Blood, reinforce the Middle Burner, expel pathogens and strengthen the body's resistance. Baihui Du 20 and Renzhong Du 26 refresh the Mind, open the sense orifices and stop spasm.

Chen Zongliang, ACUPUNCTURE AND MOXIBUSTION SECTION, HUICHANG
COUNTY PEOPLE'S HOSPITAL, JIANXI PROVINCE
(see Jianxi Traditional Chinese Medicine, Issue 4, 1985)

CASE 2

Huang, female, age 14

Case registered: 14 October 1978

History: The patient had acute rheumatoid arthritis in March 1978. She was discharged from hospital 2 months later, but continued with her medication. By the end of September of that year she began to feel cold in the knee joints and weak in all four limbs. Her reactions were dulled and she developed involuntary tremors in the limbs. She was treated with Western and traditional Chinese drugs, but did not respond. At the time of her first consultation here she had sensations of cold in the knees, weak limbs, poor appetite and sleep, and she felt faint.

Diagnosis: Tremor and dizziness: Deficiency Liver Fire causing agitation of Deficiency Wind in the Interior.

Treatment: Reinforce the Spleen Qi and soothe Wind by nourishing the Liver.

Principal Points:
1. Ganshu BL 18, Geshu BL 17, Jinsuo Du 8, Yanglingquan GB 34, Zusanli ST 36.

2. Zhongwan Ren 12, Xiaguan ST 7, Yanglingquan GB 34, Zusanli ST 36. The points were reinforced and mild moxibustion was given until the skin was red. The first prescription was given for 10 days. By this time all the patient's muscles were relaxed and the spasm in her eyes, mouth and face had improved. Treatment was continued with the second prescription. After 10 days she no longer had any tremor in her face. Another 10 treatments were given and she was completely cured. A further 10 consolidating treatments were given once every other day with moxibustion at Zhongwan Ren 12 and Zusanli ST 36.

Explanation: Involuntary dancing is categorized as tremor and dizziness in TCM. The *Shang Han Lun* (Treatise on Febrile Diseases) calls it 'tremor of muscle and tendon'. It arises from Deficient Qi and Body Fluids or Deficient Blood failing to nourish the tendons and muscles. The treatment aim is to nourish Qi, Body Fluids and Blood to soothe Wind. In this case the emphasis was put on treating the Liver and Spleen. The Liver controls the tendons and houses the Blood. The Spleen controls the muscles and with the Stomach is the source of Postnatal Qi. The prescriptions were designed to soothe Wind by nourishing Spleen Qi and the Liver.

Zhongwan Ren 12 and Zusanli ST 36 reinforce Spleen Qi, and the postnatal source of Qi. Ganshu BL 18 and Geshu BL 17 nourish the Blood and the Liver. Jinsuo Du 8 and Yanglingquan GB 34 relieve the Liver, relax the tendons to soothe Wind. When Qi and Blood are sufficient, Deficiency Wind dies down automatically. Zhongwan Ren 12 and Zusanli ST 36 were used in this case throughout the course of treatment, because they are so effective in the treatment of this illness.

> Case treated by Zhang Heyuan, case study by Liu Mingyi and Sun Hao, GUI YANG TCM COLLEGE

149. Aphonia

CASE 1

Luo, male, age 3

Case registered: 20 August 1982

History: The patient had paroxysmal spasmodic coughing for a month, which had got worse in the last 2 weeks. On 31 July he was admitted to hospital in a coma with frequent tremor of the limbs. Examination at that time revealed that the boy was in a coma, with an anal temperature of 40.4°C. His eyes were looking to the right. His alae nasae were moving slightly, he was short of breath and foaming at the mouth. His limbs tremored frequently. Lips slightly dark. Neck soft. His lungs wheezed. Kernig's sign suspected positive. Heart rate 120/min. regular, with thin sound (sic). *Blood test:* WBC 40.2 × 10^9/l, lymphocytes 86%, neutrophils 13%, eosinophils 1%. His condition was diagnosed as encephalopathic pertussis (spasmodic stage). He was treated with Western and traditional Chinese drugs for 10 days. After this he regained consciousness, but could not speak. After 20 days his condition was stable and his family requested acupuncture and moxibustion.

Examination: Anal temperature 37.4°C. The boy's hands and feet were slightly warmer in the centre. He could cry, but was unable to speak. Superficial venule of index finger light purple. *Tongue body:* red. *Tongue coating:* slightly yellow.

Diagnosis: Phlegm Heat obstructing the clear orifices.

Treatment: Refresh the Mind and open the clear orifices.

Principal Points: Lianquan Ren 23, Xielianquan (Extra, bilateral)[1], Yamen Du 15.
   Yamen was reinforced with light twirling, and the needle was not retained. Lianquan Ren 23 and Xielianquan (Extra) were given medium strong stimulation, reinforcing and reducing evenly with twirling lifting and thrusting for 2 minutes before withdrawing the needles. Treatment was given once daily. The boy was able to speak after the first treatment, though his speech was slurred. After two more sessions he was speaking easily.

Explanation: Aphonia from brain disease following pertussis is rarely seen in clinic. Most cases are caused by limited impairment of the speech centre in the brain. Pertussis or whooping cough is caused by invasion of external pathogens into the respiratory system. The pathogens and Phlegm obstruct the air ducts, resulting in impairment of the Lung. In children the organism is not strong and the Lung Qi is not sufficient. The obstruction by Phlegm transforms into Heat and Wind rising upwards, so the clear orifices become blocked. When the tongue is blocked there is aphonia.
   Yamen Du 15 refreshes the Mind and spirits. Lianquan Ren 23 and Xielianquan (Extra) resolve turbid Phlegm and relax the tongue. Good results were obtained by correct and proper treatment with the right points and the right manipulation.

---

[1]Xielianquan (Extra) is located lateral to Lianquan Ren 23.

Mao Weisong, QINGTIAN COUNTY PEOPLE'S HOSPITAL, ZHEJIANG
PROVINCE
(see Shanghai Journal of Acupuncture and Moxibustion, Issue 2,
1987)

CASE 2

Liu, female, age 7

Case registered: 25 October 1975

History: The patient had lost the ability to speak for a month after contracting toxic dysentery. She was unable even to say 'Mama' or 'Dada'. Medication had not helped; in fact, she had been sick when taking traditional Chinese decoctions.

Examination: The patient was conscious, and her temperature was normal. Pulse and blood pressure normal. Hearing normal. She was unable to say even one word. Tongue and frenulum both normal. Heart and lungs normal. Movement of limbs normal. No pathological reflex induced.

Diagnosis: Aphonia: Toxic Heat leading to obstruction of the clear orifices.

Treatment: Open the clear orifices.

Principal Points: Renzhong Du 26, Fengfu Du 16.
The points were given medium stimulation and the needles were not retained. Treatment was given daily. After three treatments the patient was able to say some simple words. After seven treatments she was able to say longer sentences. She had 12 treatments in total. Her speech was largely restored and she was discharged from hospital.

Explanation: This disease is categorized as aphonia in TCM. It is caused by invasion of virulent Heat pathogen leading to malfunction of the Zangfu and Stasis in the channels and collaterals.
Renzhong Du 26 is a meeting point of Du Mai with the Stomach and Large Intestine channels. It refreshes the Mind and opens the sense organs. Fengfu Du 26 is a meeting point of Du Mai with the Bladder channel and Yang Wei Mai. It clears Heat, resolves Phlegm and activates the Functional Qi. These two points together are effective for aphonia and semiconsciousness.

Zhang Dengbu, SHANDONG TCM COLLEGE HOSPITAL
(see Heilongjiang Traditional Chinese Medicine, Issue 4, 1983)

150. Weakness in the legs

Zhang, female, age 11, schoolgirl

Case registered: 6 June 1981

History: The patient fell sick with a cold, then developed high fever. After 2 weeks her legs became very weak. Soon she was unable to stand. Her urination was normal, but her stools were a little loose and frequent (twice a day).

Examination: She looked lacklustre. Her sensitivity to pain, temperature and pressure was reduced in her arms and legs. No pathological reflex. *Tongue body:* pale. *Tongue coating:* thin, greasy and yellow. *Pulse:* hidden, minute and rapid.

Diagnosis: Wei syndrome.

Treatment: Clear Damp Heat, activate Functional Qi of Chong Mai and the Yang Ming channels.

Principal Points: (to clear Damp Heat) Shangjuxu ST 37, Xiajuxu ST 39, Quchi L.I. 11, Sanyinjiao SP 6.
　　All the points were needled bilaterally, except Sanyinjiao SP 6, which was reinforced and reduced equally. Treatment was given once every 2 days. After 10 treatments, the Damp Heat was resolved, the functions of the Stomach and Spleen were restored, the Qi and Blood of the Liver and Kidney became full and the disease was almost cured.

Principal Points:(to regulate Chong Mai): Zhaohai KID 6, Taichong LIV 3, Taixi KID 3, Shangjuxu ST 37, Xiajuxu ST 39.
　　The points were needled bilaterally and reinforced. After 10 treatments she was moving about without difficulty. Qi and Blood in Chong Mai were now full. The stagnating pathogens were expelled, the tendons were well nourished, Yin and Yang and the Zangfu were once again regulated.

Explanation: The *Su Wen* says that Chong Mai is the Sea of the channels and is in charge of nourishing. It meets with the Stomach channel at the assembled tendons which converge at Qijie (Thoroughfare of Qi)[1]. This vessel and the Stomach channel both belong to Dai Mai and are connected to Du Mai. When the Stomach channel is Deficient, the assembled tendons become flaccid, so Dai Mai cannot contract, resulting in flaccidity and weakness of the legs. Chong Mai is the Sea of the Twelve Channels, and the Stomach is the Sea of the Zangfu. Being Yin and Yang respectively, the two govern all the channels and vessels, and meet at the genitals with the assembled tendons, then at Qijie on both sides. When Qi and Blood in Chong Mai and the Stomach channel are full and circulate around the

---

[1]Qijie: some commentators see it as synonymous with Qichong ST 30, others hold it to be between the Kidneys, one of several gathering points of energy in the body.

body, the Qi and Blood of the whole body are nourished. The converse is also true: when the two vessels are Deficient in Qi and Blood, the assembled tendons become flaccid, Dai Mai cannot contract, causing paralysis of the legs. Thus the key to Wei syndrome is treatment of Chong Mai and the Stomach channel.

Li Licheng, JINAN CENTRAL MUNICIPAL HOSPITAL, SHANDONG PROVINCE

151. Guillain-Barré syndrome

Liu, male, age 8

Case registered: 6 July 1982

History: The previous morning the patient felt weak in the limbs and was unable to stand up. By the afternoon he could not move, and by the evening his voice was hoarse, and he was choking and coughing when trying to swallow. Examination of his cerebrospinal fluid at the county hospital was normal. By the next day his arms were completely paralysed. He was restless and had no fever. In the Paediatrics department of this hospital he was given anti-inflammatory therapy, hormones, neurotrophic drugs and intramuscular stimulants, as well as oxygen and nasogastric feeding. His condition stabilized, but his limbs were paralysed and he was unable to swallow.

Examination: He was examined both in (i) the Paediatrics Department and (ii) the Acupuncture and Moxibustion Section:

(i) *Temperature:* 37.5°C. *Pulse rate:* 108/min. *Respiratory rate:* 30/min. Heart, lungs and spleen normal. Right nasolabial groove more shallow. No swallowing reflex. Lips red. Tongue purple with white coating. Hyperaemia around the throat. Abdominal and thoracic breathing weak. Flaccid paralysis of all four limbs. Grade 0 muscle power. Very slight tendon reflex in all four limbs. Coughing very weak.

(ii) The patient seemed lacklustre and his complexion was dry. Difficulty in breathing. Cyanosis. Restless. Weak cough. Restricted movement in head and neck. Obstruction of secretions in throat. Mouth and lips dry. Choking and coughing. Dribbling from the corner of the mouth. No swallowing. Facial paralysis. Flaccid paralysis of all four limbs. *Tongue body:* pale red. *Tongue coating:* slightly yellow. *Pulse:* thin, weak and rapid.

Diagnosis: Infantile Wei syndrome.

Treatment: Clear Heat, nourish Yin, dredge the channels and collaterals, strengthen the tendons and marrow.

Principal Points:

1. Jianyu L.I. 15, Quchi L.I. 11, Lieque LU 7, Hegu L.I. 4, Taiyuan LU 9, Lianquan Ren 23, Tianrong SI 17, Zusanli ST 36, Yanglingquan GB 34.
2. Zusanli ST 36, Yanglingquan GB 34, Xuanzhong GB 39, Taiyuan LU 9.

All the points in the first prescription were reduced to clear Heat except Zusanli ST 36 and Yanglingquan GB 34. As the patient improved and could swallow again, the second prescription was brought into play.

After the second treatment he could move his thumbs and his abdominal breathing was more visible. After four treatments he could move his arms a little, and his abdominal breathing was more vigorous. He dribbled less, but still could not swallow. After nine treatments he could bend his arms and move his neck and head more easily. After 10 treatments the nasogastric tube was removed and he was given glucose solution to drink. He was able to drink this with only a little coughing and choking. After this he could eat biscuits and eggs, and his appetite and spirits improved greatly. Treatment was continued for another month, when he was discharged. His paralysis was almost completely better. The case was followed up 2 months later, and he was found to be absolutely fine.

Li Shuxian, ACUPUNCTURE AND MOXIBUSTION SECTION, QINGYANG PREFECTURE PEOPLE'S HOSPITAL, GANSU PROVINCE
(*see Journal of Traditional Chinese Medicine, Issue 4, 1984*)

Editor's Note: This case of Wei syndrome was due to Liver and Kidney Deficiency. When the tendons and bones are not nourished by Qi and Blood, movement in the limbs is impaired. The doctor followed the principle, 'Treat Wei syndrome by using points solely on the Yang Ming channel'. Initially he used points on the Large Intestine channel as main points, adding Lung points to nourish Yin and clear Heat, invigorate the collaterals and Blood. The second prescription was used to activate Qi and Blood, strengthen Deficiency and reinforce the tendons and bones.

152. Torticollis (wryneck)

Zhang, male, age 4

Case registered: 16 December 1984

History: 10 days previously the boy had fallen from a tractor and scratched his forehead on the right. 3 days later he got hit in the left eye. After another 2 days he fell out of bed. These were all minor accidents and had not disturbed his play, but 4 days previously he developed a headache. He had no fever or nausea, but was restless and unable to sleep. His head and neck then began to bend over towards the right. This was tentatively diagnosed as a dislocation of the cervical vertebrae at a Laiyang hospital, but X-ray examinations later showed nothing abnormal. Laboratory examinations showed *WBC:* $9.8 \times 10^9/l$ ($9.8 \times 10^3/mm^3$), neutrophils 80%, lymphocytes 20%, haemoglobin 90 g/l (9g%). His parents were advised to take him to a hospital with better facilities, such as the one at Qingdao, but for financial reasons they brought him here.

Examination: He was conscious and articulate. His neck was bent to the right, and his jaw rested on his chest. His left shoulder was elevated and his waist was inclined to the right. He had to be supported to sit still. Movement was restricted in his left ankle, and the foot was slightly everted. He was unable to stand. There was muscular contraction in his neck on the right. The muscles in his right shoulder and the back and left side of his neck were firm.

Diagnosis: Imbalance of Yang Qiao Mai and Bladder channel.

Treatment: Regulate Yang Qiao Mai and Bladder Qi.

Principal Points: On the right side only: Jiaji (Extras) at C3, 5, 7 and T1, Jugu L.I. 16, Naoshu SI 10, Yanglingquan GB 34. On the left side only: Shenmai BL 62. Bilaterally: Xinshu BL 15, Ganshu BL 18.
  30 gauge needles were used. They were retained for 15 minutes and manipulated three times. Treatment was given daily. After five treatments the boy could lift his head but could not turn it freely. After a further five sessions he was completely cured.

Explanation: Yang Qiao Mai is in charge of Yang Qi. When Yang is Exuberant the patient is restless. Yang Qiao Mai is also a branch of the Bladder channel, so when there are problems in this vessel there will be symptoms of pain in the waist and back, and stiffness in the body. The *Nan Jing* says, 'Illness in the Yang Heel Vessel (Yang Qiao Mai) is characterized by sluggish Yin and contracture of Yang' (Chapter 29). The *Ling Shu* says, 'Exuberant Yang causes the eyes to be wide open' (Cold and Heat Diseases chapter).
  In this case local points were selected which related to Du Mai and the Bladder channel. Thus they activate and regulate Yang and the Qi of the Bladder channel. Jugu L.I. 16, Naoshu SI 10 and Shenmai BL 62 regulate the Qi of Yang Qiao Mai. Ganshu BL 18 and Yanglingquan GB 34 relieve the contracture of the tendons. Xinshu BL 15 calms the Mind to relieve the restlessness.

Li Shuquan, SHANDONG PROVINCIAL TCM SCHOOL

153. Blindness, cortical

Yang, male, age 2

Case registered: October 1979

History: The patient was admitted to hospital with hepatitis. After 9 days he developed a fever of 40°C and spasm of the whole body. The fever and spasm subsided after treatment, but in mid-November it was noticed that he was blind. His eyes were rolled up or fixed straight ahead, and he still had occasional spasms. He was examined in the Ophthalmology Section: his eyes looked normal, there were no abnormalities in the fundus, his pupils were equally dilated and round, and reacted to light. The condition was diagnosed as cortical blindness and he was treated with intramuscular injections of vitamin B_1 and B_{12}, infusions, hormones and blood and plasma transfusions, but there was no improvement. At another hospital, in addition to these treatments he was given cytochrome C, co-enzyme A, disopropylamine dichloroacetate (DADA), vitamins A, C and D and hormone injections for a month. He was also given about 40 doses of traditional Chinese decoctions but again showed no improvement. At this point his family decided to try acupuncture and moxibustion.

Examination: Blood test: WBC $6.8 \times 10^{12}/l$ ($6.8 \times 10^3/mm^3$), neutrophils 80%, RBC $3.6 \times 10^{12}/l$ ($3.6 \times 10^6/mm^3$). Routine urine and faeces tests negative.

The boy's development was normal, and his diet appeared to have been average. His sleep was poor and he looked lacklustre. He was weak in the knees and unable to walk. Bowels and urination normal. *Temperature:* 38°C. His eyeballs moved freely. *Tongue body:* red. *Tongue coating:* dry and yellow.

Diagnosis: Qing Mang, optic atrophy: Stagnation of Heat.

Treatment: Relieve Liver Heat and nourish Blood.

Herbal decoctions were prescribed, including modified Dan Zhi Xiao Yao San, and vitamins B_1 and C, but he had difficulty taking them. His medication was stopped and he was given acupuncture instead.

Principal Points: Jingming BL 1, Xiajingming (below Jingming), Qiuhou (Extra), Zanzhu BL 2, Tongziliao GB 1, Hegu L.I. 4, Shenmen HT 7, Fengchi GB 20, Taichong LIV 3.

Only one local point and two distal points were used at a time. Medium strong stimulation was used, and the needles were not retained. Birdpecking technique was used at the distal points. Treatment was given daily.

Administration: The boy was placed lying down, or in his parents' arms, so that his head was immobile. At Qiuhou (Extra), the doctor held the lower eyelid by pressing it against the boy's cheek, then inserted a 2 or 2.5 cun needle. At Xiajingming (Extra) the needle was inserted perpendicularly 0.6–0.8 cun alongside the eyeball, taking care not to damage it, then re-angled in the direction of the optic foramen to a depth of 1.0–1.5 cun. At this depth the needle could reach the optic foramen and the ciliary ganglion. Then it was twirled for about a minute before withdrawing it slowly. The point was then rubbed with sterile cotton wool. When needling Jingming BL 1 the boy was put in a sitting or lying position, with his head facing directly in front. The needle was slowly inserted perpendicularly. When it was 1 cun deep, medium strong stimulation was given with gentle twirling technique. It was withdrawn after a minute and the point was rubbed with sterile cotton wool.

After 10 treatments his vision improved. His eyelids now closed in reaction to light and he could follow the light with his eyes. His appetite was better and he could walk, although his legs were still weak. After another 10 treatments he was able to pick up sugar lumps from the table and walk up and down stairs. At this point he came down with a cold. He had a temperature of 38°C and a mild cough, which was treated with acupuncture. When he was better the previous treatment was resumed. After a further 10 treatments his vision was much better. He was able to pick up a pin from the ground and could see small coins from over 5 metres away. The case was followed up for a year, and his vision was found to have remained good.

Explanation: Cortical blindness only affects children. It can be caused by cerebritis, high fever and dysentery. It is characterized by loss of vision together with reactiveness to light and a normal fundus. In TCM it is categorised as Qing Mang: blue blindness or optic atrophy. The *Yan Ke Jin Jing* (Golden Mirror of Ophthalmology) states, 'Infantile optic atrophy is very dangerous. It is caused by Stagnation of Heat after disease, which prevents the vital essence of the Kidney from circulating through the channels and collaterals (Xiao Er Qing Mang Zheng, Infantile Optic Atrophy chapter). The *Yi Zong Jin Jian* (Golden Mirror of Medicine) says it is caused by, 'invasion by pathogenic Wind of the fetus. The pupils are normal and the eyes appear to be functioning after birth, but they cannot see. Sometimes there are other symptoms such as restless sleep and vomiting of yellow phlegm' (Xiao Er Qing Mang Zheng, Infantile Optic Atrophy chapter).

In this case the patient became blind after high fever. The Yin was impaired by Heat and Fire. As the Yin became Deficient the Fire became more Exuberant, so the Kidney Water was consumed and unable to go up to nourish the eyes. The treatment was therefore designed to nourish the Yin, clear Heat, soothe the Liver and purge Fire.

Jingming BL 1 and Xiajingming (Extra) nourish Yin and clear Heat. Taichong LIV 3 relieves Liver Fire. Qiuhou (Extra) and Tongziliao GB 1 purge Fire and clear the eyes. Hegu L.I. 4 disperses Wind and activates the collaterals. Shenmen HT 7 calms the Mind. Zanzhu BL 2 and Fengchi GB 20 relieve Wind. The disease was cured when the Pathogenic Heat was cleared and the Yin fluids were nourished.

Liu Shuding, DEPARTMENT OF OPHTHALMOLOGY, WUHAN TCM MUNICIPAL HOSPITAL, HUBEI PROVINCE
(see Journal of Traditional Chinese Medicine, Issue 4, 1982)

154. Infantile hydrocele

Dai, male, age 6

History: The patient had had swollen testes with sensations of heaviness for years. The condition was diagnosed as infantile hydrocele in several hospitals.

Examination: His testes were the size of fists, and shiny. Transillumination test positive.

Diagnosis: Infantile hernia: Invasion of Pathogenic Wind Damp Cold, Kidney Deficiency.

Treatment: Warm the Kidney and regulate the Liver, reinforce the Spleen to eliminate Damp.

Principal Points: Dadun LIV 1, Sanyinjiao SP 6.

14 moxa cones were burnt at each point, bilaterally. His symptoms improved after the first treatment. Five treatments were given in total and there was a marked improvement.

Chen Keqin, SHENXI PROVINCIAL TCM INSTITUTE
(see Journal of Tianjin TCM College, Issue 1, 1986)

Editor's Note: The *Ling Shu* states that the Liver channel 'goes around the genitals and reaches the lower abdomen' (Jing Mai, Channels chapter). The *Su Wen* says, 'All Dampness, swelling and fullness relates to the Spleen'. In TCM this case of hydrocele is classified as Shui Shan, Water hernia. The Kidney Qi was Deficient, leaving the body open to invasion by Pathogenic Wind Damp and Cold. The pathogens remained in the Jue Yin and Shao Yin channels, and the Damp reached the testes, causing the symptoms.

Dadun LIV 1, the Jing-Well point, is an important point for hernia. It regulates the Liver, activates Blood and removes Damp. Sanyinjiao SP 6 warms the Kidney, regulates the Liver and reinforces the Spleen.

155. Urinary incontinence at the sight of water

Li, male, age 13

Case registered: 6 January 1973

History: The patient's diet had been good. Over the last month he began to wet himself when he saw running water from the tap. The problem got worse, and soon he was wetting himself whenever he saw water anywhere. He was given medication, including atropine, but without effect.

Examination: He was overweight and pale. *Tongue body:* tender looking. *Tongue coating:* thin and white. *Pulse:* thin and wiry.

Diagnosis: Deficiency of Liver and Kidney.

Treatment: Tonify Kidney and regulate the Bladder.
    Principal Points: Pangguangshu BL 28, Zhongji Ren 3, Shenshu BL 23, Sanyinjiao SP 6, Zhaohai KID 6.
    Pangguangshu BL 28 and Zhongji Ren 3 were reduced, and the other points were reinforced. The disorder was cured after eight treatments.

Explanation: Shenshu BL 23 and Sanyinjiao SP 6 regulate the function of the Bladder. Pangguangshu BL 28 and Zhongji Ren 3 reinforce the Bladder. Zhaohai nourishes Kidney Water to support Liver Wood and calm the Mind.

Xia Lianqing, YIXING COUNTY PEOPLE'S HOSPITAL, JIANGSU PROVINCE
(see Journal of Traditional Chinese Medicine. Issue 12, 1983)

156. Contraction of the genitals

Zeng, male, age 10

Case registered: November 1975

History: 2 hours previously the boy suddenly developed lower abdominal pain and his penis and testes contracted.

Examination: He looked as if he was in severe pain. His complexion was pale and his limbs were cold. His genitals were contracted. *Tongue body:* normal. *Tongue coating:* thin and white. *Pulse:* deep and thin.

Diagnosis: Yang Deficiency, Pathogenic Wind Cold invading the Liver channel.

Treatment: Tonify Kidney Qi, warm the Lower Burner.

Principal Points: Huiyin Ren 1, Suoyin 1 (Extra), Suoyin 2 (Extra)[1], Shenque Ren 8.

The points were stimulated in the above order with burning lampwick[2]. At Shenque Ren 8 some salt was used as an intermediary. A thin slice of ginger would also have sufficed. The contraction was cured after only one treatment.

Shen Zhanyao, CHANGDE COUNTY TCM HOSPITAL, HUNAN PROVINCE
(see Jiangsu Journal of Traditional Chinese Medicine, Issue 2, 1985)

Editor's Note: There have been few reported cases of contraction of the genitals in children. From the pulse and symptoms it is clear the disease was caused by Yang Deficiency, a Ying–Wei (Defensive–Nutritive) imbalance, and invasion of Pathogenic Wind Cold into the Liver channel. The Liver channel goes around the genitals. When the channel is invaded by Pathogenic Cold, the genitals contract inwards. In this case moxibustion was very effective and quick-acting.

Huiyin Ren 1 is the meeting point of Ren Mai with Du Mai and Chong Mai. It is effective for diseases of the genitals. Moxibustion at Shenque Ren 8 tonifies Kidney Qi and warms the Lower Burner. The other points are local Ashi points and related to the Liver channel. Moxibustion here warms the channel Qi of the affected area.

157. Retarded development

Meng, male, age 2½

History: There were no complications when the child was born and he was fed on his mother's milk. After 6 months he was unable to sit or crawl by himself and seemed dull. He would cry restlessly after sleeping. He was unable to have any other food except breast milk, and gradually lost weight. By the time he was a year old things had not improved. He did not react to things around him, and had no control of his bowels or bladder.

---

[1]Suoyin 1 is located at the junction of the root of the penis and the scrotum. Suoyin 2 is located at the junction of the root of the penis and the pubic symphisis.
[2]Moxibustion with rush pith or lampwick: rush pith soaked in sesame oil or lampwick is lit and held briefly against the skin then pulled away. The skin should go red, but should not be burned.

Examination: The child looked pale, thin and dull. He became restless when his name was called. His limbs were cool, and he was unable to sit or stand. *Tongue body:* pale. *Tongue coating:* white.

Diagnosis: Infantile dementia: Deficiency of Qi and Blood.

Treatment: Tonify Qi, open the clear orifices, calm the Mind.

Principal Points:
1. Yamen Du 15, Lianquan Ren 23, Neiguan P 6, Hegu L.I. 4.
2. Yamen Du 15, Tiantu Ren 22, Dazhui Du 15, Zusanli ST 36.

Reinforcing and reducing evenly method was used, and the needles were not retained. The two groups of points were alternated, and treatment was given daily. A course consisted of 10 treatments, and a rest of 5–7 days was given between courses.

After one course the boy could ingest food other than breast milk. He looked less dull. After two courses he was quiet, and able to stand. After three courses he was grasping food with his hands and putting on weight. For various reasons he missed treatment at this point for a month. When treatment resumed Tiantu Ren 22 was removed from the prescription. By the time the seventh course was finished, he was looking radiant and energetic, and was walking around to find things to play with. He was learning to speak clearly and fluently. 10 courses were given altogether: by the end his intelligence and level of activity were completely normal. The case was followed up later. After 2 years at school he was getting average grades.

> Bai Shuzheng, ACUPUNCTURE AND MOXIBUSTION SECTION, YANGZHOU COUNTY PEOPLE'S HOSPITAL, SHANDONG PROVINCE
> *(see Chinese Acupuncture and Moxibustion, Issue 4, 1982)*

Editor's Note: This case is one of the five types of retarded development, and is due to Deficiency of Qi and Blood, which do not nourish the brain, leading to manifestations of dementia.

Yamen Du 15, Dazhui Du 14 and Zusanli ST 36 refresh the Mind and the sense organs, and reinforce the postnatal source of Qi. Lianquan Ren 23 and Tiantu Ren 22 open the clear orifices and activate the Functional Qi to restore the vocalizing function of the tongue. Neiguan P 6 and Hegu L.I. 4 calm the Mind. All these points together proved very effective.

158. Inappropriate laughter

Shen, male, age 9, schoolboy

Case registered: 11 May 1987

History: The boy had had fever. His eyes had rolled up and he had had spasm in the limbs. The fever was cured, but from the beginning of 1987 the boy began to laugh without cause. He would suddenly start laughing to himself for 30–60 seconds at a time. At its worst this might happen 30 times a day, or even in his sleep. In between his bouts of laughter the boy was completely normal. He was highly intelligent and got good grades at school. His appetite, bowels and urination were all normal. He was treated unsuccessfully with phenytoin sodium.

Examination: The boy was conscious and spoke fluently. Heart and lung normal. Physiological reflexes present, no pathological reflexes induced. EEG and ECG normal.

Diagnosis: Accumulated Phlegm Heat in the Heart.

Treatment: Calm the Mind, clear Heat in the Heart and resolve Phlegm.
Principal Points: Neiguan P 6 (bilateral), Jiuwei Ren 15, Renzhong Du 26, Zhongchong P 9 (bilateral).

Secondary Points: Xinshu BL 15 (bilateral), Sanyinjiao SP 6 (bilateral).
The needles at the principle points were retained for 20 minutes. Three moxa cones on ginger were burned at each secondary point.
Treatment was given once a day and the condition was cured after two sessions. The case was followed up for 6 months and there was no relapse.

Explanation: The *Nei Jing* says that laughter corresponds to the Heart, and that when the Spirit is Exuberant there will be ceaseless laughter. Here Exuberance of the Spirit means Excessive Heart Fire from accumulated Heat in the Heart channel.
Neiguan P 6, Jiuwei Ren 15 and Zhongchong P 9 clear Heat in the Heart and resolve Phlegm. Moxibustion on ginger at Sanyinjiao SP 6 and Xinshu BL 15 resolve Phlegm and calm the Mind.

Xia Lianqing, YIXING COUNTY PEOPLE'S HOSPITAL, JIANGSU PROVINCE

159. Ulcerated tuberculous nodes

Deng, female, age 8

Case registered: 4 May 1968

History: The patient had tuberculous lymph nodes on both sides of her neck. These had been ulcerous for over 6 months and would not heal. She was given intramuscular injections of streptomycin, and other medication orally, but she did not respond. She was weak, her appetite was poor and she had nightsweats and sensations of heat in her palms, soles and chest.

Examination: She looked thin and lacklustre. *Tongue body:* pale. *Tongue coating:* scanty. *Pulse:* thin, rapid and weak.

Diagnosis: Deficiency of Qi and Yin.

Principal Points: Ganshu BL 18 (bilateral).

Two moxa cones the size of an olive stone were burnt on each point. The cones were retained until the girl cried out in pain. Then two moxa cones the size of a grain of corn were burnt all the way down. The doctor protected his thumbs with thick paper and rubbed the still-burning moxa cones quickly. At this point she just had to endure the pain. When the points blistered they were pricked to discharge the fluid, then the area was covered with Yu Hong Gao or Vaseline. When the blisters had healed after 7–10 days the treatment was repeated. Four treatments were given in all, together with administration of Yu Hong Gao, Bai Jiang Dan and Zhen Zhu Shang Ji San. The course lasted roughly a month: all the ulcerated lymph nodes healed up, and her other symptoms were relieved. The case was followed up a year later and the girl was healthy.

Explanation: The use of moxibustion at Ganshu BL 18 for tuberculosis of the lymph nodes was handed down to me by my teacher the late Zhang Ziduan, the renowned TCM practitioner from Mianxian County, Shenxi Province. 52 cases with this disease were treated in this way: three cases did not continue treatment for one reason or another, and the therapeutic effect cannot be confirmed. Of the remaining 49, 43 cases were completely cured and six had some improvement. Our observations were that in less severe cases of shorter duration two treatments would normally effect a cure. In cases with a history of 6 months or more which were more severe or ulcerated four to seven treatments would normally effect a cure. In cases with ulceration, traditional Chinese herbs to dispel putrefaction and help regeneration of the tissues should also be given.

Xiao Xianggao, ACUPUNCTURE AND MOXIBUSTION SECTION, MIANXIAN COUNTY TCM HOSPITAL, SHENXI PROVINCE

Part Four
DISEASES OF THE EAR, EYE, NOSE AND THROAT

160. Optic atrophy, postoperative

Wang, female, age 5

Case registered: 17 August 1982

History: 4 months previously the patient developed paroxysmal frontal headaches in the afternoons. They would last for 20–30 minutes, and when severe she had projectile vomiting as well. The symptoms gradually got worse, and the headaches began to last longer. During an episode she would feel weak, but remained conscious and did not feel faint, but her body would bend backwards. She began to lose weight. Her hearing, vision, memory, urination and bowels remained normal. In hospital she had routine tests including thoracic puncture, X-ray examination and exploratory cranial surgery, which revealed a craniopharyngioma. The tumour was surgically removed on 28 May 1962 but after the operation she went completely blind. Tests were normal, and she was referred for acupuncture and moxibustion on 17 August 1962.

Examination: No light sense. Total blindness. Cornea normal. No light or accommodation reflex in either eye. Fundus examination showed the margins of the optic disk in both eyes were regular. The disks were pallid, and the arteries appeared abnormally narrow. The girl was intelligent. Her appetite was good, and her bowels and urination were normal. *Tongue body:* normal. *Tongue coating:* thin and white. *Pulse:* wiry and slow. Superficial venule of index finger dark purple.

Diagnosis: Optic atrophy.

Treatment: Refresh the Mind, clear the eyes, regulate the function of the Liver and Gallbladder, resolve Stasis, activate the Blood and the channels.

Principal Points:
1. Fengchi GB 20, Zanzhu BL 2, Binao L.I. 14, Taichong LIV 3.
2. Jingming BL 1, Sizhukong TB 23, Yanglao SI 6, Guangming GB 37.
    The child was comforted so that she would not be too scared of the needles and the 'painless method' was used, covering the needle with a cotton ball. The needles were twirled through 90° for 30–60 seconds

then withdrawn. Treatment was given daily and the two prescriptions were alternated. A course comprised 12 sessions, and an interval of 2 weeks was allowed between courses.

After the first course she regained light sense. After the first interval she was examined. She could make out her hand in front of her eyes and could recognize objects. There were fewer narrow arteries around the optic disk. The disks were still pallid, though this was more pronounced laterally. Retina test negative. Reflected light from the fovea centralis was slightly darker on both sides.

Secondary Points: Dagukong (Extra), Xiaogukong (Extra).

These points were added bilaterally. After six more treatments her vision improved more, and she was able to differentiate red, black and white. Her field of vision was still small and she was unable to move around by herself. She could not pick things up with any precision and her right eyeball looked slightly to one side.

During the third course her vision improved more: right side 0.1, left side 0.3. Pupils equal. Direct and indirect reaction to light present. The optic disks became darker red, and there was a further reduction in the number of thin arteries. Her field of vision enlarged. She was now moving around and able to pick things up more easily. Her right eye faced more centrally. Ganshu BL 18 was added.

After a further 12 treatments her vision was re-examined: right 0.8, left 1.0. Both optic disks were red. The medial sides were more red, and the lateral sides light yellow. The arteries were no longer abnormally narrow. Light was reflected from the central fovea. She could move around easily, see clearly and was in good spirits. The case was followed up after a year and there was no relapse.

Explanation: In this case the blindness was caused by the craniopharyngioma. Although it was removed, the focus obstructed the circulation of essential nourishment to the eyes. Secondary eye diseases are usually caused by failure of essential substances from the Zangfu to reach the eyes, or pathogens in the Liver and Gallbladder invading the eyes. Cases where intracranial lesions impair the organs are rarely seen clinically. The *Ling Shu* says, 'Liver Qi leads to the eyes. When the Liver is regular, the eyes can see the colours' (Mai Du, Length of Channels chapter). The *Su Wen* says, 'The Liver opens into the eyes' (Jin Gui Zhen Yan Lun, Golden Truths chapter). The *Zhu Bing Yuan Hou Lun* (General Treatise on the Causes and Symptoms of Diseases) says, 'When the eyes are not nourished by Qi and Blood from the organs, they look healthy but cannot see, so the illness is caused' (Mu Qing Mang Hou, Optic Atrophy chapter). The *Shen Shu Yao Han* (A Manual of Ophthalmology) says,

'When the fat in the brain goes downwards it obscures the visual spirit and causes blindness'. From these observations it is clear that the ancients could already see that vision is closely related to the organs, channels, collaterals and the brain.

Zang Yuwen, SHANDONG MEDICAL UNIVERSITY HOSPITAL

161. Blindness, cortical

Wang, male, age 6

History: 40 days previously the boy had high fever with spasm and coma. His condition was diagnosed in his local hospital as fulminating epidemic encephalitis and cerebral hernia. He was treated, and recovered sufficiently to be able to eat and move his limbs without difficulty, but he had become blind. He was referred to the Prefectural Hospital for treatment for the sequelae of encephalitis. Examination revealed that his pupils were equal. The disks had clear borders and normal colouring. The blood vessels and retina were normal. After treatment his vision improved a little, then he was referred to this hospital.

Examination: The boy was conscious and articulate. His neck was soft. His pupils were equal. Direct and indirect reaction to light. No nystagmus. No vision except light sense. Optic disks pale, especially laterally, with clear borders. There was optic atrophy in the fundus. *BP:* 14.7/9.33 kPa (110/70 mmHg). Liver palpable 2 cm below the xiphoid process, 1 cm below the ribs.

Diagnosis: Optic atrophy.

Treatment: Activate the channels and collaterals, regulate Qi and Blood.

Scalp Acupuncture: Visual area (bilateral).
    After obtaining needle sensation continuous sparse wave electric stimulation was given. The needles were retained for 60 minutes. Treatment was given daily, and a course consisted of six sessions. After two courses he could see a hand waved 10 cm in front of him. After three courses he could distinguish a grown up from a child at 50 cm, and was able to avoid walls when walking. After four courses he could tell red from green. His eyes were re-examined: outer eye negative, fundi negative. Treatment was continued for another month and his vision was restored. The case was followed up a year later and his eyesight was found to be good.

Explanation: Experience has showed that scalp acupuncture is quite effective for cortical blindness. This therapy combines point location according to Western defined anatomical structures on the cerebral cortex with traditional acupuncture. In TCM it is believed that the three Yang channels of the hand and foot all travel to the head and face, and the Liver channel 'goes along the back of the throat into the nasopharynx, joining the eyes, then meeting Du Mai at the vertex'. Scalp acupuncture at the Visual area is effective for eye diseases such as cortical blindness because it activates the channels and collaterals and regulates Qi and Blood. When the eyes are able to draw nourishment from the Blood the disease will be cured.

Wang Xianhua, ACUPUNCTURE AND MOXIBUSTION SECTION, SHANDONG PROVINCIAL HOSPITAL

162. Blindness following cerebral thrombosis

Jiang, male, age 50

Case registered: 21 October 1983

History: The patient had cerebral thrombosis with loss of consciousness and paralysis of the limbs 3 months previously. These improved after treatment, but his vision was also affected. He was given Western and traditional Chinese drugs for 2 months, but there was little improvement.

Examination: Vision: left 0.9, right 0.2. Left pupil slightly more dilated than the right, about 4 mm. *Fundus examination:* abnormal light reflection from retinal arteries. The arteries were abnormally narrow, and there was notable venous compression where the arteries crossed the veins. The right field of vision had about 15° concentric contraction. The left upper field of vision was incomplete.

Diagnosis: Sudden blindness: Stagnation of Qi transforming into Fire.
　　Treatment: Activate the channels and collaterals and regulate Qi and Blood.

Principal Points:
1. Zanzhu BL 2, Muchuang GB 16, Fengchi GB 20, Zhizheng SI 7, Sanjian L.I. 3, Guangming GB 37, Ganshu BL 18.
2. Yangbai GB 14, Toulingqi (Extra), Tianzhu BL 17, Yanggang BL 48, Yanglao SI 6, Feiyang BL 58, Danshu BL 19.
　　The two groups of points were alternated, and treatment was given daily. The needles were retained for 15 minutes, and then the points were cupped. After a course of 10 treatments there was a clear improvement in his eyesight: right eye 1.2, left eye 0.4 ± 1. After two courses: right eye 1.5, left eye 0.9 ± 2. After three courses: right eye 1.5, left eye

1.2. The field of vision in the right eye was restored, and in the left there was 15° concentric contraction in the upper part. A year later eyesight on both sides was restored. The case was followed up for 3 years and there was no relapse.

Wang Guizhi, QIDASHAN IRON MINE HOSPITAL, ANSHAN STEEL COMPANY
(see Liaoning Journal of Traditional Chinese Medicine, Issue 4, 1987)

Editor's Note: The blindness was a result of cerebral thrombosis. In TCM terms this is caused by Stagnation of Qi transforming into Fire. Blood rises up with the Fire to invade the eye.

Local points on the head and around the eye such as Zanzhu BL 2, Yangbai GB 14, Muchuang GB 16 and Toulingqi (Extra) clear the head and the eye, and regulate and activate Qi and Blood in the eye area. Back points such as Ganshu BL 18, Danshu BL 19 and Yanggang BL 48 nourish Blood and clear the eye. Zhizheng SI 7, Sanjian L.I. 3 and Feiyang BL 58 were selected as distal points according to the principle of local and distal point selection. They were used to activate the channels and collaterals, and regulate Qi and Blood.

163. Blindness, hysterical

CASE 1

Shi, male, age 51, peasant

Case registered: 29 July 1979

History: 2 months previously the patient had a gastrectomy. He was discharged from hospital after 2 weeks. One day previously he became furious over a family problem and suddenly went blind. He came to hospital the next day.

Examination: He was conscious and his limbs moved freely. His eyes were normally aligned and there was no conjunctival congestion. Cornea clear. Pupils round and equal. No light sense. Diminished light reaction.

Diagnosis: Stagnation of Liver Qi, obstructing the clear orifices

Treatment: Regulate the Liver Qi, open the clear orifices.

Principal Points: Hegu L.I. 4, Taichong LIV 3, Jingming BL 1, Guangming GB 37.

Auricular Points: Liver.

After the first treatment he was able to count the number of fingers being held up a foot in front of him, and could discern people moving from a distance of 5 metres, though details were not clear. 2 days later, at the start of a home visit he was lying in bed. He could make out the shape of the central beam going across the ceiling. After needling however, he was able to distinguish fine detail on it. His eye sight was thus restored. The case was followed up for 4 years, and his eyesight remained good.

Explanation: This case of sudden blindness was caused by emotional factors. When the Liver Qi is not smooth, Qi rises upwards and the collaterals become obstructed. This Stagnation of Qi and Blood disturbs the clear orifices so the eyes are malnourished and go blind. The *Ling Shu* says, 'Liver Qi goes to the eyes. When the Liver is in harmony the eyes can recognize the colours' (Mai Du, Length of Channels chapter).

Taichong LIV 3, the Yuan-Source point, regulates Liver Qi, and activates the Blood and collaterals. Jingming BL 1, the meeting point of the Bladder, Small Intestine and Stomach channels, and Yin and Yang Qiao Mai, dredges the collaterals and clears the eyes. Guangming GB 37, the Luo-Connecting point, sends a branch to the Liver channel. It regulates the Qi of the Gallbladder and is an important point for eye diseases. Auricular point Liver was added because 'the Liver opens into the eyes'. In this case the patient was Deficient in Qi and Blood after the gastrectomy. Hegu L.I. 4 and Zusanli ST 36 are on the Yang Ming channels, which are rich in Blood and Qi. Together they tonify Deficiency.

Xu Futian, BAOCHANG COMMUNE CLINIC, HAIMEN COUNTY, JIANGSU PROVINCE
(see Jiangsu Journal of Traditional Chinese Medicine, Issue 6, 1985)

CASE 2

Zhang, female, age 42

Case registered: 17 September 1982

History: The patient had previously been healthy, but she became very distressed when her house was burgled. By the time she had cried herself to sleep it was 3.00 a.m. the next morning. When she woke up she was blind. Examination revealed her eyes to be normal, but she was completely blind. Her condition was diagnosed as 'hysterical blindness' and she was given intravenous glucose cytochrome C, intramuscular vitamin B_1 and B_{12}, oral Phenergam (promethazine) and diazepam. She was also prescribed Xiao Yao San (Free and Relaxed Pills) and Shi Hu Ye Guang Wan (Dendrobrium Moniliforme Night Sight Pills) for 10 days. There was no improvement so she was referred for acupuncture and moxibustion on 28 September 1982.

Examination: She was average sized and seemed to have had an average diet. She looked depressed. No light sense. Eyes normal. Blood and urine normal. *Tongue body:* red. *Tongue coating:* thin and dry. *Pulse:* wiry and slippery.

Diagnosis: Sudden blindness: Stagnation of Liver Qi, Blood Stasis obstructing the collaterals.

Treatment: Disperse Wind and Heat, activate the channels and collaterals.

Principal Points: Jingming BL 1, Chengqi ST 1 through to Neijingming (Inner Jingming, Extra).

Secondary Points: Hegu L.I. 4, Tai Yang (Extra) through to Jiaosun TB 20.
The patient lay on her back. Jingming BL 1 was needled to a depth of 1 cun. The doctor pressed laterally on the eyeball with his left index finger while inserting the needle. When needling Chengqi ST 1 the patient was asked to roll her eyes up, then the doctor used his left index finger to displace the eyeball upwards. A 1.5 cun needle was inserted perpendicularly to a depth of 0.1 cun, then angled horizontally towards Neijingming (Extra). At Tai Yang (Extra) the needle was inserted horizontally towards Jiaosun TB 20. At Hegu L.I. 4 the needle was inserted perpendicularly to a depth of 1 cun. The needles were retained without manipulation for 10 minutes. After withdrawal the patient was able to see dimly. She could discern her husband standing by her side, though she could not make out his face. She was advised to close her eyes and rest for 10 minutes. After this rest she could see more clearly, and differentiate the colours on the walls. After 40 minutes her vision in both eyes was 0.9. Tests at midday and in the afternoon of the next day showed her vision in both eyes was 1.5, and her eyesight was back to normal.

Explanation: This disorder is categorized in TCM as sudden blindness. The *Zheng Zhi Zhun Sheng* (Standards of Diagnosis and Treatment) says that, 'The person is normally healthy. There is no external injury to the eyeballs, no impairment of the visual spirit, but the person suddenly goes blind'.
In this case the disease was caused by emotional factors leading to Stagnation of Liver Qi and Stasis of Blood obstructing the collaterals. Wind and Fire in the Liver channel rise upward and assault the eyes, which are then not nourished by Blood, leading to blindness.
Jingming BL 1 and Chengqi ST 1 soothe Wind, activate the collaterals and open the eyes. Tai Yang (Extra) and Hegu L.I. 4 enhance this effect.

Case treated by Tang Fangtian, case study by Luo Zhenfa and Yun Zhiyou, QINGFENG COUNTY PEOPLE'S HOSPITAL, HENAN PROVINCE *(see Journal of Traditional Chinese Medicine, Issue 6, 1983)*

164. Oculomotor paralysis, post-traumatic

Tian, female, age 30, worker

Case registered: 11 April 1984

History: The patient was injured by a cart on 13 January 1984. She was admitted to hospital in a coma, with projectile vomiting, facial paralysis and haematoma around the left eye and on the head. X-rays revealed 'multiple fracture of the skull'. Cerebral angiography showed no intra-cranial haematoma. Her condition was diagnosed as contusion and laceration of the brain. She was given intravenous mannitol and cytidine diphosphate choline for 14 days. She gradually revived, but suffered from heaviness and pain in her left eye, with restricted movement and occasional double vision. She also developed headaches and faintness. Her reactions were slower and her memory was worse. She was able to move her limbs without difficulty. She was given further treatment with pyrithioxine hydrochloride (pyritinol) and vitamins, but she did not improve. At the time she was referred to the Acupuncture and Moxibustion Section, she had double vision, tinnitus, poor memory, spontaneous sweating, general weakness, headache and faintness. Her appetite and sleep were normal, but her stools were dry.

Examination: BP: 13.3/9.33 kPa (100/70 mmHg). She was conscious but looked lacklustre. Her reactions were slow but she was articulate. The area around her left eye was purple and swollen. Her left eye was cast obliquely down to the left. The movement of the eyeball was restricted, and her left upper eyelid was hanging down. Her left pupil was dilated, with no reaction to light or accommodation. Her right eye was normal. Her hearing was good in both ears. Heart and lungs normal. Movement of limbs normal. No pathological reflexes induced. *Tongue body:* pale red. *Tongue coating:* thin and white. *Pulse:* deep, weak and a little slippery.

Diagnosis: Double vision: Stasis of Qi and Blood causing malnourishment of the eyes and brain.

Treatment: Dredge the channels, invigorate the circulation of Blood.

Principal Points: Fengchi GB 20, Tai Yang (Extra), Zanzhu BL 2, Sibai ST 2, Hegu L.I. 4.

All the points were needled on the left with reinforcing and reducing evenly method. The needles were retained for 30 minutes. Treatment was given daily. After 15 sessions she had less headaches and faintness. Her left eyeball moved more freely and her eyelid lifted, but she still had double vision. The prescription was modified.

Principal Points: Yangbai GB 14 through to Yuyao (Extra), Qiuhou (Extra), Hegu L.I. 4.

This new prescription was given once a day. The points were needled on the left, and the needles were retained for 20 minutes. After a week she was able to move her eyeball without difficulty and her double vision improved. The prescription was modified again.

Principal Points: Fengchi GB 20, Tai Yang (Extra), Jingming BL 1, Sibai ST 2, Waiguan TB 5, Zhongzhu TB 3, Guangming GB 37.

The points were needled on the left and retained for 30 minutes. Treatment was given daily. After 2 weeks all her symptoms had gone and the disease was cured.

Explanation: In this case trauma to the brain damaged the blood vessels. Stagnation of Qi and Blood led to malnourishment of the brain and eyes, causing the headaches, double vision and poor memory. Treatment was designed to activate the Blood and channel Qi in the head area, and to resolve Stasis.

Jingming BL 1, Qiuhou (Extra), Sibai ST 2 and Zanzhu BL 2 activate the flow of Blood in the eyes. Fengchi GB 20, Tai Yang (Extra) and Hegu L.I. 4 refresh the eyes and head and regulate Qi and Blood. Waiguan TB 5, Zhongzhu TB 3 and Guangming GB 37 are distal points. They refresh the Mind, clear the eyes and activate the functional Qi and are important points for eye diseases.

Zhang Dengbu, ACUPUNCTURE AND MOXIBUSTION SECTION, SHANDONG TCM COLLEGE HOSPITAL.

165. Strabismus (squint)

Zhang, male, age 77

Case registered: 3 February 1983

History: The patient had a past history of arteriosclerosis and was diabetic. Over the last 2 weeks his eyesight got increasingly worse, and he developed amblyopia.

Examination: Tests revealed partial paralysis of the lateral rectus and monocular diplopia (sic), especially on the left.

Diagnosis: Double vision: Qi and Blood Deficiency, Fire in the Gallbladder.

Treatment: Activate the channels and collaterals, regulate Qi and Blood, clear Fire from the Gallbladder.

Principal Points: Tongziliao GB 1, Sibai ST 2, Yuyao (Extra), Guangming GB 37.

Guangming GB 37 was needled on both sides, the other points were needled on the affected side. The needles were first twirled to reduce, then to reinforce, then retained for 30 minutes with manipulation every 15 minutes. Treatment was given once every other day. After four treatments the patient's symptoms improved, and after nine he was completely cured: the position of his eye was normal, and he could move it in any direction without difficulty. The double vision had gone. The case was followed up a year later and there was no relapse.

Explanation: Medication is not as effective for double vision as acupuncture. The *Shen Shi Yao Han* (Valuable Manual of Ophthalmology) says, 'Double vision arises from Deficiency, defects or obstruction in the eyes. The root cause is disease in the Liver and Kidney, which are unable to supply the eyes with vital substances'. In this case the patient was an old man with a long history of other diseases. Thus the double vision was mostly due to Deficiency of Qi, Blood and Body Fluids. Yuyao (Extra) is an empirical point for eye diseases. The other points were used to activate the channels and collaterals, regulate Qi and Blood, and clear Fire from the Gallbladder.

Liu Cailan, SHENXI PROVINCIAL INSTITUTE OF TCM HOSPITAL
(see Shenxi Traditional Chinese Medicine, Issue 4, 1985)

166. Superior orbital fissure syndrome

Sun, male, age 48, cadre

Case registered: 19 May 1982

History: The patient had allergic rhinitis for 5 years. Over the last 3 years he also suffered from asthma. He was treated without effect with desensitization and electrocautery. On 3 May 1982 he was admitted to this hospital and had the pterygoid nerve surgically removed. He developed superior orbital fissure syndrome after the operation, which was thought to be caused by heat during the procedure. He was given hormones and co-enzyme A for 2 weeks with little effect, so he was referred for acupuncture and moxibustion.

Examination: He was unable to lift his right eyelid and had restricted movement in his right eye. His vision was blurred. The pupil was dilated. He had a headache on the right. *Tongue body:* slightly dark with purple patches. *Pulse:* deep and thin.

Diagnosis: Heat flaring upwards, Blood Stasis with obstruction of the collaterals.

Treatment: Invigorate the Blood by resolving Stasis, dredge the collaterals and clear the eyes.

Principal Points: Yangbai GB 14 through to Yuyao (Extra), Zanzhu BL 2, Tongziliao GB 1, Jingming BL 1, Xiangu ST 43.

All the points were needled on the right, with strong stimulation at Xiangu ST 43 and gentle stimulation at all the others. The needles were retained for 20 minutes. Treatment was given once every 3 days. After two sessions his headache improved and he was able to lift his eyelid a little. The prescription was modified by the addition of Chengqi ST 1. After 10 sessions he could keep his right eyelid open and move the eye in any direction without difficulty. The pupil gradually contracted and his field of vision became normal. He still had double vision when looking down or to the sides. Guangming GB 37 was added to the prescription, and treatment was continued once every 3 days. After a further seven treatments he had no further difficulties and was discharged as cured. The case was followed up for 6 months and there was no relapse.

Explanation: The *Su Wen* says, 'All the vessels belong to the eye' (Wu Zang Sheng Cheng, Growth of the Five Zang chapter). This means the eyes are closely related to the organs and the vessels. This disease was caused by excessive heat from the surgery causing Stagnation of Qi and Blood and impairing the channel tendons.

Zanzhu BL 2, Yangbai GB 14, Tongziliao GB 1, Jingming BL 1 and Chengqi ST 1 are points on all three leg Yang channels. They invigorate the Blood and collaterals, and remove Heat and Stasis. Jingming BL 1 is a meeting point of the Bladder with the Small Intestine and Stomach channels, and Yin and Yang Qiao Mai. It is particularly effective for eye diseases. Yuyao (Extra) is located on the orbital muscle. It therefore can aid the eyelid to stay open. Guangming GB 37, the Luo-Connecting point, clears Liver Heat and refreshes the eye, and is effective for double vision. Xiangu ST 43 nourishes and raises the Yang to clear the eye.

Chen Weicang, ACUPUNCTURE AND MOXIBUSTION SECTION, SHANGHAI MEDICAL COLLEGE NO. 2 HOSPITAL, REIJIN
(see Journal of Traditional Chinese Medicine, Issue 6, 1985)

167. Colour blindness

Liu, male, age 14, schoolboy

History: The patient was discovered to be colour blind in November 1981. He did not respond to medication and was brought for acupuncture and moxibustion.

Examination: He could only distinguish three colour test cards.

Diagnosis: Colour blindness: Liver and Kidney Deficiency.

Treatment: Reinforce Liver and Kidney, regulate Liver Qi, regulate Qi and Blood, refresh the eyes.

Principal Points:
1. Fengchi GB 20, Zanzhu BL 2, Tai Yang (Extra), Zusanli ST 36.
2. Sibai ST 2, Hegu L.I. 4, Guangming GB 37, Sizhukong TB 23.
3. Yuyao (Extra), Chengqi ST 1, Taixi KID 3, Sanyinjiao SP 6.

The points were needled with reinforcing and reducing equally method and the needles were retained for 20–30 minutes. Treatment was given once every other day. After six treatments he could distinguish the colours on seven cards. After 20 sessions he could distinguish the colours on 17, and after 30 treatments he could distinguish the colours on 25. He was given 36 sessions in total, and could eventually identify all the test cards. He was re-examined after 6 months, and colour sense was undiminished.

Explanation: The eye is closely related to the Zangfu. The *Ling Shu* says, 'The five Zang and the six Fu all supply essential substances to the eyes'. The Liver and Kidney have the closest relation to the eyes.

Taixi KID 3, the Yuan-Source point, regulates and reinforces Kidney Qi. Sanyinjiao SP 6, the meeting point of the Liver, Spleen and Kidney channels, nourishes the Liver and Kidney, reinforces the Spleen and Stomach, regulates Qi and Blood, and activates the channels and collaterals. Fengchi GB 20 is the meeting point of the Gallbladder and Triple Burner channels and Yang Wei Mai. Guangming GB 37, the Luo-Connecting point, sends a branch to the Liver channel. Sizhukong TB 23 is where the channel Qi of the Gallbladder and Triple Burner originates.

Sun Qingyun, Yezenggui and Dou Huifang, INSTITUTE OF ACUPUNCTURE AND MOXIBUSTION, CHINA ACADEMY OF TRADITIONAL CHINESE MEDICINE
(see Journal of Traditional Chinese Medicine, Issue 9, 1984)

168. Night blindness

Li, male, age 38

Case registered: 7 September 1979

History: The patient suffered from xerophthalmia (dryness of the eyes) and blurred vision at night. During the day his eyesight was normal. Treatment with Western drugs had no effect. He also felt weak, had little appetite and had lumbar pain.

Examination: He was thin. *Tongue body:* pale. *Tongue coating:* white. Pulse: thin and weak.

Diagnosis: Deficiency of Liver Blood.

Treatment: Nourish Kidney Water, promote Liver Wood, readjust Liver Qi.

Principal Points: Jingming BL 1, Guangming GB 37, Taichong LIV 3.
    The needle at Jingming BL 1 was twirled gently, and the other points were reduced and reinforced equally. Treatment was given daily. After four treatments his night vision improved, but the xenophthalmia was unchanged. This is because the Liver and Kidney were not yet fully revitalized. Further treatment was given to nourish and tonify the two organs, omitting Taichong Liver 3 and adding Shuiquan KID 5. After five more sessions all the symptoms were gone and the disorder was cured.

Explanation: The Liver opens into the eye. Night blindness is caused by Deficiency of Liver Blood, which is unable to nourish the eyes. The Kidney has the same origin as the Liver and so is also a source of visual spirit. Treatment was therefore aimed at reinforcing these two organs.
    Jingming BL 1 is a meeting point of the Bladder, Small Intestine and Stomach channels, and Yin and Yang Qiao Mai. The *Su Wen* says, 'All the vessels belong to the eyes' (Wu Zang Sheng Cheng, Growth of the Five Zang chapter). Jingming BL 1 nourishes the Liver and Kidney as well as activating Qi and Blood in the local area. Taichong LIV 3 was selected to activate Liver Qi according to the principle of 'treating the Yuan-Source points for disease in the related organ'. Guangming GB 37, the Luo-Connecting point, sends a branch to the Liver channel. In this case it was used to regulate Qi and Blood in the Liver channel. Shuiquan KID 5 is the Xi-Accumulation point. When Kidney Qi is full, it feeds its child organ, the Liver.

Jiang Yunxiang, DINGYUAN COUNTY HOSPITAL, ANHUI PROVINCE
(*see Liaoning Journal of Traditional Chinese Medicine, Issue 8, 1985*)

169. Nasal polyp

Yan, female, age 62

Case registered: 1 October 1973

History: 2 years previously the patient had a nasal polyp removed. The problem recurred recently. She had a pea-sized polyp which obstructed her breathing. She was unwilling to undergo another operation so she came for acupuncture and moxibustion.

Diagnosis: Stasis of Wind, Damp and Heat pathogens in the Lung.

Treatment: Clear Wind Damp Heat and dredge the nasal passages.

Principal Points: Suliao Du 25, Hegu L.I. 4, Lieque LU 7.

Secondary Points: Fengchi GB 20, Shanxing (Extra), Yingxiang L.I. 20.
Treatment was given every 3–5 days, treating 2–4 points at a time. The polyp disappeared after a month. The case was followed up for 10 years and there was no relapse.

Explanation: Suliao Du 25 is especially effective in the treatment of polyp. Lieque LU 7 is the Luo-Connecting point of the Lung, and the Lung opens into the nose. Hegu L.I. 4 is the Yuan-Source point of the Large Intestine which is the Yang coupled organ of the Lung. The Large Intestine channel also travels up to the nose at Yingxiang L.I. 20, a local point. Hegu L.I. 4 and Lieque LU 7 are used together according to the Guest Host principle of Luo-Connecting point to Yuan-Source point. The combination enhances the effect of individual points to clear Wind Damp Heat from the Lungs. Shangxing (Extra) and Fengchi GB 20 are important points in the treatment of nasal disease, and strengthen the effect of dredging the nasal passage.

> Case treated by Zhang Zhenhui, case study by Qiang Hong and Wei Jin, FENYANG COUNTY TCM HOSPITAL
> (*see Shanxi Traditional Chinese Medicine, Issue 4, 1986*)

170. Epistaxis (nosebleeds)

CASE 1

Cong, male, age 36, worker

Case registered: June 1973

History: The patient had a sudden nosebleed 4 days previously. The blood was dark red. He immediately washed his forehead with cold water and blocked his nose with cotton wool, but blood came out of his mouth. In hospital he was given oral and intramuscular medication. This had a temporary effect, but he subsequently had frequent nosebleeds. When he came for acupuncture and moxibustion another one had just started. He also felt faint, had a dry mouth, dry stools, and sensations of heat and distress in the chest.

Examination: His nose was blocked with cotton wool. *Tongue body:* red. *Tongue coating:* dry and yellow.

Diagnosis: Epistaxis: Exuberant Heat in the Lung and Stomach burning the nasal passages and impairing the vessels.

Treatment: Purge Heat in the Lung and Stomach, cool the Blood and stop bleeding.

Principal Points: Shangxing Du 23, Weizhong BL 40, Hegu L.I. 4, Shaoshang LU 11, Qihai Ren 6, Zusanli ST 36.

　　Shangxing Du 23 and Shaoshang LU 11 were bled, then Shangxing Du 23 and Hegu L.I. 4 were reduced. The needles were retained for 20 minutes. Next the cotton wool was removed from the patient's nose, which was no longer bleeding. Qihai Ren 6 and Zusanli ST 36 were needled next, and the needles were again retained for 20 minutes. After this the patient felt invigorated. The disorder was cured. The case was followed up for a month and there was no relapse.

Explanation: Clinical experience has shown that acupuncture is sometimes more effective in such cases than haemostatic drugs such as ethamsylate. In TCM terms the disease is caused by Heat in the Blood and Rebellious Qi. The *Su Wen* says, 'Epistaxis is caused by Heat invading the Stomach channel. The Heat causes the Blood to move recklessly causing bleeding' (Ji Yuan Bing Shi, Exploration of Causes of Disease chapter).

　　Shanxing Du 23 purges Pathogenic Heat, regulates the nose, soothes the vessels and stops bleeding. Du Mai controls all the Yang and passes through the nose. In clinical practice this point has been found to constrict the vessels of the nasal mucosa. It is an important point for nasal disease. Hegu L.I. 4, the Yuan-Source point, is related to Qi. It disperses pathogens and sends down Rebellious Qi in the Stomach and Lung. The *Bai Zheng Fu* (Verses of the One Hundred Diseases) says, 'Hegu L.I. 4 is effective for nosebleeds'. Shaoshang LU 11, the Jing-Well point, clears Heat and regulates the orifices. Weizhong BL 40, the He-Sea point, clears Heat and relaxes the vessels so Blood circulates normally.

Case treated by Xie Linyuan, article by Xie Leye, WENDENG COUNTY BONE SETTING HOSPITAL, SHANDONG PROVINCE
(see Shandong Journal of Traditional Chinese Medicine, Issue 1, 1984)

CASE 2

Wang, male, age 60, retired worker

Case registered: 26 April 1984

History: 3 days previously the patient had a nosebleed. Plugging his nose and applying a cold towel to his forehead did not help. In hospital he was given nasal drops of adrenaline, but this, together with other Western medication and more cotton wool plugs was ineffective. He came for acupuncture and moxibustion with his nose full of cotton wool and blood coming out of his mouth. He had no previous history of injury to the nose or haematological disease. He had been overworked and had quarrelled with his wife. He was upset and had a bitter taste in his mouth.

Examination: He was still bleeding. *Tongue body:* red at the tip and edges. *Pulse:* wiry and rapid.

Diagnosis: Epistaxis: Liver Fire rising up to push the Blood from the vessels.

Treatment: Clear Liver Fire.

Principal Points: Taichong LIV 3 (bilateral).
   The points were reduced. The bleeding stopped after 5 minutes. After 10 minutes the cotton wool was removed and there was no new bleeding. The needles were retained for 20 minutes. The next day the treatment was repeated to consolidate the effect. He had no further nosebleeds.

Explanation: The *Su Wen* says, 'When there is anger Qi rises' and 'Anger causes Qi to rise adversely, causing vomiting up of Blood or diarrhoea containing undigested food' (Ju Tong Lun, Pain chapter). In this case the patient had Heat in the Interior caused by fatigue. His anger impaired the Liver, so Blood was carried up with Qi to impair the vessels in the nose, causing the nosebleeds. Reducing Taichong LIV 3, the Yuan-Source point, purges Liver Fire and induces the Blood to come down. It has proved very effective clinically for nosebleeds caused by Liver Fire.

Zhang Zhenbang, FENGZHOU CLINIC, BAOJI RAILWAY HOSPITAL, SHENXI PROVINCE
(see The New Chinese Medicine, Issue 2, 1986)

171. Pain in the lung on inhalation

Liu, female, age 28

History: The patient had severe pain in her left lung when she inhaled cold air through her left nostril. The problem was more severe in winter.

Examination: She was stoutly built. Her voice was thin and timid. She gasped and sighed frequently.

Diagnosis: Lung Qi Deficiency.

Treatment: Warm and strengthen Lung Qi.

Principal Points: Feishu BL 13.

Five moxa cones on ginger were burnt on the left Feishu BL 13. Her symptoms were relieved after one treatment. A week later there had been no relapse.

Chen Keqin, SHENXI PROVINCIAL TCM INSTITUTE
(see Tianjin Journal of Traditional Chinese Medicine, Issue 1, 1986)

Editor's Note: The *Ling Shu* says, 'Lung Qi leads to the nose. When the Lung Qi is regulated the nose can recognize the smells' (Mai Du, Length of Channels chapter). Thus the nose is closely related to the Lung in health and disease. When the patient's Lung Qi was Deficient her nose was unable to warm the air, and the cold air in turn impaired the Lung. The moxibustion on ginger warmed the Lung and tonified the Qi. When the Qi was sufficiently strong the nose was able to perform its normal function.

172. Hysterical aphasia

CASE 1

Fei, female, age 45, peasant

Case registered: 19 May 1974

History: The patient had found herself unable to speak that morning. She was able to mime that she had distress in the chest.

Examination: No abnormal findings in the mouth and throat. No facial paralysis, mouth and eye were positioned normally. No paralysis. *Axillary temperature:* 36.5°C. *Pulse rate:* 80/min. *Respiration:* 22/min. *BP:* 16.5/10.7 kPa (124/80 mmHg). Heart and lungs normal. Abdomen soft. Liver and spleen not palpable. Range of movement in limbs normal. Neck soft. Trachea central. *Tongue body:* red. *Tongue coating:* thick and greasy. *Pulse:* wiry and slippery.

Treatment: 'The tongue is a manifestation of the Heart' so Neiguan P 6 was selected. The points were manipulated strongly at 5 minute intervals. After 20 minutes there was no improvement so the needles were removed and

Shenmen HT 7 was needled, again with strong stimulation every 5 minutes. After 20 minutes there was still no improvement so the needles were withdrawn and Yongquan KID 1 was selected. The needles were inserted to a depth of 0.2 cun and twirled strongly. After about 1 minute the patient cried out, 'It's too painful!', so the needles were immediately withdrawn. She was now able to describe how she had woken from a nightmare at about 2.00 a.m. She felt distress in the chest and restless, but was unable to speak. When Yongquan KID 1 was needled she felt a sensation like electricity travelling up her legs to her chest. She immediately felt comfortable and was able to speak.

Explanation: The *Ling Shu* describes how the Kidney channel 'starts from under the fifth toe, goes at an angle through the middle of the sole ... passing the centre of the back and connecting with the Bladder. The main pathway goes straight from the Kidney to the Liver, the diaphragm, into the Lung, up along the throat to the base of the tongue. A branch from the Lung goes around the Heart and then into the chest'. Yongquan KID 1 therefore regulates Liver Qi, facilitates Lung Qi, eases the diaphragm, and relaxes the throat. Neiguan P 6 and Shenmen HT 7 probably had a preparatory effect which was not immediately evident.

> Xiao Jinshun, YANGHENAN DRILLING TEAM CLINIC, XUANHUA COUNTY, HEBEI PROVINCE
> *(see Shanghai Journal of Acupuncture and Moxibustion, Issue 3, 1982)*

CASE 2

Lu, male, age 36, peasant

Case registered: November 1969

History: The patient was in an argument 10 days previously. He was pushed to the ground, and afterwards was unable to speak. His eyes and mouth remained closed and he did not eat or drink. He was given supporting therapy in hospital and small doses of tranquillizers, but after 7 days his condition was unchanged and he was referred for acupuncture and moxibustion.

Examination: The patient looked lacklustre. There were no visible signs of injury. Routine blood, faeces and urine tests were normal. CSF normal. Chest X-ray clear; lungs, heart and diaphragm normal. Temperature normal.

Treatment: Open the orifices, calm the Mind.

Principal Points: Yamen Du 15, Dazhui Du 14.

At Yamen Du 15 the needle was inserted slowly to a depth of 1.3 cun and twirled slowly at intervals through a small angle. After 10 minutes the patient opened his eyes. When asked if he was in pain he answered 'Yes'. The needle was retained and Dazhui Du 14 was needled with medium strong stimulation. After 20 minutes he was in good spirits and speaking fluently. After the needles were removed he was given a bowl of millet porridge and kept in overnight for observation. He was able to eat about half of the porridge. He was discharged as cured the next day. The case was followed up for 14 years and there was no relapse.

Explanation: In this case emotional factors disturbed the Functional Qi of the Zangfu. Yamen Du 15 is also called Yinmen (Gate of Aphasia). It is a meeting point of Du Mai and Yang Wei Mai. It leads to the root of the tongue, and activates the vessels in the orifices and calms the Mind. It treats contracture of the tongue and aphasia arising from Heat or Cold. Dazhui is a meeting point of the Yang channels and Du Mai. It is effective in all consumptive and Deficiency disease. It generates Yang and calms the Mind, and is an important point for readjusting the functions of the whole body.

Xu Futian, BAOCHANG COMMUNE CLINIC, HAIMEN COUNTY, JIANGSU PROVINCE
(see Jiangsu Journal of Traditional Chinese Medicine, Issue 6, 1985)

173. Dysphagia

Bai, male, age 91, retired worker

Case registered: 20 August 1987

History: For the last month the patient had choked and had difficulty in swallowing at mealtimes. The problem started with headaches and sensations of heaviness on the left side of his body, then he started to choke when he swallowed food or water. CT scans found no signs of brain disease. After a month of treatment with Western drugs and nasogastric feeding he was referred for acupuncture and moxibustion.

Examination: He was conscious, thin and pale. He was unable to swallow. His throat was red but not swollen. Pharyngeal reflex dulled. No atrophy of the tongue muscles. Uvula central. *Tongue body:* pale. *Tongue coating:* thin and white. *Pulse:* deep and thin.

Diagnosis: Inflammation of the throat: Kidney Yin Deficiency, Exuberant Liver Yang.

Treatment: Nourish Kidney Yin, relieve inflammation.

Principal Points: Tiantu Ren 22, Lianquan Ren 23, Yinxi HT 6 (bilateral), Zhaohai KID 6 (bilateral).

The points were reduced with lifting and thrusting technique and the needles were retained for 20 minutes. Treatment was given once a day. After four treatments he was able to drink water slowly. After eight treatments he could manage liquid food. After 13 treatments the nasogastric tube was removed and he was able to eat soft cakes without choking. Three more consolidating treatments were given. The case was followed up for 2 months and there was no relapse.

Explanation: The patient was very old, and his Kidney Yin was Deficient. The Kidney channel goes up to the root of the tongue. When Kidney Essence is Deficient it cannot support and nourish the organs in the upper part of the body. Tiantu Ren 22 and Lianquan Ren 23 ease the throat by relieving inflammation. Yinxi HT 6 and Zhaohai KID 6 nourish Kidney Yin.

Ji Qingshan, ACUPUNCTURE AND MOXIBUSTION SECTION, CHANGCHUN TCM COLLEGE

174. Uranoplegia (paralysis of palate)

Ma, female, age 13

Case registered: 9 March 1977

History: For the last 5 days the patient's speech had been blurred. Her voice was very nasal. When she drank water it would come out of her nose. Her condition was diagnosed in a local hospital as uranoplegia (paralysis of the muscles of the soft palate).

Examination: The patient was conscious but seemed dull and lacklustre. Her reactions were slow. Her voice was thin and nasal and her words were indistinct. The palatal arch was asymmetrical, being broader and softer on the right. Movement was not dynamic when making sounds. The uvula was not central but slanted to the right. *Tongue body:* pale. *Tongue coating:* thin and white. *Pulse:* deep and thin.

Diagnosis: Aphasia.

Principal Points: Hegu L.I. 4, Shanglianquan (Extra), Waijinjin (Extra), Waiyuye (Extra).

The needles were removed after sensation was obtained. Treatment was given once every 2–3 days. After three treatments she could drink water properly. She was able to speak more clearly and the uvula returned to the central position. After the fourth session she was normal again, except for some dizziness on getting up. This was treated with Baihui Du 20, and she was given two more consolidating treatments. The case was followed up for 2 months and there was no relapse.

Explanation: This disease was caused by impairment of the vagus nerve, but because of the presentation it is classified in TCM as aphasia. The *Nei Jing* says, 'The Lung opens into the nose' and, 'The Lung is in charge of making sounds'. 'The Kidney channel . . . goes up from the Kidney, through the diaphragm to the chest, up along the throat to the root of the tongue'. These excerpts show that speech is closely related to the Lung and the Kidney. 'The Lung is the gate of sounds, the Kidney is the root of sounds'.

The Large Intestine is the Yang coupled organ of the Lung. Hegu L.I. 4 is the Yuan-Source point. Waijinjin (Extra) and Waiyuye (Extra) are on the Kidney channel, which has two vessels under the tongue as its Biao-branches (Jinjin (Extra) and Yuye (Extra)).

Chen Keqin, SHENXI PROVINCIAL TCM INSTITUTE

175. Angioneurotic oedema

CASE 1

Wang, male, age 61

Case registered: 30 November 1975

History: 2 hours previously the patient noticed his lower lip swelling. It felt heavy and numb, and within an hour the sensation spread to his chin and cheeks, at which point it impaired his speech. He had no recollection of trauma, insect sting, eating anything unusual or taking any medication, but had held a bus ticket in his lips about 10 minutes before the swelling started.

Examination: He was conscious and generally healthy. Temperature normal. Upper lip normal. His lower lip was twice the size of his upper lip, and his chin and cheeks were noticeably swollen. The skin was shiny but not red, firm or tender. He had restricted movement of the lower lip.

Diagnosis: Urticaria.

Principal Points: Chengjiang Ren 24, Lianquan Ren 23, Daying ST 5 (bilateral), Hegu L.I. 4 (bilateral).

The points were strongly reduced and the needles were retained for an hour. He felt strong needle sensation, especially at Hegu L.I. 4. He reported feeling a sensation like a thick cotton thread passing slowly up his arm along the Large Intestine channel to his shoulder, neck and cheek, mouth and lips. After continuous stimulation for roughly 10 minutes the contracture, numbness and stiffness began to feel better. After 30 minutes the oedema began to subside, and he could move his lip slightly. The skin in his chin and lip felt markedly less stiff. After an hour the swelling was mostly relieved, he could move his lips without difficulty and speak normally.

Ma Dingxiang, DEPARTMENT OF STOMATOLOGY, ARMY UNIVERSITY NO. 4
(see Shenxi New Medicine, Issue 5, 1977)

Editor's Note: Angioneurotic oedema is classified as urticaria in TCM. It can be caused by Blood Deficiency, Heat in the Blood, Damp in the skin and muscles, Stagnation of Qi and Blood due to invasion of Pathogenic Wind, Accumulated Heat in the Stomach and Intestines which, together with Pathogenic Wind or Wind Heat, lodges in the skin. It is also related to general health, and intake of certain foods causing a Ying–Wei imbalance and accumulation of Damp Heat in the Interior. In this case it is possible that contact with the bus ticket might have caused the symptoms. Chengjiang Ren 24, Lianquan and Daying ST 5 activate the vessels and relieve Wind and Damp. The propagation of sensation along the channel from Hegu L.I. 4 contributed to the prompt relief of the symptoms. The *Nei Jing* says, 'In acupuncture it is important to propagate needling sensation to the affected area'.

CASE 2

Zhang, male, age 37, worker

Case registered: 16 July 1985

History: For the last week the patient had been very emotional after a quarrel. On the same day as the quarrel his lower lip started to tingle and became red and swollen. 2 days later he had the same symptoms in his upper lip.

Examination: His lips were everted, and very red and swollen. His face was ashen. *Tongue body:* red. *Tongue coating:* white. *Pulse:* wiry and rapid.

Diagnosis: Liver Qi Stagnation transforming into Fire, permitting Pathogenic Wind Heat to invade the Liver channel.

Treatment: Purge Heat, reduce swelling.

Principal Points: Hegu L.I. 4.

Secondary Points: The highest points of the swelling.

Hegu L.I. 4 was reduced strongly, and the other points were bled. The swelling improved, and the patient was cured in an hour.

Explanation: The Liver channel goes through the inside of the lips. In this case emotional factors transformed into Fire, causing a Ying–Wei imbalance, and leaving the Liver channel open to invasion by Pathogenic Wind. This resulted in Stagnation of Qi and Blood. Bleeding the affected area purged Heat and relieved the oedema. Hegu L.I. 4 is an important point for face and mouth problems. Reducing it clears Wind and Heat and activates the vessels.

Zhao Tingbai, TAIYUAN HEAVY MACHINERY WORKS HOSPITAL, SHANXI PROVINCE
(see Shanxi Traditional Chinese Medicine, Issue 6, 1986)

176. Protrusion of the tongue

CASE 1

Wang, female, age 46

Case registered: 5 October 1963

History: The patient and her husband had had a row. He explained that her tongue began to feel numb afterwards and she had difficulty speaking. Soon her tongue was protruding out of her mouth. She was unable to put it back in or curl it, and had difficulty talking, eating or drinking. She salivated constantly and was dribbling as a result.

Examination: She was restless and thin. Her tongue was slightly swollen, and protruded 5–6 cm out of her mouth. *Tongue body:* dark red. *Tongue coating:* slightly yellow and greasy. *Pulse:* wiry, slippery and a little rapid.

Diagnosis: Stagnation of Qi and Phlegm transforming into Fire.

Principal Points: Lianquan Ren 23, Yongquan KID 1, Danzhong Ren 17.

The points were reduced with lifting, thrusting and twirling technique. Her tongue started to retract after about 2 minutes. When the needle at Lianquan Ren 23 was removed, she spat out about 50 ml of white phlegm, and asked for some water. By the time she had drunk three glasses all her symptoms had gone. The case was followed up for more than 2 years and there has been no relapse.

CASE 2

Zhang, female, age 51

Case Registered: 4 August 1984

History: The patient's son reported that his mother had had a family quarrel 2 days previously. Afterwards she lay on her bed and refused food and water. The next day her tongue protruded out of her mouth and she dribbled at the mouth. She rubbed her chest as if she felt considerable distress there. She held her tongue with a towel, which was wet.

Examination: *Tongue body*: pale. *Tongue coating*: thin, white and greasy. *Pulse*: wiry and slippery.

Diagnosis: Stagnation of Qi and Phlegm transforming into Fire.

Principal Points: Yongquan KID 1, Lianquan Ren 23, Danzhong Ren 17.
    The first two points were needled with lifting thrusting and twirling technique. After 4–5 minutes her tongue withdrew into her mouth, but she still had distress in the chest and belching. Danzhong Ren 17 was added and the disorder was cured. The case was followed up for 3 years. She had a relapse in April 1986 after another emotional upset, which was cured with the same treatment.

Explanation: Although this is a very rare disease to encounter in clinic, it is recorded in the *Ling Shu*: 'For protrusion of the tongue and involuntary drooling treat the Kidney channel' (Han Re Bing, Cold and Heat Diseases chapter). I have treated seven cases, all women who developed the condition after a period of emotional upset or fatigue. It can be compared to melancholia in TCM, or hysteria in Western medicine, a kind of paroxysmal neurosis. Emotional upset causes Stasis of the Functional Qi and Phlegm, which transforms into Fire rising upwards to assault the base of the tongue.
    The Kidney channel goes through the throat to the tongue. Yongquan KID 1, the Jing-Well point, invigorates the Qi in the channel, clears the throat and tongue and relieves the cheek. Lianquan Ren 23 is also called She Ben (Root of the Tongue). The *Qian Jing Fang* (Golden Prescriptions) says, 'It is effective for swelling under the tongue, protrusion of the tongue and involuntary drooling'. It removes Phlegm, activates the channels and restores the function of the tongue. Danzhong Ren 17 activates Qi, removes Stasis and restores the function of the tongue.

    Zhou Dingxing, HEZE PREFECTURAL TCM COLLEGE, SHANDONG PROVINCE

CASE 3

Zhou, male, age 12

Case Registered: 14 February 1975

History: The patient's tongue had been protruding for 6 hours. The patient had a fever following a cold a week previously. It was treated successfully with injections and oral medication. The morning of the consultation his parents found him sitting quietly by himself. He looked dull and lifeless, and his tongue was protruding.

Examination: *Tongue body*: pale. *Tongue coating*: thin and white. *Pulse*: wiry and slow.

Diagnosis: Deficiency of Heart Qi.

Treatment: Tonify Heart Qi.

Principal Points: Laogong P 8 (on the left).
    The point was reinforced, then the patient's tongue was tucked back into his mouth. It was normal after this.

Explanation: 'The tongue is a manifestation of the Heart', and 'Heart Qi leads to the tongue'. In this case the boy had had a fever which had left the upper part of the body malnourished and his Heart Qi Deficient. Reinforcing Laogong P 8, the Shu-Stream point, regulates Heart Qi and activates the collaterals. Reducing the point is effective for sores on the tongue and in the mouth arising from Heart Fire. The *Ling Shu* says, 'The same point can have different effects when treated with different methods' (Zhang Lun, Abdominal Distension chapter).

> Case treated by Zhang Zhenhui, case study by Zhang Hong and Wei Jin, FENYANG COUNTY TCM HOSPITAL, SHANXI PROVINCE (*see Shanxi Traditional Chinese Medicine, Issue 4, 1986*)

CASE 4

Wang, female, age 40, saleswoman

Case Registered: 25 December 1967

History: The patient had fallen on the ground in a rage 2 days previously.

Examination: She was restless and upset. Her tongue protruded out of her mouth. It was not red or swollen, but dry, and impaired her speech. *Pulse*: wiry and thin.

Diagnosis: Stagnation of Liver Qi, Heart vessel failing to contract.

Treatment: Regulate Liver Qi, calm the Mind.

Principal Points: Taichong LIV 3, Tongli HT 5.
    Taichong LIV 3 was reduced, Tongli HT 5 was reinforced. After the

needles were retained for 10 minutes the patient was calmer. Next the tip of her tongue was punctured quickly with a 28 gauge 0.5 cun needle. She cried out and her tongue withdrew instantly. Her speech was restored along with normal movement of her tongue.

Explanation: The *Ling Shu* says, 'The Liver is where the tendons join ... and connects with the root of the tongue. Reducing Taichong LIV 3, the Yuan-Source point, regulates Liver Qi' (Jing Mai, Channels chapter). In the same chapter it also says, 'The Heart channel has a branch called Tongli ... when it is deficient the person cannot speak'. Reinforcing Tongli HT 5 calms the Mind. The tongue is controlled by the Heart. Needling the tongue refreshes the Heart and restores the sensory organs.

Guan Zunhui, KUNMING MUNICIPAL HOSPITAL, YUNNAN PROVINCE
(see Journal of Traditional Chinese Medicine, Issue 11, 1985)

177. Swelling and rigidity of the tongue

Liu, female, age 21, peasant

Case Registered: 18 November 1964

History: The patient was admitted to this hospital with a pulmonary abscess. The foci in her right lung improved with treatment. After 2 months however, she suddenly felt numbness in the root of her tongue. The mobility of her tongue was impaired, her speech was slurred and she felt disoriented. She was given acupuncture, which restored her speech and consciousness, but she relapsed 10 minutes after the needles were removed. She was given acupuncture again and once more improved. This time, however, when the needles were removed her tongue protruded from her mouth and she was unable to withdraw it. Her tongue was swollen and filled her mouth.

Examination: The patient was nervous and worried. *Temperature:* 37°C. *Pulse rate:* 100/min. *BP:* 16.0/9.33 kPa (120/70 mmHg). Heart beat regular. There was systolic murmur at the cardiac apex, and wet rales over the right lung. Respiratory sound weak. Her tongue was swollen and protruding. *Tongue body*: dark red, with venous engorgement on the inferior surface.

Diagnosis: Exuberant Heat in the Heart and Spleen causing Blood Stasis.

Treatment: Clear Pathogenic Heat, resolve Blood Stasis.

Principal Points: Jinjin (Extra), Yuye (Extra).
  The patient was reassured first of all. She was asked to sit still, open

her mouth as wide as possible and try to curl her tongue upwards. Some gauze was wrapped around the tip to pull it upwards. On the inferior surface the veins on either side of the frenulum were thickened. The points were bled with a three-edged needle, then she was given some saline solution to gargle with to stop the bleeding and help the tongue contract. The disorder was cured.

Explanation: Sun Simiao of the Tang Dynasty wrote, 'Sudden swelling of the tongue like an inflated pig's bladder obstructs the respiration and can kill the patient if not treated promptly. Prick the two large vessels on either side of the frenulum' (Qian Jin Yao Fang, Golden Prescriptions for Emergencies). Jing Dongyang of the Qing Dynasty also wrote, 'A rigid tongue is also swollen. It looks like a pig's liver and cannot move freely, or fills the mouth, preventing the person from eating. It is from Stagnation of Heat in the Stomach and Spleen. The first thing to do is bleed the tip or the two sides of the tongue'. The Heart channel passes through the tongue, and the Spleen channel passes through the mouth. A vessel from it connects to the root of the tongue and disperses on the inferior surface.

Bleeding Yuye (Extra) and Jinjin (Extra) clears the Heart and purges the Spleen. When the Heat is cleared and the Blood Stasis is resolved, unblocking the vessels, Qi and Blood will circulate and the disease will be cured.

Wu Jingfu, XONGYUE HOT SPRING SANATORIUM, YINGKOU, LIAONING PROVINCE
(see The New Chinese Medicine, Issue 6, 1977)

178. Tongue rigidity following a stroke

Lei, male, age 68, worker

Case Registered: 6 May 1985

History: The patient had a previous history of hypertension. In 1982 he was admitted to hospital with cerebral thrombosis, and was paralysed on the right. After treatment he became able to look after himself, but in May 1985 he had numbness and tremor in his right hand, stiffness of the tongue, slurred speech, choking and coughing while drinking, difficulty in swallowing, and dribbling from the mouth.

Examination: BP: 21.3/13.3 kPa (160/100 mmHg). He was paralysed on the right. His tongue was stiff, and he was unable to protrude it. His speech was indistinct. *Tongue coating*: yellow and greasy. *Pulse*: wiry and slippery.

Principal Points: Taixi KID 3, Zhaohai KID 6, Taichong LIV 3, Laogong P 8, Fengchi GB 20, Lianquan Ren 23.

Tongue points: Heart, Liver, Kidney, Juquan.

Taixi KID 3 and Zhaohai KID 6 were reinforced. Taichong LIV 3, Laogong P 8 and Fengchi GB 20 were reduced. Warm needle was used at Lianquan Ren 23, using a GZH unit.

The tongue points were reduced with mild twirling. The needles were inserted superficially, and were not retained.

After 24 treatments the tongue was completely normal. His speech was clear, he had no dribbling, choking or coughing at meals. The case was followed up after 8 months and there was no relapse.

Explanation: The *Ling Shu* says, 'When the Five Zang are ill, needle the related Yuan-Source points' (Jiu Zhen Shi Er Yuan, Six Needlings, Twelve Source Points chapter). Reinforcing Taixi KID 3 and reducing Taichong LIV 3, both Yuan-Source points, strengthens Kidney Water to support Liver Wood. Laogong P 8 was reduced to activate the Heart vessel, because 'the Heart opens into the tongue'. According to the *Ling Shu*, 'The Heart channel has a branch . . . leading to the root of the tongue . . . The Liver is the convergence of the tendons . . . and has vessels connecting to the root of the tongue . . . The Kidney channel goes into the Lung, through the throat into the root of the tongue' (Jing Mai, Channels chapter). The Heart, Liver and Kidney are all treated at the same time. Zhaohai KID 6, the Confluent point of Yin Qiao Mai, readjusts the Yin of the whole body. The tongue points were selected according to the principle of combining outer points with inner points.

Guan Zunhui, KUNMING MUNICIPAL HOSPITAL, YUNNAN PROVINCE
(see Journal of Traditional Chinese Medicine, Issue 11, 1985)

179. Tongue paralysis and numbness

Yin, female, age 30, school teacher

Case Registered: 24 September 1982

History: The patient was caught in heavy rain on 8 June 1982. She had fever and aversion to cold afterwards. She was given medication and the fever abated, but she now had left-sided headaches, sensations of heaviness and pain in the eyes, and numbness on the left of her face. She was treated for 2 months, but would still get paroxysmal headaches. Her hearing was impaired, and her tongue was numb, making it difficult for her to eat.

Examination: Her tongue was angled to the left. There was some muscular atrophy, impairing her speech, and diminished sensation. *Tongue body*: pale and dry. *Tongue coating*: thin and yellow. *Pulse*: thin and choppy.

Diagnosis: Retained External Pathogen in Shao Yang.

Principal Points: Waiguan TB 5, Tongli HT 5, Tianzhu BL 10, Fengchi GB 20, Yifeng TB 17, Yamen Du 15, Lianquan Ren 23.

Tongue Points: Heart, Liver, Gallbladder, Spleen, Juquan.
   The body points were stimulated with Yin hidden in Yang technique, and the tongue points were punctured superficially with a 1 cun No. 3 needle which was not retained. Warm needling was given at Lianquan Ren 23, Tianzhu BL 10 and Fengchi GB 20,using a GZH unit. After 20 treatments her headache was gone, her hearing on the left was restored, and her tongue was more central. After 72 treatments the disease was cured. The case was followed up a year later and she was found to be good health.

Explanation: The disease started in the Tai Yang stage, with fever and aversion to cold. The symptoms of headache and ringing in the ear were caused by Stagnation of External Pathogens in the Shao Yang channel. The *Ling Shu* says, 'The Heart channel goes . . . to the root of the tongue' (Jing Jin, Channels and Tendons chapter). Warm needling at Lianquan Ren 23, Tianzhu BL 10 and Fengchi GB 20, a combination of front and back points, sends warmth directly into the affected parts to warm the channels and regulate the functions of the tendons. The tongue points enhance this effect and help the restoration of the tongue body.

Guan Zhunhui, KUNMING MUNICIPAL HOSPITAL, YUNNAN PROVINCE,
(see Journal of Traditional Chinese Medicine, Issue 11, 1985)

180. Contraction of the tongue

Wang, male, age 38

Case Registered: 11 November 1979

History: The previous day the patient had an emotional upset and then diarrhoea, which was treated with antibiotics. The next day he began to feel faint and had headache, nausea and sore throat. The symptoms were better after eating. At about 3.00 p.m. they got worse, and his tongue contracted, impairing his speech and eating. By 10.00 p.m. the contraction was so severe that he was afraid he would swallow his tongue and he had to keep pulling it out with his hand.

Examination: The patient had a normal build and seemed to have had an average diet. He was conscious but in pain. *Temperature:* 36.8°C. *BP:* 16.0/ 9.33 kPa (120/70 mmHg). Speech indistinct. *Tongue body*: dark red. *Tongue coating*: thick and white. *Pulse*: wiry and rapid.

Diagnosis: Exuberant Fire in the Heart and Liver.

Treatment: Clear Heart Fire, relieve Liver Heat, regulate the flow of Qi, open the clear orifices.

Principal Points: Renying ST 9, Lianquan Ren 23, Neiguan P 6, Taichong LIV 3.
  Renying ST 9 was needled with reinforcing and reducing evenly method. Lianquan Ren 23 and Taichong LIV 3 were reduced. Neiguan P 6 was reinforced. After the needles were inserted the patient felt his tongue pushed out of his throat with a thud, and his symptoms improved immediately.

Secondary Points: Xinshu BL 15, Shenshu BL 23.
  The next day these points were added. Xinshu BL 15 was reduced, Shenshu BL 23 was reinforced. The disorder was cured with two treatments. There has been no relapse.

Explanation: Renying ST 9 regulates the Qi of the Five Zang. Neiguan P 6, the Luo-Connecting point, regulates the Upper Burner, relieves the chest, calms the Mind and activates the collaterals. Taichong LIV 3 soothes Liver Wind. Lianquan Ren 23 is effective for contraction of the tongue. Xinshu BL 15 also calms the Mind and regulates Qi. Shenshu BL 23 nourishes Kidney Water to support Liver Wood. This approach treated both the cause and the symptoms.

Chen Huaying, CENTRAL HOSPITAL, YANZHOU COAL COMPANY HOSPITAL, SHANDONG PROVINCE
(see *Shandong Journal of Traditional Chinese Medicine, Issue 6, 1986*)

181. Involuntary movement of the tongue

CASE 1

Wu, male, age 22

Case Registered: 15 September 1976

History: The patient had been distressed after some bad news 3 days previously. His tongue started to move about involuntarily. His condition was diagnosed as neurosis, and he was given acupuncture at Neiguan

P 6, Shenmen HT 7 and Zhongwan Ren 12, and electro-acupuncture, as well as intramuscular injections of Luminal (phenobarbitone) and chlorpromazine but nothing really helped.

Examination: The patient was generally in good condition but was obviously restless and in pain. His tongue was moving around and making sounds. His speech was impaired and indistinct. *Tongue body*: red. *Tongue coating*: dry. *Pulse*: wiry and rapid.

Diagnosis: Emotional upset transforming into Fire assaulting the Pericardium and disturbing the Mind.

Treatment: Clear Heat, open the clear orifices.

Principal Points: Zhongzhu TB 3 (bilateral).
    The patient sat down with his palms on a table. The points were needled with 28 gauge needles, which were twirled through a wide angle. He was asked to make an 'Ah!' sound during the treatment. The involuntary movement stopped as he made the sound, and the disorder was cured.

Explanation: In this case emotional upset transforming into Fire assaulted the Pericardium and disturbed the Mind. The Pericardium and the Triple Burner are a Yin–Yang pair. The Triple Burner channel leads to Danzhong Ren 17 and goes around the Pericardium. Zhongzhu TB 3 clears Heat, opens the clear orifices and regulates the Functional Qi of the Three Burners. Reducing this point was quickly effective.

Xu Defeng, JINXIAN COUNTY PEOPLE'S HOSPITAL, LIAONING PROVINCE
(see Journal of Traditional Chinese Medicine, Issue 7, 1981)

CASE 2

Wang, female, age 41

Case Registered: 26 December 1982

History: The patient had tremor of the tongue for over a month after arguing with her husband. She also had headaches and faintness, oppression in the chest, restlessness and insomnia, a bitter taste in the mouth and a dry throat. Her condition was diagnosed as neurosis, but treatment with this approach was ineffective. She was then given traditional Chinese drugs and acupuncture at Shenmen HT 7, Sanyinjiao SP 6, Qimen LIV 14 and Hegu L.I. 4. All her symptoms cleared except the tremor of the tongue.

Examination: Her tongue trembled up and down constantly, impairing her speech. *Tongue body*: red. *Tongue coating*: thin and yellow. *Pulse*: wiry and rapid.

Diagnosis: Stagnation of Liver Qi transforming into Fire causing Wind to move upwards.

Principal Points: Taichong LIV 3, Zhongzhu TB 3.
   The points were needled with a 28 gauge needle. Strong stimulation was given, twirling the needles through a large angle and retaining them for 30 minutes. Treatment was given daily. The tremor stopped after three sessions.

Explanation: Wind rose up invading the Pericardium and disturbing the Mind. Taichong LIV 3, the Yuan-Source point, calms the Liver and suppresses Exuberant Yang, clears Heat and relieves Wind. The Pericardium and Triple Burner are a Yin–Yang pair. The Triple Burner channel passes through Danzhong Ren 17 and connects with the Pericardium channel in the chest. Zhongzhu TB 3 clears Heat, opens the clear orifices and regulates the functions of the Triple Burner.

Wan Liangzheng, JINGDIZHEN MUNICIPAL TCM HOSPITAL, JIANGXI PROVINCE
(see Jiangxi Traditional Chinese Medicine, Issue 2, 1982)

182. Painful tongue

Liang, female, age 38, cadre

Case Registered: 16 April 1974

History: In February 1972 the patient got scared and fainted during an accident at work. Towards the end of that year she began to feel discomfort in her throat and tongue. The symptoms were intermittent, and as they were not severe she did not seek help. Late at night on 24 March 1974 she developed tingling pains in the tongue. She was given many examinations but nothing abnormal was found. The pain got gradually worse till it was difficult for her to eat or sleep, and she was relying on sedatives and sleeping pills. At this point she was recommended acupuncture and moxibustion by some friends.

Examination: She looked yellow and emaciated, and was obviously in pain. Her lips and fingernails were somewhat livid. No fever or cold. *Tongue body*: red at the tip, with one dark purple patch on the left. Venous engorgement on the inferior surface. *Pulse*: wiry and tight.

Diagnosis: Heart Qi and Yin Deficiency, Blood Stasis in the channels and collaterals.

Treatment: Readjust Yin and Yang, invigorate the Blood and resolve Stasis.

Principal Points: Quchi L.I. 11 (right), Sanyinjiao SP 6 (left), Neiguan P 6 (left), Zusanli ST 36 (right), Tianzhu BL 10 (bilateral).

The pain improved considerably after the treatment. She had been able to sleep a little, and had managed a little food. The next day she was given acupuncture at Quchi L.I. 11 (left), Sanyinjiao SP 6 (right) Neiguan P 6 (right), Zusanli ST 36 (left), Tianzhu BL 10 (bilateral) and Lianquan Ren 23 (bilateral).

All the points were reinforced, except Tianzhu BL 10 and Lianquan Ren 23. Her pain improved some more. The condition was cured with one course of six daily treatments. Another course of consolidating treatment was given, and she returned to work. The case was followed up in May 1975, and there was no relapse.

Explanation: From the severe pain and the dark purple patch on the tongue it is clear that the Qi and Yin of the Heart were impaired. The *Su Wen* says, 'Alarm causes the Qi to be disturbed' (Ju Tong Lun, Pain chapter). When Qi is disturbed it becomes impaired, causing Rebellious Qi and Blood Stasis, leading to obstruction of the Heart channel. 'The tongue is a manifestation of the Heart.' Heart Fire blazes upwards and combats with the Stasis at the clear orifices, causing severe pain. The pain is persistent because Qi is obstructed and Blood is not nourished.

Case treated by Yuan Hanxong, case study by Yuan Nansheng, CHENGDU MUNICIPAL HOSPITAL OF ACUPUNCTURE, MOXIBUSTION AND MASSAGE
(*see Journal of Traditional Chinese Medicine, Issue 7, 1984*)

183. Itching on one side of the tongue

Li, female, age 43

Case Registered: July 1985

History: The patient had severe itching on the right side of her tongue for over 7 months. She saw many doctors but no specific disease was diagnosed. Treatment with vitamin B_1, B_{12}, oryzanol and cimetidine did not help.

Examination: There was no ulceration, fissure or lump on the tongue. Sensitivity to touch and taste sensation normal. There were no differences in colour or shape between the two sides of the tongue. Movement was normal. *Tongue body*: pale. *Tongue coating*: thin and white.

Electro-acupuncture: The point 1.5 cun posterior to Baihui Du 20.

The point was needled and given sparse-dense wave stimulation for 20 minutes. Treatment was given daily. Her symptoms improved a little after the first treatment. There was considerable improvement after the fifth session, and the condition was completely cured after 10 treatments.

Ma Dingxiang, STOMATOLOGY DEPARTMENT, ARMY UNIVERSITY NO. 4

Editor's Note: The *Su Wen* says, 'All aches, itching and soreness belong to the Heart' (Zhi Zhen Yao Da Lun, The Truest and Most Important chapter). The *Nan Jing* observes that, 'Itching is Deficient and aching is Excessive'. The Heart opens into the tongue. Itching of the tongue must be due to Heart Deficiency. The point used was probably effective because it is near the upper part of the Sensory area in scalp acupuncture.

184. Cavernoma on the tip of the tongue

Huang, female, age 46

History: For the last 5 or 6 years the patient had had a peanut-sized lump on the tip of her tongue. It was diagnosed in the Stomatology Department of her local hospital as a cavernous haemangioma (strawberry naevus), but she did not respond to treatment.

Examination: On the tip of her tongue, slightly to the right, there was a lump measuring 0.6 cm by 0.6 cm. It was purple and firm to the touch. Immobile. Not tender.

Diagnosis: Stagnation of Heart Blood.

Treatment: Move Stagnation, regulate Blood.

Principal Points: Shenmen HT 7, Neiguan P 6, Taichong LIV 3.
  Shenmen HT 7 and Neiguan P 6 were needled bilaterally, and the needles were retained for 15–30 minutes. Taichong LIV 3 was added after the third treatment. Treatment was given daily, and the lump disappeared after 11 treatments. The case was followed up for 6 months and there was no relapse.

Explanation: In TCM theory the tongue is closely related to the Heart, which is said to open into the tongue and manifest in the tongue. In clinic, petechiae or ecchymoses have frequently been observed in patients with Stagnation of Heart Blood. Shenmen HT 7, the Yuan-Source point, and Neiguan P 6, the Luo-Connecting point, were selected for this reason. Blood Stasis also relates to the Liver, so Taichong LIV 3, the Yuan-Source point, was added. The selection of points was proved correct by the rapidity of the cure.

Chen Zuolin, ACUPUNCTURE AND MOXIBUSTION SECTION, SHANGHAI RAILWAY CENTRAL HOSPITAL
(see Shanghai Journal of Traditional Chinese Medicine, Issue 6, 1980)

185. Sublingual cyst

Wang, male, age 62, peasant

Case Registered: 8 July 1968

History: The patient had stomach pain, poor appetite, asthma and cough for 2 years. Over the last year a cyst had formed under his tongue. Eventually it was so big it looked like an extra tongue, and it prevented him from eating and speaking properly.

Examination: The frenulum of his tongue leant slightly to the right. There was a chestnut sized cyst under his tongue. It was smooth, soft and shiny, not bleeding or ulcerous. *Tongue body*: normal. *Tongue coating*: slippery and greasy. *Pulse*: slippery.

Diagnosis: Double tongue: Stagnation of Phlegm Heat.

Treatment: Clear Phlegm, move Stagnation, tonify Spleen.

Principal Points: Fenglong ST 40, Neiguan P 6, Zusanli ST 36.
   During the first treatment Fenglong ST 40 was needled with Yin hidden in Yang method (reinforcing then reducing), and the cyst was pricked with a 28 gauge needle to let out some mucus. The next day it was smaller. Then it was lanced with a No. 9 syringe needle and mucus was drawn out until it was flat. Neiguan P 6 and Zusanli ST 36 were reinforced. After three treatments the patient could move his tongue easily. He was able to eat and speak normally, and his asthma also improved.

Explanation: The *Ling Shu* says, 'The Spleen channel . . . goes to the root of the tongue and disperses over its lower surface' (Jing Mai, Channels chapter). When the Spleen does not function properly, Damp accumulates and transforms into Heat and Phlegm, forming the double tongue. The cyst was drained according to the principle of 'removing what is stagnant'. The prescription removes Phlegm, reinforces the Spleen, strengthens the Qi of the Middle Burner and activates the vessels.

Guan Zunxian, KUNMING MUNICIPAL HOSPITAL, YUNNAN PROVINCE
(see Journal of Traditional Chinese Medicine, Issue 11, 1985)

186. Deaf-mutism

Wang, male, age 64, disabled soldier

Case Registered: 1 August 1987

History: The patient had been deaf mute for 34 years. He had always been very emotional. 34 years previously he got in a rage and heard a roaring sound in his ears afterwards. This affected his hearing, but his speech was not impaired. Later he developed a fever for several days. Afterwards he lost his hearing and speech. His current symptoms included feeling faint, occasional headaches, bitter taste in the mouth, dry throat, poor appetite, sensations of oppression in the chest and dark yellow urine.

Examination: *Tongue body*: dark red. *Tongue coating*: thin and white. *Pulse*: wiry and rapid.

Diagnosis: Deaf-mutism: Liver Fire rising to obstruct the clear orifices.

Treatment: Soothe Liver Fire to open the clear orifices.

Principal Points:
1. Xiaguan ST 7, Tinghui GB 2, Zhongzhu TB 3, Taichong LIV 3, Zulinqi GB 41.
2. Tinggong SI 19, Yifeng TB 17, Anmian 2 (Extra), Waiguan TB 5, Yanglingquan GB 34, Xingjian LIV 2, Xiaxi GB 43.

    The points were reduced with lifting thrusting and twirling method, then the handle of the needle was scraped. Electro-acupuncture was given for 15–20 minutes, and the needles were retained for 30 minutes. The two groups of points were alternated and treatment was given daily. A course consisted of 10 treatments, and an interval of 2–3 days was allowed between courses. After 10 days he suddenly felt itching and a sensation of gas rising up in his throat. He coughed up a mouthful of phlegm and immediately felt refreshed; then his speech and hearing came back. He was able to speak clearly, but his voice was relatively very weak.

Explanation: **The** Kidney opens into the ear, and the Gallbladder connects to the ear. When Kidney Qi is full and the Gallbladder Qi is clear, a person's hearing will be good. If the Kidney Qi is Deficient, and Fire from the Liver and Gallbladder rises upwards there will be roaring in the ears and deafness. Most cases of deafness are related to malfunctioning of the Kidney and Gallbladder. The *Su Wen* says, 'When the Liver is diseased and Deficient, the eyes cannot see and the ears cannot hear . . . When Qi rises adversely there is headache and deafness' (The Five Zang and the Four Seasons chapter). Zhang Zhong Jing wrote, 'When the Liver Qi rises adversely there is headache and deafness'.

    In this case, Stagnation of Liver Qi transformed into Fire, which rose to obstruct the ear. The Triple Burner and Gallbladder channels go through the ear, so Yifeng TB 17, Tinghui GB 2, Zhongzhu TB 3 and

Yanglingquan GB 34 were selected to dredge the Shao Yang channel Qi and restore the function of the ear. Taichong LIV 3, Zulinqi GB 41, Xiaxi GB 43, Xingjian LIV 2 and Waiguan TB 5 were used to purge Fire in the Liver and Gallbladder.

Sun Xuequan, MENGYIN COUNTY TCM HOSPITAL, SHANDONG PROVINCE

187. Objective tinnitus

Xing, male, age 10

Case Registered: 15 July 1982

History: The boy had objective tinnitus for over a month. He had measles on 10 June 1982 and fever for 10 days. After the fever he had tinnitus, a rhythmical sound like the clicking of a clock. His other symptoms were restlessness, general weakness and poor appetite.

Examination: External ear and tympanic membrane on both sides normal. Mastoid process negative. No nystagmus.Throat normal; tonsils not swollen. His hearing was normal, and his answers were to the point. Auditory threshold normal on both sides. The doctor could hear a clicking sound in both ears which was not matched to the boy's heart rate.The tinnitus could be temporarily checked by eye blowing stimulation.

Diagnosis: Heat in the Gallbladder channel affecting the ear.

Treatment: Dredge the channel Qi around the ear, purge heat in the Shao Yang channels.

Principal Points: Tianjing TB 13, Yangfu GB 28, Xingjian LIV 2.
    The points were needled bilaterally. The tinnitus was cured after two treatments.

Leng Yanyun, Kang Deyi et al, JIUXIANQIAO WORKERS' HOSPITAL,
BEIJING
(see Beijing Journal of Traditional Chinese Medicine, Issue 4, 1983)

Editor's Note: Objective tinnitus is also known as oscillating tinnitus and is rarely seen in clinic. It is characterized by the fact that the sound, usually clicking or pulsing, is clearly audible to the observer. Clicking is caused by spasm of the tensor palati, tensor tympani and stapedius muscles, while pulsing is often related to arterio-venous shunt or tumour of the jugular.

Part Five
DISEASES AFFECTING THE CHANNELS

188. Chong Mai pathology

CASE 1

Tian, male, age 70, retired worker

Case registered: 18 September 1983

History: For the last year the patient had sensations of gas rising up from the lower abdomen to the throat, accompanied by contracture and pain. He did not respond to medication. The symptoms occurred mostly at night, when he had fullness in the chest and throat, and contracture and pain in the chest, abdomen and throat. His sleep and appetite were both poor. He sometimes had cold sensations in his back, like cold gas rising and rushing from his back to the top of his head. Sedatives did not help.

Examination: *BP*: 20.0/12.0 kPa (150/90 mmHg). *Tongue body*: red. *Tongue coating*: thin and white. *Pulse*: wiry and thin.

Diagnosis: Chong Mai pathology: Deficiency of Kidney Qi causing Rebellious Qi in Chong Mai.

Treatment: Nourish the Liver and Kidney to redirect Rebellious Qi downwards.

Principal Points: Yongquan KID 1 (bilateral), Lianquan Ren 23, Dadun LIV 1 (bilateral), Yutang Ren 18.
   The points were reinforced and the needles retained for 20 minutes. Treatment was given daily. His symptoms improved after the second treatment. After four more sessions all his symptoms went. The case was followed up for 3 years and there was no relapse.

Explanation: The *Su Wen* says, 'Chong Mai pathology has symptoms of Rebellious Qi and contracture inside'. This is because, 'Chong Mai goes through the navel and up to the chest, so when it is not clear Qi is obstructed causing contracture in the chest and abdomen' (Gu Kong Lun, Interstices of the Bones chapter). Zhang Jiebin of the Ming dynasty observed that, 'The root of the illness is Kidney Qi Deficiency, which causes Rebellious Qi in Chong Mai'. Ye Tianshi wrote, 'Pains caused by Chong Qi rising rebelliously up the back is disease of the Du Mai. Treat the Shao Yin channels. Pain going up the abdomen is disease of Chong and Ren Mai. Treat the Jue Yin channels'. Thus the disease should be treated by using points on the Liver and Kidney channel. The *Ling Shu* says, 'The Kidney channel has its root in Dadun LIV 1, and ends at Yuying or Yutang Ren 18' (Root and End chapter). These two points nourish the Liver and Kidney and redirect Rebellious Qi in Chong Mai downwards. The treatment addressed the cause and the symptoms.

> Zhang Dengbu, ACUPUNCTURE AND MOXIBUSTION SECTION, SHANDONG TCM COLLEGE HOSPITAL
> (see *Shandong Traditional Chinese Medicine,Issue 2, 1985*)

CASE 2

Male, age 58, foreigner

Case registered: 17 February 1981

History: For the last year the patient had sensations of cold gas rushing from his lower abdomen to his chest and throat, and in his back from the perineum to the top of his head. He also felt faint, and suffered from headaches. Tranquillizers and sedatives did not help. His sleep, appetite, bowels and urination were normal.

Examination: Spinal column and limbs normal. *Tongue body*: red. *Tongue coating*: thin and white. *Pulse*: wiry and tight.

Diagnosis: Chong Mai pathology: Deficiency and Cold of Chong Mai causing the vessel Qi to rush upwards.

Treatment: Warm and regulate the Qi of the Middle Burner to redirect Rebellious Qi downwards.

Principal Points: Danzhong Ren 17, Neiguan P 6, Qihai Ren 6, Baihui Du 20, Sanyinjiao SP 6, Houxi SI 3.
   The points were needled bilaterally, and at Qihai Ren 6 moxibustion was given after insertion. The points were reinforced and the needles were retained for 15 minutes. Treatment was given daily. After three treatments he felt an improvement in the sensation of gas rising upwards, but he still had headaches and felt faint. For the next three treatments moxibustion was added at Baihui Du 20. All his symptoms were cured. The case was followed up for a year and there was no relapse.

Explanation: Chong Mai originates from the lower abdomen, exiting from the perineum and rising in two branches, anterior and posterior. In this case the symptoms conformed with the vessel pathways. From the symptoms and pulse it is clear this disease was caused by Deficiency and Cold in Chong Mai.

Danzhong Ren 17, the Hui-Convergence point of Qi, was needled obliquely downwards to regulate Qi and redirect Rebellious Qi downwards. Neiguan P 6, the Luo-Connecting point, connects with Yin Wei Mai. It enhances the effects of Danzhong Ren 17, relieving the chest and regulating the flow of Qi. Acupuncture and moxibustion at Qihai Ren 6 tonify Yang in the Lower Burner and warm Chong Mai. Sanyinjiao SP 6, the meeting point of the three leg Yin channels, affects Liver Yin and Kidney Yang. Chong Mai is closely related to these two organs, so indirectly Sanyinjiao SP 6 reinforces Chong Mai. Baihui Du 20 and Houxi SI 3 regulate Rebellious Qi in the back.

Zhang Dengbu, SHANDONG TCM COLLEGE HOSPITAL
(see Shenxi Traditional Chinese Medicine, Issue 8, 1985)

CASE 3, HYDRONEPHROSIS

Zhang, male, age 12, schoolboy

Case registered: 20 June 1978

History: The boy had sensations of heaviness in the legs and a dull pain in the left abdomen for over a year. His parents did not take him to a doctor because it did not seem to affect his daily life or studies. On 10 June 1978 he had a sudden pain around the navel which made him cry out and turn pale. It lasted for about 5 minutes, then he vomited. The next day the condition was diagnosed in hospital as hydronephrosis. Routine blood and urine tests were all negative. Ultrasound examination, barium meal and plain abdominal X-ray showed hydronephrosis on the left. The symptoms became more severe, and he would have pain 1–2 times a day. In addition he had loose stools and clear and copious urination.

Examination: He looked ashen and nervous. Pitting oedema in the legs. Lower abdominal fullness, with occasional bowel sound. *Tongue body*: pale and moist. *Tongue coating*: thin and white.

Diagnosis: Chong Mai pathology: mass in the Lower or Upper Burner.

Treatment: Warm Chong Mai, disperse Cold, consolidate Chong Qi to relieve pain.

Principal Points: Taichong LIV 3 (left), Zhaohai KID 6 (left), Qihai Ren 6, Guanyuan Ren 4.

The points were needled with reinforcing and reducing evenly method, and the needles were retained. Moxibustion was applied for 15 minutes, and the points were massaged after the needles were removed. After 15 treatments his symptoms were much better. The oedema was better, his stools were firm, urination was normal and his abdominal pain had gone. Re-examination with ultrasound showed the left renal pelvis was normal. He was prescribed Gui Fu Di Huang Wan to consolidate the result.

Explanation: This case of hydronephrosis is categorized as Fu Liang (mass in the Lower or Upper Burner) and is caused by Stagnation of Pathogenic Cold. If the Kidney is not warmed and Chong Qu is not consolidated, the Qi rebels upwards causing periumbilical pain. If Wind and Cold stop Water in Chong Mai, there will be pitting oedema in the hips, thighs and tibia. According to the *Su Wen* this 'cannot be treated by inducing diuresis to reduce oedema. Treated in this way the problem will turn into water retention' (Qi Bing Lun, Peculiar Diseases chapter). This is because, according to Wang Bing, 'Chong Mai starts at the Kidney and exits from Qi Jie. The branch that goes upwards starts from the lower abdomen, while the branch that goes downwards leads to Guanyuan Ren 4 below the navel. Thus treating the problem with purgation method could cause water retention'. When treating Fu Liang, the purgation method is therefore not desirable. In this case the treatment principle was to warm the channels and disperse Cold, astringe the Qi of Chong Mai and relieve pain. Points on the Kidney and Liver channels and Ren Mai were selected. This was both a Deficiency and Excess condition, so reinforcing and reducing evenly method was used, followed by moxibustion.

Acupuncture with moxibustion at Taichong LIV 3, the Yuan-Source point, warms the Qi of Chong Mai and disperses Cold. It is effective for Jue (syncope) Qi. Guanyuan Ren 4[1], the Front-Mu point of the Small Intestine, is a meeting point of Chong and Ren Mai; in fact, Chong Mai starts from this point. The *Yi Jing Jing Yi* (Essence of the Medical Classics) states that Guanyuan Ren 4 'is where Primordial Yin and Primordial Yang meet'. Qihai Ren 6 is described in the *Zhen Jiu Da Cheng* (Great Compendium of Acupuncture and Moxibustion) as 'The Sea of Primary Qi', and the *Zhi Bing Yao Xue* (Important Acupuncture Points) says it 'is in charge of all Qi diseases'. Together Qihai Ren 6 and Guanyuan Ren 4 are where Primordial Qi converges. Needling them with reinforcing and

---

[1]Guanyuan means 'Gate to Original Qi', indicating that it stores Original Qi, and is related to the Origin of Life.

reducing equally method followed by moxibustion restores Yang to warm the Kidney and astringe Chong Mai.

Zhaohai KID 6 is the starting point of Yin Qiao Mai. The channel and vessel go through the legs and hips. The Kidney and Bladder are a Yin–Yang pair. Acupuncture with moxibustion here warms Kidney Yang and helps the Bladder to turn Water into Qi, thus 'helping the Source of Fire to transform Yin'.

Li Licheng, JINAN MUNICIPAL CENTRAL HOSPITAL, SHANDONG PROVINCE

189. Yang Ming pathology

Cheng, male, age 48, peasant

Case registered: 9/July 1976

History: 3 days previously the patient developed a fever, with headache and aversion to cold. He did not sweat and felt a sensation of contraction all over his body. He did not have any treatment. On the third evening he developed a high fever with profuse sweating. He was very thirsty and craved cold drinks. His urine was reddish yellow and scanty, and he was restless and panting.

Examination: *Temperature*: 38.9°C. Lungs normal. Heart rate regular, 98/min. Mild hyperaemia at the throat. No other abnormal findings. *Tongue body*: red and quite dry. *Tongue coating*: white. *Pulse*: full and strong in all six positions.

Diagnosis: Heat in Tai Yang transmitted to Yang Ming.

Treatment: Clear Heat in Yang Ming.

Principal Points: Hegu L.I. 4, Fuliu KID 7, Dazhong KID 4.

Hegu L.I. 4 and Dazhong KID 4 were reduced by obtaining sensations of cold, and Fuliu KID 7 was reinforced by obtaining sensations of heat. After 30 minutes all his symptoms improved. By the afternoon of the same day his temperature was 37.6°C and he was sweating slightly. He was still thirsty for cold drinks. His tongue was unchanged. *Pulse*: rapid and weak.

The same treatment was repeated. The next morning his temperature was normal. *Pulse*: normal. His symptoms were all gone, but he felt weak.

Secondary Points: Zusanli ST 36, Neiguan P 6.

The points were reinforced with mild twirling to consolidate the cure and strengthen his Vital Qi.

Explanation: In this case untreated Heat in Tai Yang was transmitted to Yang Ming. The Lung and the Large Intestine are an Interior–Exterior pair. Reducing Hegu L.I. 4, the Yuan-Source point, activates the Qi of all the channels, clears Heat in the Large Intestine channel and promotes the flow of Lung Qi. The Kidney and Bladder are an Interior-Exterior pair. Reinforcing Fuliu KID 7 regulates Kidney Yin, nourishes Kidney Qi and promotes the production of Body Fluids. Dazhong KID 4 connects with the Bladder channel. When reduced it joins the Exterior channel with the Interior channel, so that pathogens in Yang Ming can be expelled from Tai Yang.

Wang Kan, SHANDAN COUNTY TCM HOSPITAL, GANSU PROVINCE
(see Shenxi Traditional Chinese Medicine, Issue 6, 1985)

190. Abnormal sensations along a channel

CASE 1, STOMACH CHANNEL

Li, male, age 23

Case registered: 3 April 1978

History: 10 weeks previously the patient had two upper incisors removed after being injured in a ball game. The night after the operation, in addition to the pain, he felt sensations of numbness and slight pain travelling from the lower border of the orbits of the eye down along the sides of his nose to Renzhong Du 26, then around the mouth, joining in the lower lip. Other sensations travelled in a line along the border of the mandible up in front of the ears to the temple, going off at an angle into the forehead. Two more lines started from the lower lip, travelling down on either side of the larynx to the supraclavicular fossa, to the nipples, down both sides of the navel to the groin, down the anterior aspect of the thighs to the knees. From the knees they passed along the lateral border of the tibia to the dorsum of the feet. Here they divided into two branches, one going to the big toe, the other to the second toe. The lines of sensation were 1–1.5 cm wide, and the sensation was continuous, day and night.

He also had noisy bowel sounds, alternating dry and loose stools, frequent nosebleeds, dry mouth, sores on the lips, and a sore and swollen throat. He was faint and nervous. He had already had acupuncture and moxibustion, but they had not helped.

Examination: *Tongue body*: red at the tip. *Tongue coating*: scanty coat. *Pulse*: wiry and thin.

Diagnosis: Abnormal sensations along the Stomach channel.

3 April 1978
Principal Points: Renzhong Du 26, Zhongwan Ren 12, Neiting ST 44.
The needles were retained for 20 minutes, and manipulated twice during that time. The sensations improved during treatment.

5 April 1978
Principal Points: Chengqi ST 1, Zhongwan Ren 12, Lidui ST 45.

8 April 1978
His symptoms were much better, but he still had bowel sounds and a sore throat.
Principal Points: Shaoshang LU 11, Shangyang L.I. 1, Zusanli ST 36, Neiguan P 6, Neiting ST 44.
Shaoshang LU 11 and Shangyang L.I. 1 were bled.

13 April 1978
The bowel sounds and sore throat were relieved, but the linear sensations and nervousness were still present.
Principal Points: Chengqi ST 1, Neiguan P 6, Baihui Du 20.
Further treatment at these points cured the condition.

CASE 2, HEART CHANNEL

Geng, male, age 40

Case registered: 15 December 1977

History: The previous summer the patient took a cold bath in hot weather. Afterwards he began to feel discomfort and aversion to cold, and he felt a band of sensation travelling from the palmar side of his fourth and fifth fingers along the ulnar border of his arms into the axilla. From the axilla the sensations went to his waist and back, then down the front of his thighs to his knees. He had heavy sensations in the waist, slight numbness in the pubic region and gastrocnemius muscle. This caused him difficulty in walking steadily, and he fell down frequently. He also felt faint and tired, and sweated spontaneously and at night. He had palpitations, insomnia and his appetite was poor.

Examination: Tendon reflexes hyperfunctional in both arms and legs. Hoffmann's sign positive. Ankle clonus positive. X-ray examination of the spine showed hyperplasia from C4 to C6. *Tongue body*: normal. *Tongue coating*: thin and white. *Pulse*: thin and weak.

Diagnosis: Abnormal sensation predominantly along the Heart channel.

Treatment: Invigorate Functional Qi of Heart channel to relieve numbness and calm the Mind.

15 December 1977
Principal Points: Tongli HT 5, Neiguan P 6.
  The needles were retained for 5 minutes after needle sensation was obtained.

16 December 1977
  The numbness had improved, and he had slept better the previous night.
Principal Points: Tongli HT 5, Neiguan P 6, Shenshu BL 23.
  Shenshu BL 23 was added to nourish and strengthen Kidney Qi.

18 December 1977
  All his symptoms were much better.
Principal Points: Tongli HT 5, Neiguan P 6, Shenshu BL 23, Zhibian BL 54.
  The Kidney and Bladder channels are an Interior–Exterior pair. Zhibian BL 54 was added to treat his difficulty with walking.

22 December 1977
  His symptoms improved further.
Principal Points: Tongli HT 5, Shaohai HT 3, Biguan ST 31.

Chen Keqin, SHANXI PROVINCIAL INSTITUTE OF TCM
(see Liaoning Journal of Traditional Chinese Medicine, Issue 2, 1981)

Editor's Note: In these two cases there were abnormal sensations travelling along the pathways of the Stomach and Heart channels. The trajectories and clinical symptoms conform to those recorded in the *Ling Shu* (Jing Mai, Channels chapter). This corroborates TCM channel theory. The symptoms improved quickly or were relieved after points on the respective channels were needled. This again confirms that points on a channel can treat diseases on a channel.

191. Pain along the Liver channel

CASE 1

Qiu, female, age 51

Case registered: 1 November 1979

History: The patient had spasmodic pain in her feet for over 6 months. The pain was on the dorsal surface between the first and second metatarsals. She would wake up 3–4 times a night, and then the pain would start.

Examination: *Tongue body*: dark red patches on the edges. *Tongue coating*: thin and white. *Pulse*: wiry and thin.

Diagnosis: Blood Stasis in the Liver channel.

Treatment: Move Liver Qi and disperse Blood Stasis.

Principal Points: Taichong LIV 3, Qimen LIV 14, Yanglingquan GB 34.
   Her symptoms improved after two sessions: the pain only came once a night. After four sessions all her symptoms went and she had no discomfort at all.

Explanation: Blood Stasis in the Liver channel is rarely seen in clinic. The Liver ensures the free and easy movement of Qi. It likes movement. When the Liver Qi is Stagnant, Qi in the body cannot disperse, and Qi and Blood do not circulate. This caused the pain along the Liver channel.
   Qimen LIV 14 and Taichong LIV 3 resolve Blood Stasis in the Liver channel. The Liver is in charge of the tendons. Yanglingquan GB 34, the Hui-Converging point of tendons, relaxes the tendons and relieves pain. The Liver and Gallbladder channels are an Interior–Exterior pair. Yanglingquan GB 34 is also the He-Sea point, and so assists the Liver to ensure the free flow of Qi.

> Chen Zuolin, SHANGHAI RAILWAY BUREAU CENTRAL HOSPITAL
> *(see Shanghai Journal of Acupuncture and Moxibustion, Issue 1, 1982)*

CASE 2

History: 2 days previously the patient was hit on the big toe of his right foot by a falling iron bar. At first the pain was localized. After a few moments his toe became red and slightly swollen. The pain travelled up along the medial aspect of his leg, passing Ligou LIV 5 and Ququan LIV 8, to the groin and around the genitals. The next day the redness and swelling were less marked, but the pain in his leg got worse, affecting the lateral part of the buttock (Huantiao GB 30) and he developed dull pains in the right side of his body.

Examination: There was no redness or swelling in the painful area. Inguinal lymph nodes normal.

Diagnosis: Pain in the Liver channel caused by injury to the big toe.

Treatment: 'Treat channel diseases with points on the channel.'

Principal Points: Dadun LIV 1, Taichong LIV 3, Ququan LIV 8, Yinlian LIV 11, Huantiao GB 30.

A G6805 unit was used to give electrical stimulation. The pain was greatly relieved immediately after treatment.

Explanation: According to modern neurophysiology, pain in the proximal part of a limb can develop to affect the lower part, whereas illness and pain in the lower part of a limb does not generally develop to affect the upper part. This is therefore quite a rare case.

Dadun LIV 1, the site of the injury, is the Jing-Well point. Injury here caused pain in the channel, so according to TCM channel theory points along the channel were used to cure the pain.

Li Zhenlin, PLA NANJING POLITICS INSTITUTE CLINIC
(see Shanghai Journal of Acupuncture and Moxibustion, Issue 4, 1986)

192. Pain along the Spleen channel on palpation of a point

Yin, male, age 30, peasant

Case registered: 11 March 1983

History: 9 days previously the patient felt sudden pain and numbness in his left leg before going to bed. He took a couple of antipyretic painkillers and slept. The pain came again the next morning. He massaged his leg, and noticed that when he applied pressure on the medial anterior part of the ankle he had tingling pain which radiated to his big toe and along the medial aspect of his leg. The pain was like a thread, but was lessened immediately if he released the pressure. When the pain stopped he felt numbness, cold, heaviness and weakness in the leg. He also felt generally weak and faint and his appetite was poor. He had a previous history of Hot and Cold diseases.

Examination: He was generally quite healthy. His left leg was normal in colouring, but slightly cooler than the healthy side. When Shangqiu SP 5 was pressed he cried out. The pain radiated down in a line to the medial tip of his big toe, and up through Sanyinjiao SP 6, along the posterior border of the tibia, the medial aspect of the knee and thigh, and disappeared at the groin. The movement of the pain was timed. From Shangqiu SP 5 it took 12 seconds to go to Chongmen SP 12, and 3 seconds to Yinbai SP 1. When the pressure was released the pain would gradually disappear. Other points along the Spleen channel were palpated, but no other pain on pressure was discovered.

Diagnosis: Pain along the Spleen channel on palpation: Invasion of Pathogenic Cold.

Treatment: Dredge the channel, invigorate the flow of Qi and Blood, stop pain.

Principal Points: Yinlingquan SP 9.

   The point was reduced. When the needle was inserted he reported sensations of soreness and heaviness rushing up and down, which he found very comforting. The needle was retained for 20 minutes. After the treatment the same spot on his ankle was pressed. There was no pain moving upwards, and the pain going downwards had improved. The next day his faintness and fatigue were much better. His appetite was better, and he had no more pain, heavy sensations, numbness or tenderness. He was still slightly numb on the inside of his ankle to the big toe. Gongsun SP 4 was reduced, and the needle was retained for 20 minutes. The condition was cured afterwards.

Explanation: Pain, numbness and erythema along a channel have been discussed in medical texts as old as the Ling Shu, which has been proved correct by numerous cases in clinic. This particular disorder is quite rare. The Su Wen says, 'When Cold invades the vessels, the body's Qi is obstructed causing sudden pain' (Ju Tong Lun, Pain chapter). Yinlingquan SP 9 and Gongsun SP 4 dredge the channels, invigorate the circulation of Qi and Blood and relieve pain.

Hao Shanjie, SHENXI PROVINCIAL TCM INSTITUTE HOSPITAL
(see Shenxi Traditional Chinese Medicine, Issue 8, 1984)

193. Papular eruption along the Kidney channel

Zhang, female, age 46

History: For the last 6 months the patient had papular eruptions on her left leg. They started at the sole of her foot, and continued along the medial aspect of her leg to the top of her thigh. She had heaviness and discomfort in the waist and sacral area, and frequent urination (10 times a day. She had no other discomfort except itchiness along the affected area.

Examination: The distribution of the eruptions was mostly similar to the trajectory of the Kidney channel on the leg. The eruptions were pale red, prominent and had clear borders. From the sole to the ankle they merged and were not very visible, but from her ankle to thigh they were evenly distributed and clearly visible.

Diagnosis: Papular eruptions along the Kidney channel: Kidney Qi Deficiency.

Treatment: Reinforce Kidney Qi, dredge the channels and collaterals, resolve Stasis, regulate Qi and Blood.

Principal Points: Taixi KID 3.

The point was needled on the affected side and sensation was propagated along the leg to the thigh. She felt these sensations for over 24 hours, as if the needle was still in place. The next time she came the eruptions had subsided considerably, and were only visible on the inside of her thigh. The treatment was repeated, and she had the same sensations. On her third visit the eruptions were completely gone. After 4 sessions her urination was normal, and she had no lumbar pain.

Explanation: In TCM theory the skin on the Exterior and the organs on the Interior are closely connected by the system of channels and collaterals. Illness in the Interior organ can be transmitted to the Exterior skin, and vice versa. This is a typical case of illness in the Kidney being transmitted to the skin through the channel. The Ling Shu says, 'When the organs are ill, treat the respective Yuan-Source points' (Jiu Zhen Shi Er Yuan, Six Needlings Twelve Source Points chapter). The Yuan-Source points are where the Qi of the Zangfu passes or resides. Taixi KID 3, the Yuan-Source point, reinforces Kidney Qi and dredges the channel. The disease will be cured when the Kidney Qi is sufficient, the channel Qi is restored and Qi and Blood are regulated.

> Zhang Fengrun, ACUPUNCTURE AND MOXIBUSTION SECTION, SHENXI PROVINCIAL TCM INSTITUTE
> *(see Shenxi New medicine, Issue 1 1978)*

194. Linear warts along the Pericardium channel

Zhang, male, age 18, student

History: 2 weeks previously the patient noticed a line of white eruptions on his right arm from the wrist to the elbow. They were about 1 mm in size, and itchy. The itchiness got worse if he scratched. After 4 days he was prescribed chlorpheniramine and ABOB (moroxydine) for 4 days but there was no improvement. Over the next 4 days he used tincture of iodine, which eased the itching but burnt the skin. When a piece of skin came off the eruptions were worse over the new skin. He then tried dexamethasone but also without success.

Examination: There was an irregular line of warts along the course of the Pericardium channel from Daling P 7 to Quze P 3. The size of the warts varied from 1–6 mm across. They were greyish brown, and firm and rough to the touch. Some of the lesions were fissured.

Diagnosis: Linear warts along the Pericardium channel: Deficiency in the Small Intestine Luo-Connecting channel.

Treatment: Dredge the channels and collaterals, regulate Qi and Blood.

Principal Points: Neiguan P 6, Quze P 3, Zhizheng SI 7.

The points were needled on the right, and treatment was given daily. The needles were retained for 20 minutes, and manipulated at 5 minute intervals.

After a week there was no more itching, and the skin lesions were reduced by a third. Another area of dense red spots appeared on his palm however. The area was the size of a small coin. It was prominent and itchy. Daling P 7 was added to the prescription. After 15 treatments the warts all came off and the eruptions were cured. The case was followed up for 6 months and there was no relapse.

Explanation: This disorder is a manifestation of channel and collateral pathology. Neiguan P 6, Quze P 3 and Daling P 7 are on the channel and were selected to dredge the channel Qi, and regulate Qi and Blood in the channel. Zhizheng SI 7 is the Luo-Connecting point. The *Ling Shu* says, 'The Small Intestine channel branches at Zhizheng, which is 5 cun above the wrist. The branch connects transversely with the Shao Yin channel, and passes through the elbow to Jianyu L.I. 15. When it is exuberant the joints become flaccid and the elbow is weak: when it is deficient warts will develop like scabies. To treat this take the point where the branch starts' (Jing Mai, Channels chapter). Zhizheng SI 7 can therefore be used to treat warts.

Li Shuquan, SHANDONG PROVINCIAL SCHOOL OF TCM.

195. Herpes zoster along the Gallbladder channel complicated by sciatica

Liu, female, age 59, worker

Case registered: 15 September 1987

History: A month previously the patient had burning pain in the left lumbar region followed by a line of herpes down the lateral aspect of her left leg which reached the antero-lateral part of her ankle. The condition was diagnosed as herpes zoster in a local hospital, and treated with Western and traditional Chinese drugs. The herpes were reduced by the treatment, but recently she had rushing pains in her left leg which were aggravated at night and affecting her sleep. They were getting worse, and sedatives did not help. She had no previous history of injury to the lumbar area.

Examination: She was elderly. Her temperature, pulse and blood pressure were normal. Heart and lungs negative. Unable to palpate liver and spleen. Spine negative. Straight leg lifting test positive at 30° on the left. Dorsiflexion test of left foot positive. Left Achilles tendon reflex dulled. Right leg tests negative.

There were scattered herpes and spotted pigmentation on her waist on the left, on her left hip, the lateral aspect of the leg and the antero-lateral aspect of the ankle. *Tongue body*: red. *Tongue coating*: yellow. *Pulse*: wiry and slippery.

Diagnosis: Damp Heat in the Liver and Gallbladder.

Treatment: Clear Damp Heat in the Liver and Gallbladder, activate the collaterals and stop pain.

Principal Points: Huantiao GB 30, Fengshi GB 31, Yanglingquan GB 34, Fenglong ST 40, Juegu GB 39, Qiuxu GB 40, Xiaxi GB 43.

The points were all needled on the left and reduced. The needles were retained for 20 minutes and manipulated at 5 minute intervals. Treatment was given daily.

After a week the pain was much improved, the herpes were mostly gone, but the spotted pigmentation remained. After a month the herpes were completely gone, and the pain was almost gone. Straight leg lifting test on the left negative. Dorsiflexion test on the left negative. 2 more weeks of consolidating treatment were given and the patient was cured and discharged.

Explanation: This is a rarely seen condition. From the signs and symptoms it is clear that the cause is exuberant Fire in the Liver and Gallbladder with Accumulation of Damp heat inside and invasion of Toxic Heat from the outside. The sciatica was caused by Toxic heat invading the channels and collaterals, and Blood Stasis . Treatment was designed to clear Damp Heat in the Liver and Gallbladder, activate the collaterals and relieve pain.

The points selected were mainly on the Gallbladder channel. Huantiao GB 30, Fengshi GB 31, Yanglingquan GB 34 and Juegu GB 39 purge Wind and Heat Toxins from the Liver and Gallbladder and activate the channels and collaterals. Reducing Xiaxi GB 43, the Yong-Spring point, purges Excess Fire in the Liver and Gallbladder. Fenglong ST 40, the Luo-Connecting point, helps to clear Damp Heat.

Zhang Dengbu, shandong TCM COLLEGE HOSPITAL.

196. Vitiligo along the Pericardium and Lung channels

He, male, age 6

History: A year previously the skin on the patient's right arm began to turn white.

Examination: There was a band of white skin 1.0–1.5 cm wide on his arm which mostly followed the trajectory of the Lung channel, extending to Dazhui Du 14. Another band followed the course of the Pericardium channel into the axilla and the upper part of the chest.

Principal Points: Hegu L.I. 4 through to Laogong P 8.

The point was needled on the right and the needle was withdrawn immediately. Treatment was given once every other day. His skin was much better after 8 treatments. The bands of white skin became broken up into scattered areas, and his skin was darker.

> Chen Keqin, SHENXIN PROVINCIAL INSTITUTE OF TCM
> (*see Meridian Sensitive Subjects, Meridian Transmission, Renmin Weisheng Press, 1979*)

197. Lichen planus along a channel

CASE 1, HEART CHANNEL

Mao, female, age 39

History: 2 months previously the patient had a cholecystectomy. The day after the operation she developed a skin rash on the anterior aspect of her left wrist, at Shenmen HT 7. Over the next few days the rash extended up her anterior arm and elbow in a band 2–5 mm wide. It continued over the anterior axillary fold, over the chest to about 5 cm lateral to the nipple. Another line extended downwards from the wrist, through the hypothenar eminence, to the ulnar border of the palm, and continued into the radial border of the little finger and the ulnar border of the ring finger. The rash was very itchy.

Examination: The skin lesions were very dark. The rashes were continuous, and there were no clear borders between them.

Diagnosis: Lichen planus along the Heart channel.

Principal Points: Shenmen HT 7.

The point was needled on the right and the needle was retained for 10–20 minutes. Treatment was given once every other day. After 70 treatments there was no more itching, and the lesions were mostly gone, leaving behind only a few spots of pigmentation.

CASE 2, BLADDER CHANNEL

Zhang, male, age 2

History: The child had lichen on his left leg. The lesions were in a line, starting at the heel, and going up through gastrocnemius, the popliteal fossa, the posterior aspect of the thigh to the hip, terminating to one side of the sacrum.

Examination: The area of skin lesion was wider towards the top, and narrower near the foot. 5 cm above the transverse gluteal crease the band of lichen measured 0.3–0.5 cm. The eruptions were slightly prominent, and light brown in colour.

Diagnosis: Lichen planus along the Bladder channel.

Principal Points: Kunlun BL 60.
   Rapid needling technique was used. Treatment was given once every other day. After 24 treatments the eruptions had gone, leaving behind only a few pigmented spots.

> Chen Keqin, SHENXIN PROVINCIAL INSTITUTE OF TCM
> (*see Meridian Sensitive Subjects, Meridian Transmission, Renmin Weisheng Press, 1979*)

Editor's Note: These cases are channel phenomena. In the first case the lesions extended along the Heart channel and was cured by the use of the Yuan-Source point Shenmen HT 7. In the second case the lesions extended along the Bladder channel and were cured by the use of the Ching-River point of the channel.

Appendix

Biochemical values

Venous blood: approximate adult reference values

Analysis	Reference values	
	S.I. units	Other units
Alanine aminotransferase (ALT)	10–40 i.u./l	
Aspartate aminotransferase (AST)	10–35 i.u./l	
Bilirubin (total)	2–17 µmol/l	0.3–1.0 mg/dl
Cholesterol (fasting)	3.6–6.7 mmol/l	145–270 mg/dl(??)
Creatinine	55–150 µmol/l	0.6–1.7 mg/dl
Glucose (fasting)	3.9–5.8 mmol/l	70–110 mg/100 ml
Immunoglobulins (Ig): IgA	0.5–4.0 g/l (40–300 i.u./l)	
IgG	5.0–13.0 g/l (60–160 i.u./l)	
IgM – males	0.3–2.2 g/l (40–270 i.u./l)	
– females	0.4–2.5 g/l (50–300 i.u./l)	
Potassium	3.3–4.7 mmol/l	
Proteins – total	62–82 g/l	6.2–8.2 g/dl
– albumin	36–47 g/l	3.6–4.7 g/dl
– globulins	24–37 g/l	2:4–3;7 g/dl (??:)
Thymol Turbidity Test (TTT) (Maclagan)	1–4 units	

Miscellaneous approximate adult reference values

Cerebrospinal fluid (Lumbar puncture)
Chloride: 120–170 mmol/l
Glucose: 2.5–4.0 mmol/l (45–72 mg/dl) – 50 to 70% of plasma concentration
Protein (total): 100–400 mg/l (10–40 mg/dl)
Pressure: 5–15 cmCSF

Hormone concentrations in plasma; approximate adult reference values
Peptide hormone concentrations vary between different assays according to the standards used. The following values are based on the current WHO international reference preparations

Analysis	Reference values	
	S.I. units	Other units
Plasma-bound iodine (PBI)	mg%??	
Thyroxine (T4)	70–150 nmol/l	5.5–12 µg/1100 ml
Triiodothyronine (T3)	1.1–2.8 nmol/l	70–80 ng/100ml

Urine (specific gravity = 1.000–1.032): approximate adult reference values

Analysis	Reference values	
	S.I. units	Other units
Daily output (in urine)		
17 hydroxycorticosterone	2–8 mg/24 h	
17 ketosteroid	6–15 mg/24 h	
Creatine	0–60 mg/24 h	
Creatinine	1–1.8 g/24 h	
Protein		

Haematological values

	S.I. units	Other units
Erythrocyte sedimentation rate (ESR) (Westergren)		0–6 mm in 1 h normal
(Figures given are for patients under 60 years of age. Higher values in abnormal older persons are not necessarily abnormal)		7–20 mm in 1 h doubtful >20 mm in 1 h
Haemoglobin – men	130–180 g/l	13–18 g/dl or g %
– women	115–165 g/l	30–200 mg/dl or g %
WBC – adults	4.0–11.0×10^9/l	4000–1000/µl 4.0–11.0×10^3/mm^3
Differential white cell count		
Neutrophil granulocytes	2.5–7.5×10^9/l	40–75%
Lymphocytes	1.0–3.5×10^9/l	20–45%
Eosinophil granulocytes	0.04–0.4×10^9/l	1–6%
Platelets	150–400×10^9/l	150 000–400 000/µl or /mm^3
RBC count – men	4.5–6.5×10^{12}/l	4.5–6.5×10^6/µl or /mm^3
– women	3.8–5.8×10^{12}/l	3.8–5.8×10^6/µl or /mm^3

Subject index

Points index